For Churchill Livingstone:

Commissioning editor: Ellen Green
Project manager: Valerie Burgess
Project development editor: Valerie Bain
Design direction: Judith Wright
Project controller: Derek Robertson
Copy editor: Sue Beasley
Indexer: Tarrant Ranger Indexing Agency
Page layout: Kate Walshaw
Sales promotion executive: Hilary Brown

Research Mindedness for Practice

An Interactive Approach for Nursing and Health Care

Edited by

Pam Smith MSc, PhD, BNurs, DNCert, HVCert, RGN, RNT
Visiting Research Fellow, School of Health, University of Greenwich, London

Foreword by

Jennifer M. Hunt MPhil, BA(Hons), RGN, FRCN
Director, Nursing Research Initiative for Scotland,
Glasgow Caledonian University, Glasgow

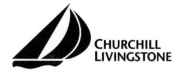

CHURCHILL LIVINGSTONE

NEW YORK EDINBURGH LONDON MADRID MELBOURNE SAN FRANCISCO AND TOKYO 1997

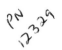

PN
12329

CHURCHILL LIVINGSTONE
Medical Division of Pearson Professional Limited

Distributed in the United States of America by Churchill Livingstone,
650 Avenue of the Americas, New York, N.Y. 10011, and by associated
companies, branches and representatives throughout the world.

© Pearson Professional Limited 1997

First published 1997

ISBN 0 443 05293 X

British Library Cataloguing in Publication Data
A catalogue record for this book is available from the British Library.

Library of Congress Cataloging in Publication Data
A catalog record for this book is available from the Library of Congress.

Medical knowledge is constantly changing. As new information
becomes available, changes in treatment, procedures, equipment and
the use of drugs become necessary. The editors/authors/contributors
and the publishers have, as far as it is possible, taken care to ensure
that the information given in this text is accurate and up to date.
However, readers are strongly advised to confirm that information,
especially with regard to drug usage, complies with the latest
legislation and standards of practice.

WT 24
NURSING RESEARCH

The
publisher's
policy is to use
**paper manufactured
from sustainable forests**

Produced through Longman Malaysia, PP

Contents

Contributors

Charmagne S Barnes BSc(Nurs) DPSN PGDE RGN RSCN RNT
Senior Lecturer – Paediatrics, School of Midwifery
and Family Health, Middlesex University, London

9 Critiquing the research literature

Veronica Corben BSc(Hons) DPSN PGDE RGN
Senior Lecturer, Faculty of Health Care and
Social Services, University of Luton, Luton

5 Phenomenology

Julie Cumpper BA PGDE RSCN RGN RM
Senior Lecturer, School of Paediatric Nursing and
Child Health, South Bank University in association
with Great Ormond Street Hospital for Children
NHS Trust, London

3 Experimental methods

Wladyslawa Czuber-Dochan MSc DipN PGDE RGN RNT
Nurse Tutor, School of Nursing and Midwifery,
University of Nottingham, Nottingham

7 The media and research

Benny Goodman BSc(Hons) PGDE CertEd RGN
Academic Co-ordinator (Camborne), Institute of
Health Studies, University of Plymouth, Plymouth

6 Ethnomethodology

Margaret Harper BA(Hons) PGDE RGN RM RSCN ENB 405
Senior Lecturer, Paediatric Nursing,
South Bank University, London

2 Research paradigms

Nina Hartman BA MA PGDE
Lecturer, City University, London

2 Research paradigms

Donna Marie Lewis BSc(Hons) PGDE
Senior Lecturer, School of Multi-professional
Health Care, Middlesex University, London

9 Critiquing the research literature

Joy Lyon BNSc(Hons) PGDE SRN ENB 100
Lecturer Practitioner, Cardiothoracic Nursing,
School of Nursing and Midwifery,
University of Southampton/Cardiothoracic Unit,
Southampton General Hospital, Southampton

10 Ethical issues

Linda McBride BSc MSc PGDE
Senior Lecturer, Professional Studies in Nursing,
Faculty of Science and Health,
University of East London, London

7 The media and research

Janet Kinnaird Moir BA(Hons) MSc PGDE
Health Visitor, Southern Birmingham Community
NHS Trust, Birmingham

8 Literature reviews

Stevan Monkley-Poole BSc(Hons) MSc DPSN PGDE RN
Research Leader – Mental Health and Learning
Disabilities, Division of Social Work, Counselling,
Learning Disabilities and Mental Health,
University of Hertfordshire, Hatfield

11 Research proposals and funding

Jane E Say BSc(Hons) PGDE RGN RNT
Senior Lecturer, University of Hertfordshire, Hatfield

3 Experimental methods

Teresa Smart BSc(Hons) MSc
Senior Teacher, Director of Mathematics and IT,
John Kelly Girls' Technical College, London

4 Data analysis

Pam Smith MSc PhD BNurs RGN DNCert HVCert RNT
Visiting Research Fellow, School of Health,
University of Greenwich, London

1 Setting the scene
12 Epilogue

Frank Strange BSc(Hons) MA PGDE RGN ENB124
Lecturer in Health and Community Studies,
North Devon College, Barnstaple

6 Ethnomethodology

C Nina Stephenson BSc(Hons) MSc DipN PGDE RGN RNT
Lecturer/NVQ Co-ordinator,
University of Hertfordshire, Hatfield

5 Phenomenology

Caroline Walker BA(Hons) PGDE RGN RHV
Lecturer Practitioner, Health Visiting,
Oxford Brookes University/Oxfordshire Community
Health NHS Trust, Oxfordshire

10 Ethical issues

Julie Wilson BSc(Hons) MSc PGDE RGN DNCert RDNT
Lecturer, Department of Nursing Studies,
King's College London

7 The media and research

Foreword

In 1972, the Briggs report stated that 'Nursing should become a research-based profession'. Twenty-four years later we are a long way from achieving that aim. There are still many nurses—in education, practice and in management—who appear frightened of research, lack knowledge about it, and do not give very much support to those who want to get involved in it, either as doers of research or as users of research findings.

Nurses have been hampered in developing research mindedness by the way research has developed in the UK, with:

- slower growth of research into nursing practice—the fundamental core of nursing—compared to research about nurses and nursing education
- time wasted on debating whether qualitative rather than quantitative methodology should be at the foundation of nursing research
- lack of coordinated clinically based nursing research programmes
- lack of sufficient skilled researchers and teachers of research, and
- association of research with academic elitism.

As a result, unfortunately, there is still a somewhat uneasy relationship between what many nurses do in their day-to-day work and nursing research—research has become surrounded by mystique. I am not saying that research should be taken on board lightly, but I do believe that nurses, midwives and health visitors have categorized research as an extremely complex, intellectually demanding exercise, which is beyond the capabilities of most of them. As a result, too few nurses are involved in the research process and in research utilization.

The current climate, however, *demands* that nurses become research minded. The whole 'evidence-based practice' movement has changed the environment in which we now work in health care. Research mindedness is no longer a luxury, an 'add-on' extra, but has to be an essential component of our day-to-day practice. This offers nurses new opportunities for getting involved in research, not only because of the emphasis on evidence-based practice but also because of the changes in funding.

It is, therefore, more important than ever that nurses become knowledgeable about research, that they find research interesting, exciting and useful, and that they lose their apprehension about research. To do this, nurses need the right sort of tools and the right information, presented in a way which meets their needs and is congruent with their experiences as nurses.

This book takes on board many of these issues and concerns about research, and provides a fresh and innovative approach to enabling nurses to develop their knowledge about this important subject. It contains the 'meat' of the research process, such as research methodologies and issues like ethics, so providing a sound introductory text, but, unlike many other textbooks on research, it places these firmly within the context of clinical practice which is the real life of nursing.

The other very different aspect of this book is the way that it draws upon the experiences of those learning about research, not only drawing upon them but also using those involved as contributors, which ensures that what is said has a relevance and freshness which is very appealing.

Research is about extending the boundaries of knowledge and meeting such a challenge is not always a comfortable process. We all have to learn to become more research minded without simply accepting research uncritically. We have to learn to distinguish between good and poor research, and such critical appraisal is time consuming, resource intensive and intellectually demanding. This book will help nurses and others to understand research, to critique, and to learn how research can be of benefit to them and, through their increased knowledge, to their patients and clients.

J.M.

Acknowledgements

This book could not have been completed without the help and support of all the authors, and in many cases their families. However, I would like to give a special mention to the following contributors. In the early stages, the idea for the book was enthusiastically supported by Linda McBride and Janet Moir. Two other contributors, Julie Cumpper and Julie Wilson, undertook to read the draft manuscripts and make editorial suggestions after agreement with their colleagues. Their role was invaluable in preparing a user-friendly text. I would also like to say a special 'thank you' to Teresa Smart, the author of Chapter 4, who stepped into the breach at the last minute when the original author had to pull out.

In the Introduction, I mention that the student teacher group who produced this book, comprised 19 experienced nurses, midwives and health visitors. In the event, Jackie Lewis and John Gordon were unable to make a written contribution. Their original participation in the seminars, however, was important to the book's development. Joe Hanlon also provided invaluable advice.

I was particularly pleased that Professor Jennifer Hunt, Director of the Nursing Research Initiative for Scotland, accepted the invitation to write the Foreword. She has a long history of, and current commitment to, patient-focused research.

Finally, I would like to thank all the staff at Churchill Livingstone for their help and support.

Introduction

HOW THIS BOOK CAME ABOUT

The process of writing this book has been as important as the final product. It began life as a module on teaching research with postgraduate education students at the Royal College of Nursing's Institute of Advanced Nursing Education. The course, entitled 'Promoting Research Mindedness', was an 18-week module with a particular purpose. The aims of the module were as follows. Students would build on their existing knowledge and experience of research. They would also identify their interests from the prescribed content as well as requesting lecturer-led sessions. In this way they would gather ideas for their own teaching and facilitation of research with nursing students and practitioners.

The module students, who were half-way through their teaching diploma, included 19 experienced nurses, midwives and health visitors with a variety of academic and professional backgrounds. Although many of them had some research experience, usually associated with academic study, others regarded themselves as 'beginners' in this field.

The module leader had taught research for 10 years to nurses, midwives and health visitors and had experienced a range of results. At best, students were challenged and liberated by research; at worst, they found it less stimulating than 'a damp squib'.

The students admitted they were not looking forward to the module, partly because of past negative experiences of research teaching. In order to avoid the 'damp squib experience' it seemed vital to acknowledge the students as valuable resources and equal partners in the module and to put the module leader's experience of teaching research under scrutiny. Sessions were to be seen, not as giving the ultimate word in teaching research, but as a process to be taken apart and put together again. It was decided therefore that the early sessions would be presented as 'demonstrations' by the module leader to be followed up by student-led sessions on topics chosen for interest from the course content. This approach to teaching research worked well and quickly became a collaborative enterprise, generating a unique energy and interaction that has since been translated over a number of months into this book. In the process, module students and leader became the collective 'we' referred to below.

From teaching to text

When we first considered translating our classroom experiences into text, our original intention was to write for nurse teachers who would be engaged in teaching a range of pre- and post-registration students in nursing, midwifery and health care topics. Our original intention was to use each session as the basis of a chapter in which we could present our ideas for promoting research mindedness in the classroom. In the process of writing, however, we realized the need to extend our examples beyond the classroom to the practice setting where the majority of nurses, midwives, health visitors and others are engaged in delivering frontline health care.

To some extent, the content of the book reflects the course aims and proposed content, which included broad topics such as research paradigms, philosophies, methodologies and the stages of the research process. We were able, however, to choose our topics for the sessions and interpret them in our own way. The uniqueness of the chapters comes in the opportunity to explore the meaning of research mindedness and its relationship to seeing, thinking and knowing as practitioners and teachers using different research approaches and techniques.

We are aware that some of these terms may mean very little to you at the moment. Indeed many of us were in this situation at the beginning of the module, condemning the use of such terms and terminology as 'elitist research jargon'. As the module progressed, however, we realized that familiarization with the language of research and its origins was part of becoming research minded. This in turn helped us to see how research contributed to nursing knowledge and practice and gave us more confidence to discuss and express our ideas in our own terms.

Our intention in the book is to take you through a similar process of becoming more research minded. The chapters are designed to assist you to explore and explode some of the myths associated with research and to show you how it can be used to increase your confidence about what you already know, as well as to inform your teaching and practice.

The earlier chapters look at the theoretical perspectives which inform research approaches whilst those that follow consider techniques associated with the research process. Chapters have a similar format in that we look in each at the theory associated with the topic, its role in promoting research mindedness and its application to teaching and practice through case studies and reflections based on our experience. Each chapter, while contributing to an integrated whole, can also be read independently, which enables the reader to dip in and out of the text selectively.

Chapter 1 sets the context for the book. Based on sessions led by module leader, Pam Smith, we explore terms and terminology such as 'research mindedness', 'research awareness', 'research appreciation' and 'the research process'. We also examine the Department of Health's research and development strategies and the Taskforce on Nursing, Midwifery and Health Visiting Research in the context of market-led health care.

In particular, we explore the relationship of research mindedness and the research process to the role of the practitioner and their relevance for practice. These issues are re-visited in subsequent chapters.

In Chapter 2, Margaret Harper and Nina Hartman explore the values and assumptions or world-views that underpin the main approaches currently used in nursing and health care research.

The chapter encourages readers to reflect on their own views of the research process and how it relates to nursing knowledge and practice. The chapter aims to do this by presenting readers with ideas that will stimulate them to enter into dialogue with themselves, their colleagues and clients about the nature and purpose of research. The importance of learning through stories is emphasized.

The main viewpoints or 'paradigms' that underpin research are identified and their association with the natural and social sciences explained. These viewpoints include 'positivism', 'interpretivism', 'critical theory' and 'feminism'. The authors illustrate the benefits and limitations of each viewpoint and their association with the natural and social sciences, using examples from clinical and teaching practice.

In Chapter 3, Jane Say and Julie Cumpper deepen the reader's understanding of the positivist paradigm through a closer look at experimental methods in classroom and clinical settings. They show how the skills associated with the experimental research process, such as a systematic, critical and enquiring approach, are not just reserved for the laboratory but can be extended to the classroom and practice setting.

Chapter 4 is a visual and verbal tour of some of the important issues surrounding study design, and statistical data analysis. Teresa Smart shows the need to consider methods for recording, storing, handling and analysing data from the outset rather than at the end of the research. She also demonstrates how statistics as a discipline provides us with 'tools' to condense and make sense of what we observe and record within our research and everday practice.

Nina Stephenson and Veronica Corben's discussion in Chapter 5 of phenomenology as a novel approach to research, builds on Chapter 2 by showing how it is inspired by the interpretive paradigm or viewpoint. Both authors have undertaken research using phenomenology and draw on their respective studies to illustrate the approach. They also demonstrate how its underlying philosophy and methods can be used to promote research mindedness in practitioners and teachers and challenge stereotypes. The authors use art and literature to take the reader through the phenomenological experience.

In Chapter 6, Benny Goodman and Frank Strange combine interpretive and critical research paradigms to consider the contribution of ethnomethodology to the study of nursing and health care. The authors show the relevance of the specific approach by introducing readers to sociological studies in order to encourage a re-examination of what they take for granted in their everyday world.

In Chapter 7, Wladyslawa Czuber-Dochan, Linda McBride and Julie Wilson describe a seminar in which they presented a television programme on AIDS as a way of promoting research mindedness. They also found the programme led them to explore the relationship between investigative journalism and the research process. They did this by judging the programme on the basis of quantitative research criteria and found that its emotional content challenged their assumptions that research equals objective science. Throughout the chapter, the authors draw on examples from print as well as television journalism to discuss the media's impact on health care practice and research.

In Chapter 8, Janet Moir uses everyday examples to demonstrate problem-solving strategies and their application to searching and reviewing the literature. She gives the reader helpful tips on how to identify topics and clarify concepts as a prelude to getting started and accessing material from libraries and databases. She also shows the various ways in which the literature review is used according to the different research approaches and their underlying philosophies. Finally, Janet Moir advises the reader on organizing information and writing up the review.

Chapter 9, written by Donna Lewis and Charmagne Barnes, serves two purposes. The first is to introduce readers to the nature of the 'critiquing' process as key to promoting research mindedness; the second is to give them the opportunity to revise their understanding of the research process. The authors use Jill Macleod Clark and colleagues' popular study on nurses and smoking to guide readers through the critiquing process. They provide helpful reading tips and criteria with which to evaluate research articles and assess their relevance for teaching and practice.

In Chapter 10, Joy Lyon and Caroline Walker look at the ethical issues surrounding research, including the knowledge and philosophy on which ethics are based, how they are interpreted through government policy and ethics committees and their application to nursing research and practice.

Stevan Monkley-Poole's Chapter 11, on writing proposals and funding, draws together some of the practical applications of research mindedness in taking ideas forward. The relationship between research, teaching and higher education in the light of the research assessment exercise, is discussed.

Chapter 12 concludes by summarizing the book's content and reflecting on the collective writing process. Suggestions are made for how the book can be used in classroom and clinical settings.

If you are new to research, we suggest you start by reading Chapters 1 and 2. It will probably be necessary to read Chapter 2 more than once because it explores the theoretical aspects of research and may contain ideas that are new to you. Both Chapters 1 and 2, however, provide a good foundation for the other chapters in the book where you will re-visit a number of issues from a variety of perspectives.

Because we enjoyed our explorations to become more research minded, we hope you will too.

Enjoy!

Setting the scene

1

Pam Smith

PREAMBLE

'Promoting research mindedness' was the title of the 18-week module which was the inspiration for this book. During our first session we decided to explore the term and check our understanding of it. Very quickly we realized that we did not share a common definition. Some people were more familiar with the terms 'research appreciation' and 'research awareness'. Others were concerned that a module promoting research mindedness drew a false distinction between thinking about and doing research. To some extent this discussion reflected the prior experience of the group. Like the readers of this book, they were coming from varied educational, clinical and research backgrounds. While most of them were familiar with the world of practice and teaching, many regarded themselves as beginners when it came to research. The module therefore gave them the opportunity to acquire new knowledge as well as build on their existing knowledge and experience in order to gather ideas for how to promote research mindedness in teaching and practice. We hope that you will be able to use this book in the same way.

RESEARCH AWARENESS AND RESEARCH MINDEDNESS

Origins of the terms

In this chapter we begin with an investigation of the origins of the terms 'research mindedness' and 'research awareness'. We refer to articles from the nursing press, curriculum documents from the statutory bodies, the Royal College of Nursing (RCN) and government reports in order to gauge the language and rhetoric of research. We also compare these definitions with those presented in a textbook for social workers, explicitly committed to promoting the research-minded practitioner.

For nurses and midwives, the roots of research mindedness can be traced to the famous Briggs' report (DHSS 1972). In that report, nursing and midwifery were exhorted to become research-based professions.

The report also stated: 'While in other professions the active pursuit of serious research must be limited to a minority in the profession ... a sense for the need for research should become part of the mental equipment of every practising nurse or midwife' (p. 370).

It is interesting to note that the Briggs' committee membership included Sue Pembrey and Christine Hancock. Sue Pembrey went on to initiate practice development in Oxfordshire Health Authority and was the founder of the National Nursing Institute. Christine Hancock as Chief Nurse of Bloomsbury Health Authority in the early 1980s set up a nursing research network as a basis for practice development. More recently, however, as General Secretary of the Royal College of Nursing she was a member of the Taskforce, looking at a strategy for nursing, midwifery and health visiting research (DoH 1993).

Following the Briggs report, one step that was taken to enable nursing to become a research-based profession was the setting up in 1977 of the Joint Board of Clinical Nursing Studies (whose responsibilities for post-basic education were later taken over by the English National Board for Nursing, Midwifery and Health Visiting). The reason why the Board contributed to nursing's quest to become a research-based profession was that it included in its syllabuses the 'promotion of research awareness' (Hunt & Hicks 1983). The Board made clear (like the Briggs' report before them) that their aim was not to produce 'nurse researchers' but 'to promote the concept of research-mindedness—that is, the development of an inquiring attitude of mind, a logical approach to problems relating to nursing, an awareness of the existence of research reports and the ability to read, evaluate, select and make use of relevant findings'.

Even post-basic courses such as 995, superseded by 870, were specifically committed to the understanding and application/appreciation of research, not the doing of it. Rather, students were to be enabled to understand and appreciate the value and implications of research for their practice.

However, the expectation over the years was for generations of post-basic students on these courses to undertake small-scale projects. The response to this endeavour has been equivocal, as the following statement from the recent Taskforce on the Strategy for Research in Nursing, Midwifery and Health Visiting (DoH 1993, p. 6) suggests:

> *Such work is to be commended when it is undertaken with due regard for practical and ethical considerations and within a good supervisory and supportive research structure. However, it must not be seen as a substitute for the generalisable and cumulative research which we would place at the heart of a strategy for advancing research in nursing.*

It is clear therefore that the Taskforce does not expect every nurse and midwife to undertake research, especially without adequate resources and structures. Rather they recommend the integration of research processes and findings into everday teaching and practice, re-affirming the Briggs' recommendation that research 'become part of the mental equipment of every practising nurse or midwife'.

Similarly, when at the beginning of the module we examined the aims of current educational programmes we found that the promotion of research awareness and/or mindedness rather than the doing of it, remain relevant today. These aims are reflected in both pre- and post-registration educational programmes. For example, Project 2000 (Dip HE) students are expected to 'demonstrate an appreciation of research and relevant literature as an aid to practice' (GB Statutory Instrument 1989), while one of the 10 key characteristics for Higher Award Students is to demonstrate: 'The ability to use research to plan, implement and evaluate concepts and strategies leading to improvements in care' (ENB 1991). We were struck by the similarity between this statement and the four stages of the nursing process in which care is assessed, planned, implemented and evaluated by nurses and other health workers. Drawing on familiar experiences in this way helped us to make connections between practice and research and to feel less daunted by it.

We also recognized that making such connections dispelled some of the fears associated with research. We agreed with Rees (1992) that 'teachers have to be competent in these [research] skills themselves before they can help to develop them in students'. Dispelling our fears was a prerequisite for acquiring those skills and part of becoming research minded. We also agreed that Rees' observation was equally relevant to the classroom-based teacher and to the practitioner who works alongside students to make research-based thinking and practice a reality. Clifford (1993) in recent research, however, found that: 'Although the notion of practice being "research-based" is a widely used term it is not one that has been rigor-ously explored'.

We hope that our book through promoting research mindedness as part of rigorous exploration will contribute to research-based practice.

Definition of terms

In the literature some authors use the terms 'research awareness' and 'research mindedness' interchangeably. We found that as a group we varied. Some of us used the terms interchangeably while others preferred to make the distinction between 'awareness' and 'mindedness'. It was argued that individuals could be aware of research in a passive way, whereas mindedness required action. In order to resolve our dilemma we turned to the Chambers English Dictionary. There we found the following distinction: *aware* was defined as 'informed', 'conscious of'; *minded* on the other hand was defined as 'inclined', 'disposed', suggestive of an attitudi-nal change.

We pondered on this idea of being 'inclined' or 'disposed' and someone recalled that it reminded her of a definition she had read in a popular research textbook for nurses and health workers which talked about a 'research stance' (Sapsford & Abbott 1992).

Sapsford & Abbott say 'we have tended to talk on occasions, as every-one does, as if "research" were a set of skills to be brought out and applied to the particular problem. This is true of course but a training in research entails more than this … the "research stance" is more a frame of mind, an openness and neutrality at the point of immediate argument, a kind of imagination' (p. 16).

We decided therefore that the research 'stance' seemed to have some commonality with being research 'minded', 'inclined' or 'disposed'. Indeed one student suggested that an alternative title for the module might have been 'Adopting the research stance'.

The definition of research mindedness that most people were familiar with was that of the Royal College of Nursing's Research Group (RCN

1982). In a policy statement, the Group defined research mindedness as implying 'a critical and questioning approach to one's work, the desire and ability to find out about the latest research in the area and apply it as appropriate'. We agreed that this was a useful working definition and contained many of the elements of research mindedness identified by the Joint Board of Clinical Nursing Studies.

We also discussed a chapter on research that I had written as part of a general textbook for Project 2000 students (Smith 1992a). The aim of the chapter was to assist 'beginning' students to become 'research aware'. I summarized the components of research awareness as:

- developing the confidence to have ideas and ask questions about nursing
- becoming familiar with research methods and techniques
- being able to critically assess research reports
- being able to incorporate research methods and findings into knowledge and practice.

In discussion we concluded that my definition of research awareness was more akin to promoting research mindedness and showed us the fine dividing line between the meaning of the two terms. On the basis of this discussion, I decided to change the aim of my chapter in a second edition of the book to assist students to become research 'minded' rather than just 'aware' (Smith 1996).

Finally, we looked at a definition in a textbook for social workers, which described the characteristics of research-minded practitioners in the following way:

- [they] will be constantly defining and making explicit their objectives and hypotheses;
- [they] will treat their explanations of the social world as hypotheses—that is, as tentative and open to be tested against evidence;
- [they] will be aware of their expertise and knowledge and that of others;
- [they] will bring to the fore theories that help make sense of social need, resources and assist in decision making with regard to strategies;
- [they] will be thoughtful, reflecting on data and theory and contributing to their development and refinement;
- [they] will scrutinize and be analytical of available data and information;
- [they] will be mindful of the pervasiveness of ideology and values in the way we see and understand the world.

We liked the definition of research mindedness adopted by these authors (Everitt et al 1992) because of the integrated approach they took to research-based practice. The emphasis for them was clearly not on doing research but on using its theoretical perspectives and methods to think analytically about and inform practice. Research mindedness also allowed practitioners to identify their own knowledge and expertise which would otherwise go unrecognized and undetected.

We concluded that one way to solve the dilemma (some would say 'tyranny') of deciding on which terms to use seemed to be to review them all and devise our own working definitions.

You might at this point like to write down your own definition of 'research mindedness' to compare it with each author's understanding and use of the term as discussed at the beginning of each chapter.

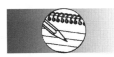

Your definition is likely to include some of the following elements: thoughtful; questioning; enquiring; analytical; making two-way links between theory and practice.

KNOWLEDGE FOR PRACTICE, EDUCATION AND RESEARCH

As the discussion progressed, 'knowledge' emerged as an important topic for discussion. Since one of the purposes of research is to produce new knowledge, we agreed it was important to have reached a working understanding of what it was. For most of us knowledge was synonymous with the facts and theories we drew on to teach and practice.

In order to consider further the relationship of knowledge to facts and theories, we discussed the results of a survey on scientific knowledge conducted in 1990 (Laffan 1993). The survey was based on the responses of a representative sample of 2000 Britons who were over 18. The findings showed that the majority of the respondents expressed an interest in science and thought it was important. But when it came to specific questions about scientific facts there were a few surprises: 34% knew that the earth orbits the sun once a year; 50% knew that electrons were smaller than atoms and another 50% knew that antibiotics were ineffective against viruses. Whilst in the first instance we expressed dismay at the poor state of scientific knowledge of the average Briton, we then began to ask questions. Who for example had decided that knowing about viruses and electrons was important for every Briton? What was the value of possessing knowledge if it could not be applied to daily life? What counted as 'knowledge' and what did not? Who decided? Research in the 1970s showed that women recognized mothering and housewifery as a set of skills (Oakley 1974). But did those skills require knowledge as defined by the survey or 'just common sense'? These questions mirror the debates around the relative status of medical and nursing knowledge.

For example, when I observed an auxiliary community nurse on her rounds, I noted that she was very skilled in bathing patients in their own homes. Each bath was 'tailor-made' to patients' individual conditions and circumstances, leaving them not only clean and comfortable but also satisfied. But how would that auxiliary's skill be rated against 'knowing' scientific facts about medical diagnosis and treatment for the conditions that some of her patients were suffering from? The answer depends on how we define knowledge, scientific fact and theory.

Several members of the group identified Carper's framework of knowledge (Carper 1978) as useful for looking at the patterns or processes by which nursing knowledge is produced. Carper describes four patterns of knowing for nursing. These are:

- the formal approaches associated with traditional scientific methods which she refers to as 'empirics' or 'empirical' as in the sense of systematic, scientific observation
- the knowledge associated with the art of nursing, described as 'aesthetics', of which empathy is a key component
- the personal knowledge unique to each individual and the use of 'self' in our relationship with others
- the knowledge that is associated with moral decision making and ethics.

It is clearly important for practitioners to think about the different types of knowledge and how they are valued. In the case of the auxiliary nurse, for example, Carper's framework makes it possible to identify the knowledge she brings to bathing patients and the quality of the personalized relationships with them as both aesthetic and personal knowledge.

Carper's framework can also be applied to an analysis of the following incident recounted by the sociologist Ann Oakley (1986, p. 182). Oakley, whose work on housework has already been referred to, also studied health care. The incident illustrates how even a feminist sociologist sensitive to women's issues can fail to recognize nurses, their knowledge and skills. In a 15-year career as a health service researcher, Oakley admits, she hardly noticed nurses at all and took their presence for granted. It was only as a patient that she came to recognize nurses' knowledge and skill. She was undergoing cancer treatment in radioactive isolation when a nurse noticed that she looked distressed. Instead of donning protective clothing and staying the maximum recognized time of 10 minutes, the nurse sat down with Oakley and talked her through her feelings for nearly an hour. Oakley never saw the nurse again but she attributed her survival to her caring intervention.

In the incident described by Oakley, it was only through her intense personal experience rather than as an 'objective' researcher that she was able to recognize what nurses know and do. Using Carper's framework, we can identify that the nurse was drawing on her 'aesthetic' knowledge to comfort Oakley. In risking her own safety, the nurse may have also been drawing on her ethical knowledge to make a moral decision to put the patient's needs above her own.

Traditionally, however, scientific or empirical knowledge (such as that defined in the science survey) and which predominates in medicine, is often more highly prized than aesthetic or personal knowledge common among nurses. One reason for the high status of scientific knowledge is its association with facts and theories. But on closer scrutiny these facts and theories are not immutable and can change. Rees writes: 'We must accept that the information and research we talk about today is based on yesterday's understanding' and he urges teachers 'to encourage students to understand the limitations of our present knowledge and provide them with the skills to evaluate new information and research findings and to apply this to tomorrow's situations'.

Research with nurses, midwives and health visitors into the health-based curriculum (Lask et al 1994) illustrates the relevance of Rees' observations. Risk factors associated with disease were identified by respondents as an important aspect of the knowledge base required for health education. Many of them also expressed concern that these risk factors appeared to change as new research evidence came on stream. They felt insecure at the prospects of giving health advice that might be already out of date. They appeared to lack the research skills to help them break through the limitations inherent in seeing knowledge as immutable or unchanging facts.

'Epistemology' was another word that kept cropping up in our discussions about knowledge and you will find that some of the authors of subsequent chapters refer to it. For the purposes of clarification we defined it as 'theories of knowledge' which can be illustrated in Carper's four ways of knowing. For example, on the one hand the epistemology that underpins scientific knowledge is assumed to be objective and pure; on the other hand, as the Oakley incident implies, subjective emotions may affect our moral decisions.

Just as you wrote down your own definitions of 'research mindedness' you might now like to do the same for 'knowledge' using examples from your own experience. Think of examples that demonstrate the different types of knowledge you use in everyday practice. If Ann Oakley had been your patient, for example, in addition to the aesthetic, personal and ethical knowledge required to care for her, you might have also drawn on the 'scientific' knowledge available concerning her treatment and the effects of the radiotherapy.

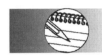

THE LINK BETWEEN KNOWLEDGE, REFLECTION AND RESEARCH

Another theme to emerge during our discussions was the link between knowledge, reflection and research. We drew on Benner (1984) and Schon (1987) to explore the close association between them. Benner's research illustrates the use of reflection in nurses' skill acquisition as they move from novice to expert (Benner 1984). According to Schon (1987), this process takes place through 'reflection in action' as practitioners develop 'professional artistry' to bridge the theory–practice gap. Reflection may also be retrospective as practitioners think back on situations after they have occurred. They may then use their feelings to evaluate the situation and gain new insights, understandings and knowledge. One way to do this is to keep a reflective diary as a record of the situations experienced and the insights gained over time. Below is an example of how a senior student nurse describes the reflective process in my research on emotional labour (Smith 1992, p. 47).

When you're on the ward you're watching people all the time and you think 'I'll remember that' or 'that's not the way I'd do it'. Then again it's almost inspirational or off the cuff. You think 'I've never met this before, I've got to act' (reflection in action). Or you go off duty and think you've handled something and sift through it (retrospective reflection).

The group were in agreement that reflective practice would assist the practitioner to become more research minded.

Similarly, we noted that researchers who use interviews and participant observation work in a reflective and analytic way, move between the field and their data to guide their future research, make interpretations and develop findings.

For example, a specialist teacher who was observing how teachers in the same speciality communicated with students in the classroom wrote:

Analysis of each week's observation furnished so much food for thought, not only concerning my future work in the field, but for interaction with my own classes as well. Trying to see ourselves as our students might be seeing us is a bit frightening, but nevertheless one of the most enlightening experiences one can have. My study helped me see what I liked and didn't like about teaching and myself as a teacher.

(Rose quoted in Ely et al 1991, p. 200)

From this extract it is possible to see how a researcher who is also a practitioner can draw insights from her own knowledge of the field both to reflect on her own practice and to develop research findings. The example would be equally applicable to a nurse or health visitor researcher observing patients and clients.

THE RESEARCH PROCESS

At the beginning of this chapter we confirmed that research mindedness was not about undertaking research but we also suggested that making the distinction between the two activities was false. Familiarity with the research process might appear to contradict the first point but confirm the second as integral to becoming research minded. The research process offers a conventional but useful framework in which to fit the theoretical perspectives, approaches and methods of research that are explored throughout the chapters of this book. It is also a useful starting point for newcomers to research.

What then is the research process?

The research process refers to the different stages involved in undertaking a research project. Like any process, however, although we represent the research as being divided into distinct stages which follow on from each other, often they are not mutually exclusive and there may be some overlap between them.

The research process involves identifying a topic, specifying underlying theories, formulating questions, selecting a suitable approach, specifying methods and devising a plan to take the study forward.

An important part of the research plan includes the careful considera-tion of time and financial budgeting, secretarial support and obtaining eth-ical clearance. Time spent resolving outstanding organizational, political and ethical issues repays itself with interest over the rest of the study.

The stages of the research process can be grouped in the following way:

- identifying the research problem
- selecting an appropriate research approach
- designing the study
- developing data collecting methods and techniques
- collecting the data
- analysis and interpretation of the data
- presentation of research findings.

The way in which researchers take the research process forward will depend to some extent on whether a qualitative or quantitative research approach is adopted. Many researchers involved in studying health and its delivery prefer to see the so-called distinction as more of a continuum in which as Bell (1993) suggests 'no approach prescribes nor automatically rejects any particular method'.

It is common in social science to see the use of a multimethod approach or 'triangulation' by which more than one method is used and/or groups of people studied within the same study. In the end, a number of factors may influence a researcher's decision to select a particular research approach.

It may be that one approach is more suitable to a particular topic than another, or researchers base their decisions on experience and preferences, the availability of a research supervisor (also with particular preferences) and practical issues of time and money.

We concluded this session by discussing research terminology and lan-guage. As mentioned in the introduction, we were keen to avoid the elitism of research jargon but realized the importance of becoming familiar with key terms. We discussed ways of introducing students to the language of research and dismissed the idea of presenting them with a glossary in the first session because we thought it might be quite overwhelming. Rather we decided it would be better to introduce them gradually to the terms as they applied to different aspects of research mindedness. This is what we have done from here on throughout this textbook. As you meet new words in a chapter, we draw your attention to them by emboldening them in the text. You will then be able to refer to them in a glossary of terms at the back of the book.

Finally, we wanted to put the study of research in a broader context and, in order to do this, we identified during our classroom discussion some of the important policy documents that have been written on health service research in general and nursing research in particular. We have summa-rized some of the key issues contained in these documents below.

KEY NURSING RESEARCH DOCUMENTS

The following key documents were identified by one of the contributors, Donna Lewis, as giving an overview of the research strategies for nursing promoted by a number of official bodies and government reports:

- Department of Health and Social Security (DHSS) 1972 *Report of the Committee on Nursing*, commonly referred to as the 'Briggs' report' after the name of the Chair, Professor (now Lord) Asa Briggs.
- English National Board for Nursing, Midwifery and Health Visiting (ENB) 1989 *Project 2000: a new preparation for practice—guidelines and criteria for course development*.
- International Council of Nurses (ICN) 1990 *How the ICN is promoting nursing research*.
- United Kingdom Central Council for Nursing, Midwifery and Health Visiting (UKCC) 1992 *Code of Professional Conduct*.
- Department of Health (DoH) 1993 *Report of the Taskforce on the Strategy for Research in Nursing, Midwifery and Health Visiting*.

Key points

Briggs committee (DHSS 1972): Recommended that nursing become a research-based profession and set the tone for future developments in nurse education and research.

ENB (1989): Recommended that 'the curriculum should reflect the integration of theory and practice underpinned by relevant research'.

ICN (1990): Stated that there is 'no health without research' and that research should be promoted in all countries; ICN is in the process of developing an international agenda which emphasizes the role of governments and professional nursing bodies in focusing on and implementing research.

UKCC (1992) Code of Professional Conduct: Emphasized the need for practice to be based on up-to-date knowledge.

DoH (1993) Taskforce report: Emphasized the need for nurses, midwives and health visitors to participate in multidisciplinary research as well as for academic nursing departments to develop research programmes in specialist fields and organize research training. The Taskforce saw their recommendations as relevant to occupational therapy, speech and language therapy and physiotherapy. The move away from small-scale projects to systematic generalizable research was recommended. The provision of dedicated monies and scholarships to fund nursing research and research training by the national research councils such as the Medical Research Council (MRC) and Economic and Social Sciences Research Council (ESRC) as well as the Department of Health was called for. The ultimate aim of research was to inform and improve practice.

A recent PREP (Post-registration Education and Practice) fact sheet on continuing education (UKCC 1995) identified research as an integral component of education and practice which contributed to and enriched advanced clinical practice as a whole. In turn, outcomes of advanced clinical practice were identified as an increase in nursing research and research-based practice.

Key NHS research and development documents

Since it is important to situate nursing research within the broader context (as we did in the classroom), we conclude this chapter with some thoughts on the Department of Health research and development strategy, launched in 1991 (DoH 1991).

The strategy marked the first national framework for setting research priorities. One of its prime aims was to promote a research culture within the NHS that moved the base of clinical practice from ritual to evidence and improved the quality of patient care. The strategy was in line with the newly organized purchaser/provider health service (DoH 1989) and the 'Health of the nation' policy document (DoH 1992) which specified five priority areas for improving the nation's health, namely: coronary heart disease and stroke; cancers; mental illness; HIV/AIDS; and accidents. Research and development programmes were set up to document and reduce the incidence within each area and investigate treatment outcomes. In turn, the findings of such investigations could be used to develop audit tools. The responsibility for these programmes was devolved to the regional health authorities, which from 1996 will be incorporated into the Department of Health.

Since we completed our classes in June 1994, further developments have taken place and will continue to do so, particularly in relation to research that contributes to 'evidence-based practice'. Health service purchasers setting up contracts with providers are more likely to 'purchase' a service or treatment if research has 'proved' its effectiveness. Systematic reviews of clinical trials including nursing interventions are being undertaken and new ones set up to provide evidence for improving health care. Centres at Oxford and York have been established to review trial findings and disseminate their results nationwide. We shall say a little more about these initiatives in Chapter 3.

Finally, the Culyer report (DoH 1994), concerned with addressing potential threats to research funding and support associated with the NHS market reforms, made proposals to prevent this happening. The report therefore recommended closer working between the NHS and the academic research community so that service-oriented research would not be squeezed out by the traditionally more prestigious medically led scientific research. One set of recommendations was specifically aimed at improving the chances of 'Cinderella settings and disciplines' (and by implication nursing, midwifery and health visiting) to secure research funding (Culyer 1995). In this way health-based research was seen as having a double benefit, by preventing people becoming clients in the first place while improving the treatment and care of those who did. Finally, it provided 'knowledge that may benefit all' (Culyer 1995).

In summary, then, what these documents and statements tell us is that research within nursing and health care is here to stay. Research in its various guises is no longer an optional extra in the new-look health service of the 1990s. Nurses, midwives and health visitors need to shape a role for themselves in order to meet both their own professional and personal needs and those of their patients and clients. Becoming research minded therefore (which this book aims to promote) is an important preparation for this role.

REFERENCES

Bell J 1993 Doing your research project. Open University Press, Buckingham

Benner P 1984 From novice to expert: excellence and power in clinical nursing practice. Addison-Wesley, Menlo Park, California

Carper B A 1978 Fundamental patterns of knowing in nursing. Advances in Nursing Science 1(1): 13–23

Clifford C 1993 The role of nurse teachers in the empowerment of nurses through research. Nurse Education Today 13: 47–54

Culyer T 1995 Cure at a cost. Synthesis, Times Higher Education Supplement, January 20, p i

Department of Health 1989 Working for patients: the health service: caring for the 1990s. HMSO, London

Department of Health 1992 Health of the nation. HMSO, London

Department of Health 1994 Support for research and development in the NHS (Chair: Professor T Culyer). HMSO, London

Department of Health (Research and Development Division) 1991 Research for health. HMSO, London

Department of Health (Research and Development Division) 1993 Report of the Taskforce on the Strategy for Research in Nursing, Midwifery and Health Visiting (Chair: Professor A Webb). Department of Health, London

Department of Health and Social Security 1972 Report of the Committee on Nursing (Chair: Professor Asa Briggs). HMSO, London

Ely M et al 1991 Doing qualitative research: circles within circles. Falmer, London

English National Board for Nursing, Midwifery and Health Visiting 1989 Project 2000: a new preparation for practice—guidelines and criteria for course development. ENB, London

English National Board for Nursing, Midwifery and Health Visiting 1991 ENB framework for continuing professional education for nurses, midwives and health visitors—guide to implementation. ENB, London

Everitt A, Hardiker P, Littlewood J, Mullender A 1992 Applied research for better practice. Macmillan, London

Great Britain Statutory Instrument 1989 Nurses, midwives and health visitors training amendment rules, Schedule 2, S.I., No. 1456, Rule 18a. HMSO, London

Hunt M, Hicks J 1983 Promoting research-awareness in post-basic nursing courses. Occasional Papers, Nursing Times (March 30): 41–42

International Council of Nurses 1990 How the ICN is promoting nursing research. International Nursing Review 37(4): 295–298

Joint Board of Clinical Nursing Studies 1977 The research objective in Joint Board courses—an introductory guide. Occasional Publications, JBCNS, London, p 3

Laffan G 1993 A new holistic science. Nursing Standard 7(17): 44–45

Lask S, Smith P, Masterson A 1994 A curricular review of the pre- and post-registration education programmes for nurses, midwives and health visitors in relation to the integration of a philosophy of health: developing a model for evaluation. ENB, London

Oakley A 1974 The sociology of housework. Martin Robinson, London

Oakley A 1986 On the importance of being a nurse. In: Telling the truth about Jerusalem: a collection of essays and poems. Basil Blackwell, New York

Rees C 1992 Practising research-based teaching. Nursing Times 88(8): 55–57

Royal College of Nursing 1982 Research mindedness and nurse education: an RCN Research Society report. RCN, London

Sapsford R, Abbott P 1992 Research methods for nurses and the caring professions. Open University Press, Buckingham

Schon D A 1987 Educating the reflective practitioner. Jossey Bass, San Francisco

Smith P 1992a Research and its application. In: Kenworthy N, Snowley G, Gilling C (eds) Common foundation studies in nursing, 1st edn. Churchill Livingstone, Edinburgh

Smith P 1992b The emotional labour of nursing—how nurses care. Macmillan, Basingstoke

Smith P 1996 Research and its application. In: Kenworthy N, Snowley G, Gilling C (eds) Common foundation studies in nursing, 2nd edn. Churchill Livingstone, Edinburgh

United Kingdom Central Council for Nursing, Midwifery and Health Visiting 1992 Code of Professional Conduct, 3rd edn. UKCC, London

United Kingdom Central Council for Nursing, Midwifery and Health Visiting 1995 PREP and you: maintaining your registration; standards for education following registration. UKCC, London

FURTHER READING

All Wales Nursing, Midwifery and Health Visiting Research Group 1994 Strategy for nursing in Wales: a framework for research and development in Wales. Welsh Office, Cardiff

Boore J 1991 A strategy for research (Northern Ireland). Nursing Standard 5 (51): 55–56

Clark M 1992 A strategy for nursing research (Scotland). Nursing Standard 6 (22): 22–23

Department of Health and Social Security 1993 A strategy for nursing, midwifery and health visiting in Northern Ireland: an action plan for nursing research and development in Northern Ireland. DHSS, Belfast

Scottish Office Home and Health Department 1993 Research and development strategy for the National Health Service in Scotland. HMSO, Edinburgh

The Welsh Office NHS Directorate 1992 Sharpening the focus: a research and development framework for NHS Wales. Welsh Office, Cardiff

Note: The Nursing Research Initiative for Scotland (NRIS) was set up in 1994 based at Glasgow Caledonian University and the Victoria Infirmary NHS Trust. The project is under the directorship of Professor Jennifer Hunt and its focus is direct patient care research.

Research paradigms

Margaret Harper _Nina Hartman_

2

KEY ISSUES

- An examination of the values and assumptions that underpin the main research approaches used in nursing and midwifery today
- The relationship of the research approach to the creation of nursing and midwifery knowledge
- Reflection on personal views of nursing and midwifery inquiry in order to achieve a deeper level of self-understanding
- Alternative ways of generating knowledge for practice
- Story telling

PREAMBLE

The challenge

This chapter explores the values and assumptions that underpin the main research **approaches** used in nursing and midwifery today. Our primary aim is to demonstrate that in the right context each research approach can create knowledge that is important for nursing and midwifery.

While reading, you may find an approach that you instinctively feel 'at home' with. This is fine, since beliefs, values and past experience help us construct a personal philosophy that gives us a particular orientation to the world we live in and influences the way we practise as nurses, midwives or health visitors. Problems only arise when personal philosophy and allegiances to certain approaches become **ideology** and the views of others are dismissed as irrelevant or unimportant.

We hope that this chapter will encourage you to reflect upon your own views of nursing and midwifery inquiry, perhaps resulting in a deeper level of self-understanding. Hopefully it will also challenge you to consider the value of different ways of generating knowledge and how they might be useful to your practice.

As you may have gathered by now, the seminars that led to the publication of this book were full of chat, critical debate, fierce challenge and shifting of deeply held beliefs. All the seminars were conducted in an atmosphere of respect, good humour and safety. We hope that you will find both the book and this chapter to be a safe place to look at your views also. We want to stimulate dialogue: with yourself, colleagues, clients and, as you read, the other chapters of this book.

INTRODUCTION

The purpose of nursing research is to develop, refine and extend the scientific base of nursing knowledge (Polit & Hungler 1989). The development of nursing knowledge is governed by philosophical viewpoints which describe the nature of human beings and the human–environment relationship (Fawcett 1993). These philosophical viewpoints are also called **paradigms**, or world-views, and are the basis of the conceptual models used in practice. The principles embedded in each of these paradigms will dictate the type of knowledge that will be generated, the criteria for establishing 'truth' and also the conduct of the research study.

The development of nursing knowledge has been influenced by the paradigms of positivism, interpretivism and critical social theory. In this chapter each paradigm is explored and the key components of knowledge, **theory**, truth and the role of the researcher discussed. We illustrate the benefits and limitations of each paradigm by using examples from our clinical and teaching practice. Feminism is used as an extension of critical social theory.

The literature suggests that many nurses and midwives still view research in terms of **quantitative** and **qualitative** data collection **methods** (Porter 1989). We discovered during the course of our seminar that our peers were no exception. The limitations of this view are examined. The value of understanding research from a philosophical, as well as a methodological, perspective is highlighted, and we describe the seminar in which we presented these perspectives to our peers. We also want to show the significance of encouraging critical and creative thinking as a way of developing research mindedness and good practice.

RESEARCH MINDEDNESS

You will read many definitions of research mindedness as you work through the chapters of this book. No doubt by the end you will have clarified your own ideas of what it means to be a research-minded practitioner. While preparing the material for this chapter, we were each exposed to separate experiences which immediately clarified for us what we think are the essential elements of research mindedness. We now each tell our stories about those experiences.

Margaret's story

What I value so much about my experience is that powerful ideas and self-understanding often come at the oddest times, when you least expect them and are not looking for them. Also, seemingly simple things can teach us so much. Some of the biggest experiences we have in practice, for example, can arise from what on the surface can be quite mundane events. Smith F (1992) believes that we learn in the form of stories and also construct stories to make sense of events. This is what I am doing here. I am using my story to represent my ideas of what research mindedness is, rather than stating someone else's. Maybe my story will help you to start thinking about your own definitions and stories.

'My blood is too rich'

I was sitting on a 134 bus; it was pouring and I was wet through. A young girl sat opposite me, dabbing at a sore on her ear with a dirty, soggy, blood-stained tissue. I offered her a clean handkerchief and asked if she had fallen and hurt herself.

'I get this sometimes when I eat certain things.'

'Oh?'

'I think I'm allergic to some things, I break out in these spots, then they bleed.'

'I'm allergic to milk, I get a patch of eczema on my leg when I take anything with milk in it.'

'It's because my blood is too rich, I get these spots when my blood is too rich.'

My eyes opened wide and my heart started to beat faster; in 17 years nobody had ever told me that they thought their blood was too rich. My German grandmother said mine was too rich when I got heatspots and my mother said my sister's was too rich when she was the only one in the house who got bitten by a flea.

The girl smiled and thanked me for the handkerchief, then got off the bus at Camden Town. I so much wanted to run after her—rain and all—and ask: 'What makes you think that your blood's too rich?'

It would have been cheeky; the context was not right. Anyway, she might have hit me with her umbrella and I would not have blamed her. I am now haunted by lay explanations of health and illness; how they go far beyond common sense and how powerful they are in shaping health beliefs and behaviour. I am working on how I can make the context right.

I cannot even sit on the bus in peace. That is what being research minded means to me.

So, for me, research mindedness is a way of being, part of the way I live my life, my dispositions or the stances I take. The dispositions or stances I value are a healthy curiosity, respect, care and concern, an openness to surprise, a sense of humour and the ability to stay wide awake—nothing mysterious.

This focus on dispositions or stances is intentional since it taps into qualities we all have, are most probably practising and which can certainly be cultivated. We can all be or become better research-minded practitioners by using the raw material that we possess as people first. It is nursing knowledge that later transforms this into something very special.

Nina's story

What being research minded means to me is encapsulated in the following quotation from the Chinese-American writer, Maxine Hong-Kingston (1975), who says: 'I learned to make my mind large, as the universe is large, so that there is room for paradoxes'. Hong-Kingston, with her emphasis on making our minds large to take in the largeness of the universe in order to make room for paradoxes (contradictions), reflects my complex attitude to research and research mindedness. As a midwife working in midwifery and nursing education, with a commitment to practice, I know what my attitude to research is 'supposed' to be. However, the truth is that I am not always sure what we mean by research mindedness, and sometimes feel that I do not want to know either. Part of the reason for this is precisely what this chapter is about, that for most of our professional history the predominant **philosophy** in nursing and midwifery did not allow us to discover diverse, alternative forms of knowledge contained in our practice. One of the keystones of critical social theory and feminism (which we talk about later in this chapter) is to allow those diverse, alternative forms of knowledge to be discovered, so making our minds large and making room for paradoxes.

While pondering on how to reveal these awkward attitudes to my colleagues, I had an illuminating experience in the classroom. This is my story. I was teaching a group of student midwives. It was one of those normal, humdrum working days. We were discussing neonatal care and parent support as described in various textbooks and articles. In the group discussion we got on to the topic of how parenting and particularly mothering is defined.

One of the students told us that she had looked after a baby in the special care baby unit (SCBU) whose mother was labelled 'a bad mother'. The reason she had been labelled in this way was because she hardly ever visited her baby, although the baby's father came regularly. The student, who was black, sensed that there were racist overtones in the attitude of the (predominantly white) staff towards this mother, who was also black, implying that her infrequent visits were in some way associated with her racial differences. The student, as a member of a minority, felt unable to say anything to the staff because of what she experienced as the 'double jeopardy' of her student status and her race. On the occasions when the mother visited, the student observed that she seemed withdrawn and quiet. English was not her first language, though she spoke it fluently. As it turned out, the student and this mother spoke the same first language. The student told us that because they were able to communicate in their own language she discovered that the mother had had nine miscarriages prior to the birth of this premature infant. She was, of course, now afraid to invest in this new, intensely longed for, patiently, passionately awaited relationship with her tiny baby. As the student recounted the woman's story, the classroom was silent, the textbook examples set aside.

I was on the edge of my seat by now, the hairs on my body standing up. It felt as though this mother, with all her passions and fears, her intense and 'distant' mothering, was in the classroom with us. This was not 'bad mothering', this was motherhood experienced most intensely. Nor was this a humdrum working day. This emotional moment when deep connections had been made, turned my whole experience of the day, of teaching, of being a midwife, into something vibrant and meaningful all over again.

A plethora of questions jumbled into my mind as this story unfolded. How are investments in new relationships made? How are attitudes to mothering communicated to midwives, student midwives, student nurses, and new mothers? What does this say about our attitude to women? How is racism addressed in our profession? What happens when, as here, a student feels that both she and a client are being treated in a racist way? What are the implications for experienced midwives as mentors and preceptors?

This emotional connection to an experience, to a topic, is what being research minded means to me—a connection that generates questions and a desire to look at things anew.

Of course there are many attitudes to and definitions of research mindedness. Through our two very different stories we have given you examples of ours so that you can think about your own definitions and why you define them in this way.

Having told you our stories to illustrate what being research minded means for us you might like to think of some stories of your own. You might also like to consider what qualities you think are necessary for an individual to become research minded. For us, it is about using all our senses to alert us to what is going on around us. It is about having 'wide-open eyes' and the flexibility to change our ideas.

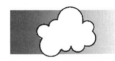

Of course we can only become research minded if the institutions we work in are willing to provide support and resources.

Make a list of what support and resources you think are required. Your list might include local nursing research staff available to support practice and education, designated thinking time for reading and reflection, opportunities to get together with colleagues to tell your stories.

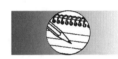

PHILOSOPHY, VALUES, ASSUMPTIONS AND APPROACHES TO NURSING AND MIDWIFERY RESEARCH

Research, like any subject, has its own language and inevitably the next section is full of words that may at this stage be unfamiliar to you. We have emboldened those words which appear in the glossary in order to make it easier for you if you need to look them up as you read through the chapter.

Philosophy

Leddy & Pepper (1993), two American nurse academics, define philosophy as 'a science that comprises logic, ethics, aesthetics, metaphysics and the theory of knowledge'. It is a reflective discipline which uses the rational process of philosophic inquiry to investigate issues of significance to humankind. So the science of philosophy is really about using disciplined thinking to explore areas of importance. During this process beliefs and values are clarified, giving purpose and direction to the focus of study.

The principal focus of the philosophy of science is exploring the nature of scientific knowledge (Suppe & Jacox 1985). It governs legitimate **phenomena** for investigation, the methods of investigation, the criteria of what constitutes knowledge and truth and the relationship between the researcher and the research subject. The assumptions that underpin knowledge and truth are known as **epistemology**, and the assumptions that describe reality, **ontology**.

The development of scientific knowledge is influenced by paradigms, or philosophical viewpoints, which provide an ontological perspective that guides epistemology and research approaches (also referred to as **methodologies**) (Newman 1992). Research contributes to the development of scientific knowledge by theory testing and theory building. In nursing, these activities are influenced by the paradigms of positivism, interpretivism and critical social theory (Lowenberg 1993). In our opinion, feminist theory develops and extends critical social theory.

We now draw on philosophy to explore the principal assumptions underpinning the three paradigms, using practical examples to illustrate them. Limitations of space preclude a more complete discussion of the rich competing perspectives both within and between the paradigms. We have summarized some of the main features of each paradigm in Table 2.1 and

Table 2.1 Belief systems of the paradigms of positivism, interpretivism and critical social theory (Sources: Newman 1992, after Guba 1990)

Ontology	Epistemology	Methodology
Positivism		
Reality is objective: exists independently of perception	Inquirer adopts an objective, detached stance	Experimental Empiric Controlled
Driven by natural laws	True belief corresponds to fact	Testing of hypotheses
Interpretivism		
Reality is mentally constructed and is socially and culturally based	Knowledge is constructed in a social and historical context	Hermeneutic Dialectic
Multiple interpretations and multiple realities accepted	Findings represent a creation of the process between the researcher and research subject	Focuses on uncovering the variety of constructions that exist among them
	Truth is based on pragmatic criteria	
Critical social theory		
Reality is constructed and influenced by societal structures	Subjective Values mediate inquiry Constructed, communal, contextual	Dialogic Critique of ideology
Human beings are capable of rational self-critique	Goal is to free participants from the effect of ideology	Reveal hidden power imbalances
	Standards of truth	Facilitate social transformation
	Meaning and truth are interpreted within the context of history	

you might like to refer to it to guide your reading. This chapter provides a useful foundation for ensuing chapters and you will probably find yourself referring back to it frequently. This is how we want you to use the chapter. Learning is cumulative, and will not be achieved just by reading through the chapter once.

For those readers seeking a more complete understanding of the philosophy of science, further reading is suggested at the end of the chapter.

Positivism

The positivist philosophy of science emerged in the 19th century and is associated with the French philosopher Comte (1789–1857). It was refined and developed in the 1920s by a group known as the Vienna Circle to become **logical positivism**.

The logical positivists believed that the only true knowledge was that which could be gained by the application of logic to data arrived at by sensory experience (Meleis 1991). Logical positivism, later known as logical **empiricism**, engendered a new certainty in the power of science to solve problems of significance to humankind. It became synonymous with the 'scientific method' (i.e. experiments) and the 'received view' of what counted as knowledge.

This view of science influenced philosophical thinking until the 1960s and shaped the development of both medicine and nursing as scientific disciplines.

Positivism maintains that there is an **objective** reality that exists independently of the observer, where phenomena are driven by natural laws that are accessible to **observation** and **measurement**. The only valid way to generate knowledge is the application of logic and experience derived from sensory data. Its epistemology demands that the researcher adopt an objective, detached stance (Newman 1992). This is based on the idea that the phenomena will then show themselves as they exist in reality, uncontaminated by any subjective **bias** that the researcher might bring to the data.

In positivist science, the principal focus of research tends to be on theory testing. Theories themselves are considered to be completed products that unify the diverse phenomena of a discipline, and the ultimate goal is toward theoretical reduction with enhanced explanatory power (Silva & Rothbart 1984).

Research is based on experimental methodology that aims to isolate cause and effect. Its focus is on controlling **variables**, testing **hypotheses** and reducing a phenomenon to its component parts as a means of understanding the whole (Newman 1992). Legitimate subjects for study are therefore restricted to those that are amenable to direct observation and measurement.

Indeed, early positivists claimed that phenomena that did not meet these criteria were not valid subjects for investigation. This detached stance is purported to yield scientific truths that, owing to their abstract, universal nature, are value-free, context independent and generalizable (Tinkle & Beaton 1983). For a belief to be true it must correspond to a fact (Meleis 1991). In other words, a study carried out in one situation giving a certain set of results ought to be completely replicable in a different situation, provided the same procedure is followed. This ability to predict and generalize has been very powerful in securing the dominant status of positivism in the generation of scientific knowledge.

This paradigm is closely associated with quantitative methods; the principles underpinning the experimental method described in Chapter 3 clearly reflect the philosophical assumptions of positivism. However, the idea that specific research methods are exclusively linked to certain paradigms, or themselves represent discrete philosophical viewpoints, is currently being questioned in the research literature and will be explored later. For now, it will be taken that the assumptions of the paradigm shape the unique character of a research study and help to clarify the knowledge generated. Depending on the philosophical viewpoint of the researcher, they may or may not dictate the method selected for data collection.

Scientists themselves (Polanyi 1958, 1967) and philosophers of science (Suppe & Jacox 1985) began to recognize that the purified, objective stance of positivism did not actually reflect the scientific process, or the context of discovery. It was acknowledged that the context of scientific discovery was characterized by a good deal more subjectivity than the rigid parameters of positivism permitted. Polanyi, a chemist and philosopher of science, discussed at length the importance of intuition in the scientific process (Polanyi 1967). He believed that the scientist's own intuition entered into every aspect of the scientific process, from its conception to its conclusion.

He also postulated that, even before the completion of the most rigidly controlled studies, scientists would often 'feel' that they knew what the result was going to demonstrate. This is obviously in direct conflict with the image of the detached scientific observer.

Khun (1962, 1970; cited in Moody 1990), who studied the natural sciences, postulated that periods of consensus in scientific thinking which he called 'normal science' only continued until overwhelming competing evidence caused a revolution in thinking, when a new period of 'normal science' ensued. Khun used this to illustrate how conflicting scientific results can be discounted as irrelevant when they contradict the dominant paradigm.

Consider the reluctance of early scientists to admit that the world was round and not flat; or the ridicule that Semmelweiss was exposed to when he suggested hand washing as a means of reducing puerperal sepsis. Once Pasteur identified the first organisms by microscopic investigation, providing the groundwork for the germ theory of disease, a new period of 'normal science' followed where the link between specific organisms and disease processes was accepted.

The positivist viewpoint has been particularly criticized for the pervasive effects it has had on the development of medical science, or biomedicine. It is postulated that the emphasis on understanding the whole through a parts perspective has led to a mechanized view of the body, which in illness is viewed as a machine to be fixed. Parts of the body tend to be seen in isolation from one another and the mind and body viewed as separate entities. The importance of objective evidence places greater weight on outward signs of disease than on the subjective beliefs of the patient. The social, cultural and historical aspects of patients' lives are often seen as less significant than the scientifically identifiable causes of disease. This viewpoint has been criticized for locating illness at the individual level, thus leading to 'victim blaming' (Gordon 1988). Its **reductionist** emphasis and marginalization of the patient's subjective experience is also viewed as dehumanizing (Gordon 1988).

It has been suggested that the increased interest in complementary therapies in the last few years has been a direct response to increasing public frustration at the unsatisfying nature of many medical encounters. It demonstrates a heightened interest in positive health and a lay recognition that the health of mind and body are inextricably linked.

The focus on reductionism and objectivity and the marginalization of context are clearly limitations of the positivist approach in nursing. There has been a growing emphasis on the value of holistic care and assessment in recent years. The context of care is also seen to be increasingly important and there is a broad recognition that it is through our own subjectivity that sensitive, high-quality care is delivered. The current emphasis on the development of reflective practice is a powerful recognition of the subjective, affective components of care.

Such individual qualities as the capacity to nurture hope, confidence or positive self-esteem may make all the difference to whether a treatment works, but may not even be considered as relevant factors in a positivist study because of the difficulty of **operationalizing** and measuring abstract concepts.

Where such difficulties arise, one must question whether this is the most appropriate perspective for their study. Clearly what the researcher conceives as important and what the patient or client sees as important may be two quite different things, but the parameters of the study will dictate the information that will be generated. Thus, vital knowledge may be lost because there is no category into which it can conveniently be fitted.

Bond (1993), however, eloquently argues the case for continued experimental research, while acknowledging that in itself it is not sufficient to generate all the types of knowledge needed for nursing practice. The notion that a theory can be proved regardless of context has been discredited, but Bond believes that empirical research may support the predictability of a theory being relevant, permitting theory-based generalizations.

Where a situation is amenable to direct observation and quantification, the case for experimental study is strong. Studying different methods of organizing and delivering nursing care may well contribute to more effective strategic planning decisions. While acknowledging the difficulty of operationalizing and controlling variables in specific caring practices, with these limitations in mind experimental studies may reveal significant differences in numerous areas such as dressing techniques, feeding regimes and the prevention and management of decubitus ulcers.

Clearly, knowledge that identifies causal relationships and enhances our ability to describe, explain and predict phenomena can improve our capacity to substantiate argument with factual evidence. Cherished rituals such as rubbing pressure sores or the stripping and fanning of febrile children were only abandoned when objective 'facts' about their potentially harmful effects were discovered. Observing responses to pain has led to the development of a variety of scoring charts for children and adults. This can lead to more effective pain management and greater feelings of confidence and empowerment for the patient.

When positivist science is used appropriately it can create extremely valuable knowledge. Many successful medical and surgical interventions have occurred as a direct result of experimental research. Objective data, such as physiological parameters under controlled circumstances, have been particularly influential in the delivery of critical care nursing. The physiological deterioration on handling exhibited by most ill premature infants has resulted in the widespread implementation of minimal handling policies.

Similarly, the observation that clustering care leads to spikes in intracranial pressure (ICP) in patients with raised ICP has led to scattering care to minimize its impact. Highly advanced, non-invasive technological monitoring is increasingly uncovering previously hidden information about the effects of caring practices, therapeutic touch and pharmacological agents, to name but a few. Experimental research provides an important means of justifying the rationale for nursing activities and can lead to a much safer environment of care.

As well as demonstrating that an intervention is effective, positivist science is also capable of measuring the relative efficacy of different treatments. The recognition that medical care was heavily based on tradition, ritual and individual bias, rather than scientifically proven evidence, led to the Department of Health's recommendation that treatments should be subjected to the scrutiny of **randomized controlled trial** (RCT). In RCTs patients are randomly assigned to a certain group without them or their doctor knowing which. The treatment(s) or **placebo** is then applied and eventually the outcome recorded. The relative effectiveness of each treatment can be charted immediately and over time to illustrate short-, medium- and long-term benefits. This is believed to provide a more objective and rational means of delivering health care and allocating scarce resources.

This form of testing has yielded valuable knowledge in many areas of health care. RCTs have demonstrated the benefits of maternal corticosteroid administration in the enhancement of fetal lung maturity (JAMA 1995) and have helped to identify the most effective breast cancer protocols (Oakley 1990). Using RCTs has also highlighted substantial cost savings in the use of antimicrobial treatment for acute cystitis in women, the cheapest drug being the most effective (Hooton et al 1995).

Positivist studies are not, however, merely restricted to experimental research. A variety of methodological tools may be employed, such as surveys, questionnaires, interviews, and descriptive research. Such techniques are today being extensively used in the health service to monitor patient satisfaction and to help in the allocation of health resources.

Some studies may be quite exploratory in nature; others may be more tightly controlled. The common denominator will be the view of reality adopted by the researcher. In a positivist study this will have been preconceived and defined by the researcher and the methods used will illustrate this. This is not to denigrate the quality or integrity of such studies but is rather to show how important the underlying philosophical assumptions are in shaping the knowledge that is generated by such studies.

Planning and monitoring health care provision

Certain surveys, for example the General Household Survey (GHS), yield important information about the general health and social circumstances of the population. While health is defined as a negative variable, i.e. absence of disease, the incidence of illness, where it is located and patterns of health service usage can be sensitively and selectively monitored. This can be helpful in targeting health resources on those in greatest need.

Such data can also identify disparities in health between areas and social classes. Identifying differences in the health experience of the general population can help to locate the most fruitful areas for research to identify the causal links in health inequalities and explore how these might begin to be addressed. One of the most damaging influences on children's health in the UK today is pervasive and unremitting poverty (Kumar 1993). The ideas of how this might be tackled vary considerably, according to the position one takes on the ideological spectrum. The links between poverty and health are currently being investigated at the University of Warwick with a view to making poverty a realistic practice issue for nurses (Blackburn 1993).

When examining studies such as the GHS, it is important to remember that figures do not speak for themselves—they demand a framework for interpretation. Such frameworks or theories will inevitably involve the reader's subjective experience and interpretive viewpoint. This questions the assertion that data are value-free by virtue of the objective stance taken. My interest in the sociology of health focuses my interest on inequalities and in particular how they are related to the social structure. A psychologist or health economist might make a completely different interpretation of the same data.

The last part of this section has focused on the importance of philosophy in the shaping and execution of a study and also on the interpretation of the knowledge generated. An awareness of the type of knowledge generated by a particular philosophical paradigm helps to inform us of how that knowledge might be used to subsequently influence our practice. The benefits and limitations of positivist science have been outlined and, clearly, the knowledge generated is that which enables us to describe, explain and predict phenomena. To be able to do this, the phenomenon should be reasonably well known and clearly delineated. When it is not, positivist science is limited in its ability to inform us. This point is fundamental; we can use knowledge in a variety of settings and adapt it in various ways. As nurses we are good at this, since much of our theory needs to be creatively applied in the practice setting. What we must not do is to expect knowledge to inform us about something it cannot; this point will be developed in the next section.

The ethos of today's market-driven health service demands that as nurses we develop some tangible means of demonstrating our value. Moves to alter ward skill mix to include greater numbers of unqualified nurses mean that we must urgently address the specific benefits that would accrue to patients and the institution of retaining higher numbers of qualified staff. It is essential that the care nurses give is delivered in the knowledge of likely outcomes; this is particularly relevant given the current economic climate where nurses are being asked to justify and defend their practice (Atwood 1984).

Performance indicators, the Patient's Charter and the quality controls built into today's contracting arrangements directly relate to target achievement and measurable outcomes.

Nursing is a broad discipline, encompassing business management and administration as well as direct care. Our strategies for generating knowledge must reflect the needs of the whole discipline. Used appropriately, positivist research studies have value for nursing and, ultimately, the recipients of nursing care.

Beyond positivism

Positivist science had a powerful impact on early research and theory generation in nursing. It was considered to be synonymous with 'good science' and was seen to be highly valued in the discovery of medicine's knowledge base. In order to gain legitimacy, nurse researchers followed this paradigm to build a sound body of knowledge for nursing. In the 1970s, however, there was increasing unease and widespread recognition that positivist research methodologies did not accurately reflect nursing's more holistic philosophical base (Munhall 1982, Tinkle & Beaton 1983, Watson 1981) and too often sacrificed 'meaningfulness for rigor' (Silva 1977, p. 633). Positivist science was seen to be limited in its capacity to illuminate information of significance to the phenomenon of caring. This paved the way for a more open view of knowledge which allowed experience, intuition and understanding to be viewed as important pathways of advancing nursing knowledge.

The interpretive paradigm

The **interpretive paradigm** emerged as a response to the limitations of positivism; particularly in the human sciences of sociology, anthropology and psychology. Its ontology is based on the premise that reality is mentally constructed and is socially and culturally based. This allows for multiple interpretations of reality, or as one researcher describes it: 'reality is seen as constantly buzzing chaos that must be interpreted cognitively, rather than an objective reality waiting to be discovered' (Lowenberg 1993, p. 65).

Knowledge is recognized as being constructed in a social and historical context (Thompson 1990) and theories are not usually tested but can be generated from the understanding gained from the study (Vaughan 1992). Theories in this tradition are more open and in process and are amenable to change (Laudan 1977; cited in Silva & Rothbart 1984). Truth is based on 'logical fit' or the practical usefulness of the findings in solving problems and rests on the scientific consensus of scholars in the discipline (Meleis 1991).

Many intellectual traditions have influenced the development of the interpretive paradigm, resulting in no single overall approach. Lowenberg (1993) separates the three methodological divisions or approaches in nursing as **phenomenology, ethnography** and **grounded theory**. While these approaches do have different epistemological assumptions, the research methodologies focus on subjectivity and on eliminating the distance between the subject and the researcher. The aim is to discover meaning and to promote understanding. Meaning is considered to be situated in a particular cultural context. The creation of meaning is seen to be an active, affective process (Denzin 1989) and the constitutive power of language in understanding meaning is recognized (Thompson 1990). Here, language is not viewed simply as a means of communicating but is rather seen as being inextricably linked with cultural practices and understandings.

However, interpretive researchers differ in their opinion as to whether language or context is the primary influence in the construction of meaning (Lowenberg 1993). The **hermeneutic** perspective emphasizes language, while symbolic interactionists and ethnomethodologists stress the importance of context (Lowenberg 1993).

The eventual interpretation of meaning is a synthesis of the process between the researcher and the research subject. This acknowledges that data will be processed through the researcher's unique frame of reference and will therefore represent a unification of meaning between the researcher and the research subject. This represents a fundamental difference from the role of the researcher as envisaged by the philosophy of positivism.

While positivism strives as far as possible to distance the researcher from the subject, the interpretive paradigm positively values the researcher's subjective involvement. Some interpretive studies attempt to retain a sense of objectivity about the subjective meanings of others by 'bracketing' their own assumptions about the phenomenon. Thus, it is argued, researchers can study subjective meaning objectively; echoing the subject–object distinction of positivism. Indeed, interpretive researchers implementing this methodology are considered to be still operating partly in a positivist way by endorsing the existence of an objective reality separate from the researcher (Nielsen 1990). Philosophers who have extended thinking in the interpretive paradigm (Heidegger 1962, Gadamer 1975) have seriously questioned the possibility of the researcher ever being able to 'bracket' assumptions in this way. They argue that we perceive, experience and interpret reality through pre-understandings or 'biases' which are so fundamental to our being that they cannot be temporarily suspended or detached.

Instead, they advocate that we acknowledge our interpretive viewpoint and its influence in the synthesis of meaning. The removal of the subject–object distinction provides a clear alternative to positivism.

To illustrate the interpretive paradigm we use Patricia Benner's (1984) study of expert nursing practice, which involved Heideggerian hermeneutics (see Box 2.1). The methodology focuses on the interpretation of the lived experience and is acknowledged to be grounded in the contemporary epistemology of the interdisciplinary interpretive movement (Lowenberg 1993).

■ **BOX 2.1**

Heideggerian hermeneutics

- Derives from the philosophy of hermeneutic phenomenology (Martin Heidegger 1889–1976).
- Goal is to discover meaning and achieve understanding.
- Focus is on interpretation of the lived experience.
- Aims to accurately describe and interpret participants' meanings and practices.
- By identifying, describing and interpreting common practices, important and hidden aspects of practical knowledge can be revealed.
- Always open to change and criticism; acknowledges that the development of knowledge is never complete.

This is an important point since the potential for knowledge to be shared across disciplines is enhanced and the potential for initiating 'learning conversations' from different interpretive viewpoints is created. With the present movement in higher education towards interdisciplinary teaching and the emphasis in the World Health Organization's policy on multisectoral working to achieve broad health aims, the potential for shared knowledge generation strategies would seem to be particularly pertinent.

The reader may wonder why the understanding of meaning is so important to nursing practice, when we emphasize the importance of empathy, take care to assess patients' needs sensitively, and constantly evaluate the effectiveness of our nursing interventions. We have many textbooks and up-to-date journals to guide our practice and ensure that we work from an informed knowledge base. The increase in awareness of the significance of the knowledge of understanding owes much to interpretive studies in the sociology of health and illness. They have emphasized the importance of the biographical and cultural contexts of illness and its management by patients and carers (Radley 1993). Beliefs and interpretations about health and illness held by the lay public can significantly affect such factors as health behaviour (Blaxter 1990), coping with illness (Benner & Wrubel 1989, Miles 1991, Radley 1993), compliance with treatment (Morgan et al 1985) and social positioning in response to illness (Morgan et al 1985, Radley 1993). These issues are of major significance to health professionals and policy makers, since the decisions the lay public make about their health, which may sometimes be highly obscure to health workers, are often very rational within their systems of meaning. Failure to understand these meanings can result in treatment regimes and health promotion activities which have little or no relevance to certain client groups. Uncovering belief systems and practices and finding culturally acceptable strategies are possibilities generated by the interpretive paradigm and necessities at a time of increasing economic constraint in health expenditure.

Within the clinical environment, having an understanding of the suffering experienced by an individual can enable us to reduce the sense of isolation and disintegration which often accompanies illness. As we care for someone struggling to make sense of and cope with an experience which is temporarily beyond understanding, it can often precipitate a questioning of our own deeply held commonsense assumptions about the world we feel we know well and negotiate daily. In the struggle, we see that there is no simple answer but a range of possibilities that may be more or less acceptable—and which are open to change. In 'being with' someone in a therapeutic sense, we learn about the experience and about ourselves as we share the experience. We can use this understanding as a powerful tool in teaching and in subsequent therapeutic interactions.

There are many areas of nursing practice at present where rapidly advancing medical techniques have outstripped our understanding of how we can best support patients and their families through distressing and painful experiences: the transplant graft donated by a sibling which has failed to 'take'; malignancies induced by immunosuppressant agents; parents who cannot give up because they profoundly hope and believe that we can give their child life again when all hope seems to have gone; the mother who takes a damaged fetus to term, despite an in utero diagnosis of the condition. These are not uncommon occurrences and yet our knowledge of how families make sense of these experiences and of how we can help them through this difficult time is inadequate. While responses are individual and often idiosyncratic, the sharing of a common language and cultural practices often illuminates greater similarities than differences in responses to illness.

Interpretive research studies, therefore, can provide knowledge which is useful beyond its immediate context, by virtue of the fact that we are human, share a language and similar culture and are undergoing a similar experience. While no interpretive scholar would attempt to suggest that the information generated is generalizable in the sense that a positivist study is, there is no doubt that it can illuminate vitally important areas of taken-for-granted practices that are relevant to others working in similar areas.

If, for example, I wanted to improve the rates of breast-feeding in a neonatal intensive care unit, I would be helped in a limited way by the knowledge that age, social class, ethnicity, level of education, maternal health and parity are factors associated with success in breast-feeding. This knowledge would help me to identify mothers who statistically demonstrate a positive orientation towards breast-feeding and might possibly benefit from focused attention. It would not help me to plan how this intervention should be carried out, or what it should consist of. To establish this, it would be much more important to understand first what the experience of breast-feeding in this unusual context might involve.

From past experience, many mothers in these circumstances express profound feelings of demoralization and humiliation about having to use an electric breast pump for protracted periods of time. Many vividly describe 'feeling like a cow' and often feel demeaned and inadequate by the small volumes they produce.

Nursing skill and knowledge must therefore revolve around humanizing this first experience and valuing the often minuscule products as a positive contribution to the baby's health (see Box 2.2).

■ **BOX 2.2**

Consider the experience of a mother in a study I undertook. She was sitting nursing her baby when a nurse came in with a tray of expressed breast milk saying: 'and what will I do with all this rubbish?'. The mother naturally felt that the ward rhetoric about the value of breast-feeding and the reality were two different things. She said that had she been less motivated she would have given up then.

The same mother, in a rather embarrassed way, told me that one of the things that had helped her to remain positive about breast-feeding success was looking at a picture book of women breast-feeding their babies that we kept on the ward. She admitted that it had made her feel sexually excited, happy and hopeful, all at the same time, and had very much helped to sustain her enthusiasm when she felt very downhearted and discouraged.

Another mother described a sequence of events that had led up to the accidental discarding of all of her milk. 9 months after the event she still blanched and wept as she said: 'Margaret, I felt as if they'd thrown me down the sink'.

These experiences, and those of many other women, helped me to come to understand deeply the vital and fragile nature of the context in which breast-feeding occurs in the neonatal unit and the importance of attitude and language. I had the most brief glimpse of something perhaps erotic, something perhaps about wish fulfilment, which is rarely addressed but might well be of the utmost importance when working with these women. I also came to see how the milk somehow represents a unique part of the woman's own life force and is intimately linked with her own self-worth.

This goes far beyond received wisdom, which says that expressed breast milk is important because it is often the only thing the mother can do for her baby. If mothers actually view breast milk as 'self', the implications are far bigger than midwifery and neonatal staff have ever imagined. These are tantalizing glimpses which I felt honoured to receive in the comfort and security of these women's own homes. It was the first time they had felt comfortable enough to share them with anyone. It was the first time anyone had asked. Although the context was a taped research interview, this was also an intimate conversation.

One of the strengths of the interpretive paradigm is that the methodologies do positively facilitate intimacy and provide a means of uncovering information that can contribute to a very profound understanding. If neonatal nurses are to develop the knowledge and skill to promote breast-feeding in a context characterized by stress, grief, confusion and feelings of low self-worth, we need to go much further in deepening our knowledge of this experience. While the example in Box 2.3 is relevant to a particular disciplinary interest, health care is full of instances where we act with an incomplete understanding of the client's perspective.

■ BOX 2.3

A mother, Anne, recently told me a story of how she had made sense of her 20-month-old infant's kidney cancer. During the acute phase, when there was a fear that Peter might lose both kidneys, she visualized his cancer as an evil captain in charge of an army that was attacking her little boy. She hated him, wanted to fight him. As Peter started his chemotherapy and subsequently lost one kidney and part of the other, she visualized the drugs weakening this captain, then killing him. She was happy. She was so glad he had died that she felt she had to get rid of the body. She thought of digging a hole in the garden and planting a bush, but decided that if the bush withered she would feel superstitious about it. So she finally decided to throw him in front of a train. She did this on a busy platform, much to the consternation of the train driver and her fellow passengers. She felt relieved, then inexplicably burdened by sadness. When she considered this, she said that she still feared for her little boy but had nobody to hate any more. She said she felt that she had lost a worthy adversary and mourned this loss for several days.

I tell this story for several reasons. Firstly, because it was just chance that I came upon it, so I might never have known about it. Secondly, because Anne could not believe that I should be interested in such a rambling tale (there was much more); she felt that people would think she was quite mad for constructing such a vivid story, so she did not share it. Thirdly, because if we had only known that an 'all clear' diagnosis can be tinged with such bitter ambivalence, we could have supported this mother much more effectively through her experience and positively affirmed her coping strategies. Military metaphors are an extremely common way of making sense of illness; what remains hidden is the way these are developed in the illness trajectory.

While this story is idiosyncratic and personal, it provides a privileged glimpse into the internal world of someone facing up to the potential loss of a loved one. It is in this story that the structure of Anne's coping is revealed. By uncovering more such stories we may begin to understand common themes which may profoundly affect the quality of caring practices.

People's stories form the basis of interpretive research studies. The researcher makes no effort to restrict the subjects to predetermined categories but rather encourages them to describe the phenomenon of interest as openly and in as much detail as they are able to. Such studies have their greatest potential in illuminating previously hidden knowledge and in so doing help us to look at familiar situations with fresh eyes. The focus on common, everyday practices often means that the knowledge gained is of immediate practical value. Some scholars believe that the methodologies of the interpretive paradigm uncover the nature of nursing itself. At the very least, phenomenological and hermeneutic methods have great significance in illuminating the lived experiences of health, illness, disease and death.

Critical social theory and feminism

We now want to introduce you to the paradigms of critical social theory and feminism for three reasons: first, because of the important role they play in encouraging and developing critical and creative thinking as part of promoting research mindedness; second, because issues such as gender, class, and inequality and associated value systems are made explicit by critical theorists and feminists; third, because critical social theory and feminism go beyond positivism and interpretivism to make us conscious of the bias and political agendas that may inform research.

How critical social theory and feminism go beyond interpretivism

Interpretivism has been embraced by many nurses and midwives as being preferable to positivism because it aims to discover meaning and promote understanding. Furthermore, the researcher's subjective involvement is positively valued. The interpretive paradigm provides health care research with increased reflectivity and improved communication, and thus a point from which to implement enhancements in care itself.

However, the interpretive paradigm does not offer an adequate way of dealing with the theoretical and practical problems that may arise with systematically distorted patterns of communication. Take for example Nina's story in which 'distorted patterns of communication' were in evidence between the mother of a premature baby and the staff of the special care baby unit. The distorted patterns of communication were fed by stereotypes of 'good mothers' and a dominant world-view that was white, professional and potentially racist. Many researchers would take these communication patterns for granted, regarding them as 'evidence'. Nor does the interpretive paradigm in itself offer an analysis of how to create the potential for improvements in the conditions revealed by the research. In the case described in Nina's story, improvements would have involved examining and restructuring the communication systems between mothers of preterm babies and unit staff.

Critical social theory and feminism therefore have the actual or potential power to improve and transform the situations under study and empower the clients and consumers of health care as well as the health professionals themselves. Improvement, transformation and empowerment are achieved by using a model of **reflexivity** in order to unmask distorted patterns of communication and underlying value systems, unlike anything used by positivists or interpretivists. In this way critical theorists and feminists aim to arrive at an 'emancipatory' version of 'the truth' (Van Manen 1977). In Nina's story, the 'emancipatory version of the truth' is represented by the midwife's account of the mother who rarely visited her preterm infant. Seen in this light, the woman was revealed as 'passionately caring' rather than 'a bad mother', the version favoured by staff. Thus rather than using research to make predictions and control or simply to understand phenomena, critical theorists and feminists aim to use it to emancipate and transform the settings and subjects under study (Humm 1995).

Critical social theory

Critical social theory and feminism share some similarities. **Critical theory** is generally acknowledged to have evolved out of a critique of the techno-logical knowledge developed by positivist science which contributed to the oppression of the working class. The focus of this work took place in Frankfurt, Germany in the late 1920s and was inspired by Marxist ideas. The group, who became known as the Frankfurt School, consisted of a range of interdisciplinary scholars, including: Erich Fromm, psychologist; Herbert Marcuse, philosopher; Max Horheimer, philosopher and social psychologist; and Friedrich Pollack, economist. Critical social theory acknowledges and integrates subjective forms of knowledge, so that both human perceptions and experiences, as well as 'objective' observations, are considered of scientific worth (Campbell & Bunting 1991, pp. 5–6).

Critical theory, like feminist theory, demands that knowledge should be used for emancipatory social and political aims. Critical theory believes that one of the prime purposes of theory making and of research is to analyse the difference between the actual and the possible. The aim of this is to provide an analysis of **ideology**, i.e. belief and value systems that are presented as 'facts' by society's most powerful groups, in order to control or exert power over other groups. Critical theory aims to neutralize or nul-lify the effects of ideology so that certain groups and eventually the whole of society can be liberated or emancipated to evaluate and improve their lot (Campbell & Bunting 1991).

Critical theory states that perceptions, social and personal truths are always related to culture and social meaning and must be interpreted within their historical context. In other words, critical theory posits that knowledge is socially constructed and not 'objective'. Therefore, an under-standing of social structures such as race or class is crucial to any research activity within the critical paradigm. Indeed, the analysis of social struc-tures is seen as more important than individual personal meanings (a key epistemological difference between critical theory and phenomenology for example). Thus the critical paradigm rejects the idea that there can be any one 'objective' knowledge.

One major shortcoming of critical social theory is that it accepts the male world-view as the social norm, taking it as the frame of reference for all research. Critical social theory, therefore, is an 'androcentric' (male-centred) paradigm that requires feminists to do the work for women that the Frankfurt School researchers began, and continue to do, for men (Speedy 1991, p. 196).

Feminist theory

Enabling 'the woman's voice' to be heard and listened to 'after centuries of androcentric din' has become integral to feminist research for moral and political as well as epistemological reasons (Lugones & Spelman 1983, p. 574). Lugones & Spelman identify two reasons for women's voices to be integral to feminist research: first, it greatly increases the chances of ren-dering more accurate accounts of women's lives; second, feminist research is able to express and publicize experiences relevant to women. The expression of experiences in a myriad ways, is among the hallmarks of self-determining individuals and communities and is particularly pertinent to researching nursing and midwifery's diverse and complex clinical and educational settings.

That feminist theory is woman-centred is a vital issue in midwifery practice and theory making. This issue is equally vital for nursing and health visiting practice and theory making. The aim of feminist theory is to research or investigate women's lives and experiences in their own terms, by creating theories grounded in the actual experiences and language of women (du Bois 1983, Humm 1995). Feminist approaches to theory and research reflect 'woman-centredness' by making women's experiences the major focus of study; aiming to see the world from the point of view of a particular group of women and improve conditions for women and for all people (Campbell & Bunting 1991). Indeed much feminist research aims to improve not only the lot of people, but all living things, including far-reaching environmental or 'eco-feminist' research approaches. Dorothy Kleffel (1991) has written persuasively on the juncture of nursing and **ecology**.

Definitions of feminisms

Many feminist researchers prefer to use the term 'feminisms' rather than feminism to indicate that neither should there nor could there be one definition. Feminists may have many differing emphases and affinities such as class, race or sexual preference (Humm 1995, Speedy 1991). Women do not necessarily experience patriarchy (male domination) in the same ways, and the subsequent divergent viewpoints are all valid. This means that one woman's 'liberation', 'empowerment', or 'emancipation' may be very different from another woman's (Campbell & Bunting 1991). In general, all feminisms incorporate both a doctrine of equal rights for women and an ideology of social transformation aiming to create improvements in the world for women that go beyond simple social equality.

We have already seen in Nina's story that racism distorted the communication patterns between staff and the mother of a preterm baby. For many feminists, racism is closely linked to gender issues. Smith (1983) makes this link very clearly when she says:

> *The reason racism is a feminist issue is easily explained by the inherent definition of feminism. Feminism is the political theory and practice to free ALL women: women of colour, working class women, poor women, physically challenged women, lesbians, old women, as well as white economically privileged heterosexual women. Anything less is not feminism, but merely female self-aggrandisement.*

Feminist research approaches

Feminist research approaches incorporate various methods of analysis but the object of generating information and knowledge is to create alternatives to oppression. Humm (1995, p. 94) says: 'Consciousness-raising is the quintessential method of feminism, and since feminism means a knowledge of existing things in a new light it needs a distinctive account of the relation of method to theory'.

Feminist approaches contain certain key aspects. We have followed Speedy's (1991) classification in dividing them into three areas. Firstly, as has been stated earlier, feminist research approaches see women and *women's experiences* as central to the research. Secondly, feminist research centralizes *intersubjectivity*, or the development of a dialectical relationship between subject and object of research. This means that both the researcher and the researched have to be involved in the ethical, social and political implications of the research. Reciprocity, reflexivity and honesty are all important issues and feminist research rejects the hierarchical, detached, anonymous style of traditional positivist research approaches (Oakley 1981, Webb 1984). Thirdly, feminist research approaches identify a need for *transformation, empowerment* or *unmasking* as a research outcome, once awareness or acknowledgement of a deficit or contradiction exists (Campbell & Bunting 1991, Stanley & Wise 1983, Webb 1984).

Humm (1995, p. 243) observes: 'Integrating personal praxis (practice) and research is not unique to feminism, but feminist theory adds the point that both the content *and* the process of feminist research must involve fresh thinking about gender'. Meleis (1987), amongst other nursing theorists, points out that nursing and midwifery research already includes topics of significance to women, such as the menopause, rape, osteoporosis, physical and sexual violence against women, childbirth, heart disease, breast cancer and lesbian health. In midwifery, the postnatal period traditionally has received the least attention in either textbooks or research studies. Yet this period is often a time when women need most support with child care, advice on breast-feeding, relief of perineal discomfort, and adaptation to role and relationship changes with their partner, friends and family. Traditionally, medical and midwifery services have often glossed over these issues, belittled or ignored them. However, with the rise of the critical and feminist paradigms in health care research, these issues are being highlighted by women themselves.

Specifying the demand for 'the woman's voice' to be heard, reveals a number of things. First, although all women have been silenced in one way or another because they are women, nevertheless some women do not and/or cannot identify themselves as women only. They are 'forced' to acknowledge their race, class, ethnicity, religion, sexual alliance, physical ability, in a way that most white middle-class, heterosexual, able-bodied women do not have to.

There are many questions raised by the challenge to racist and/or feminist theories in relation to nursing, midwifery and educational research. What do you think is the point of making theory? How can those 'making theory', i.e. the researchers, reach the meaning of women's experiences? And what is or should be the relationship between the researchers' theory and the women's meaning. In this respect, Lugones & Spelman discuss the issue of 'insider' (or 'subjective' experience) and 'outsider' (or 'objective' experience) in the business of 'theory making'. 'When the outsider makes clear that she is an outsider and that this is an outsider's account of your behaviour, there is a touch of honesty about her behaviour' (Lugones & Spelman 1983, p. 577).

The outsider's point of view has traditionally, within the **positivist paradigm**, been taken to be most objective and therefore more accurate. Feminist research has successfully challenged this, and feminist methods and methodologies are now prevalent within nursing, midwifery and health care research (Oakley 1981, Webb 1984 inter alia). Oakley has defined and demonstrated how the use of subjectivity is essential to both the interviewing process and to the production of data. 'Indeed, feminist researchers highlight the vulnerability of research subjects especially during interview, in which traditionally the researcher "takes" all the information on offer without reciprocity or responsibility' (Smith P 1992, p. 148). These issues are particularly pertinent to midwifery, where the midwives are predominantly women, and the clients are *all* women. 'Feminist research can be seen to value yet develop qualitative research traditions by making gender relations visible at the level of both researcher and researched' (Smith P 1992, p. 148).

Feminist research methods

Controversy about the use of quantitative or qualitative research methods is prevalent amongst nurse scientists and researchers just as it is amongst feminist scientists and researchers. Most feminist researchers advocate a multiparadigmatic approach, arguing that feminist research can utilize a variety of research paradigms, providing it is based on feminist principles. Thus it is not the research methods, the information gathering techniques themselves, that determine the intrinsic nature of a research investigation. Rather it is the epistemological, methodological and other paradigmatic issues that determine the nature of a research (or any other) project. Thus feminist theorists argue that quantitative research methods can be used within a feminist framework, just as much as qualitative research methods (Jayaratne 1983). Many feminist and nursing researchers argue that there are no research methods that in themselves are 'more feminist' than others; it is more about how particular research methods are employed in practice (Harding 1987, Speedy 1991).

Furthermore, research within these paradigms aims to make the research approaches accessible to questioning and (re)interpretation. Research results are published, wherever possible, in both professional and popular journals in order to increase accessibility to as many women as possible (Kleffel 1991).

It is important to note that although there are feminist theorists who argue that feminists do not have to be female, nor the subject matter have to be female but, rather, 'gender focused', in reality, the vast majority of nurses and midwives are women and, in midwifery at least, all clients are also female (Bernard 1973, Kelly 1978, Speedy 1991). This reflects part of the 'reflexive' research stance that Harding (1987) advocates; being 'research minded' means that research is not a distant 'out there' phenomenon, but is a co-participant activity between researcher and researched. The fact that most midwives and nurses are women means that we can be alienated from our gender by the traditional positivist approach, not just to health care but also to research (Campbell & Bunting 1991, Kleffel 1991).

Chinn (1985), a nurse theorist from north America, suggests that a major contribution of feminist thinking to nursing is the basic feminist concept that women are oppressed. Other nurse theorists have recommended that nursing recognize the existence of oppression and affirm not only the right of nursing and midwifery to develop their own professional destiny, but also to develop a paradigm shift in nursing and midwifery research which will make women more visible, and on women's terms (Kleffel 1991, MacPherson 1983).

Qualitative research methods have traditionally been favoured by feminists engaged in social science research, and have also traditionally been seen as more 'feminine' or 'soft' compared to the 'hard', 'masculine' quantitative approaches. Many feminist and nursing/midwifery researchers argue that qualitative research methods allow for a better reflection of the nature of women's experiences (Oakley 1981, Watson 1985). Some of the approaches compatible with feminist principles that have been suggested by nurse theorists include: participant observation; small purposive **samples**; in-depth interviewing; as well as the use of literary descriptions and analyses from literature as we describe in our case study below. Other methodological approaches include reflections on original art and its meaning as used in phenomenology, an approach taken in Chapter 5 by Stephenson and Corben, and the use of music, dance and other creative work (Kleffel 1991). Nurse researchers are already developing a distinctive feminist nursing/midwifery research methodology. Kleffel (1991) describes a number of nursing and midwifery studies that have used such approaches. These include research projects that have: addressed the issue of rigour in feminist nursing research (Hall & Stevens 1991); used a feminist perspective in fieldwork interviews on a study of diabetes (Anderson 1991); and used feminist research criteria as an empowerment model in a study of the effects of physical abuse during pregnancy on maternal–infant outcomes (Parker & McFarlane 1991).

Traditionally, feminist researchers have concerned themselves with generating theories about gender rather than race. One interesting question about theory is how and on what criteria to test it. There is already a well-established tradition amongst philosophers of pointing out that identifying a statement as true or false is only one of many possible ways of characterizing it. As Lugones & Spelman (1983) observe: 'Theories appear to be the kind of things that are true or false ... but as we know, [they] don't have to be true in order to be used to strengthen people's position in the world' (p. 578). Lugones & Spelman go on to point out that feminist theory is as susceptible to criticism as Plato's political theory or Freud's theory of female psychosexual development (p. 578).

Feminism is an ideology (beliefs and value system) and practice which acknowledges the oppression of women, and seeks to redress the situation by which theory is used to take advantage of others. In order for feminism to retain, or even regain, its cutting edge over positivism, interpretivism and critical theory, it is necessary to include a virulent anti-racist strategy within its bounds. It may be practical or preferred at times for the different movements based on gender and race to work separately from each other. However, it seems to be possible, and also desirable, that there are at least times when the differences between women are transformed into a powerful alliance.

The African-American feminist scholar, bell hooks, states:

I'm very interested in feminist theory and other progressive movements that speak to people where they are and invite people to engage in change and transformation in the concrete locations of their daily lives, as opposed to imagining that there is a top of the mountain space that is feminist consciousness, race consciousness, class consciousness—and wanting people to suddenly be at the top of the mountain rather than thinking about their lived realities, their concrete realities.

(hooks 1991, p. 12)

Note how bell hooks writes her name without any capital letters. She does this to signify her distaste for anything that smacks of hierarchy. Her writing seeks out the relationship between theory and actuality on issues of social change. She attempts to analyse our positions within a white supremacist society, guarding against racism and developing appropriate 'alternative perspectives' and anti-racist practices. This is a vital issue in nursing and midwifery and an area for further research, as recent challenges from within the profession seem poor or non-existent.

One challenge came from Pam Smith's study of student nurses which showed that: 'During their ward experiences ... students were exposed to racial stereotyping without being offered any alternative perspectives with which to challenge them. ... any racial stereotyping by either nurses or patients was left unchallenged and without appropriate consciousness raising, to be reproduced, potentially, at a later date by students' (Smith P 1992, p. 66).

Studies of NHS nurses, midwives and health visitors show evidence of discrimination and inequality with regard to career choices and promotion. Carol Baxter, reporting in 1988, concluded that because racism was so apparent among the nursing profession, 'Black nurses' as a group were an 'endangered species'.

We now want to use our seminar experience to demonstrate some of the issues we have been discussing around the different research paradigms, approaches and methods open to nurses, midwives and health visitors.

A CASE STUDY: MOLLY'S STORY

As part of the module on 'Promoting research mindedness' from which this and other chapters in this book grew, we had to present a seminar. We used an audio tape of Molly Bloom's soliloquy from James Joyce's *Ulysses*. One of the reasons we chose Molly's story was to emphasize the importance of exploring 'the woman's voice'. It is important to note, however, that Molly's soliloquy was written by a man.

The main advantages of presenting ideas in a seminar are that it stimulates and challenges the participant's powers of comprehension and evaluation. Underlying values, principles and assumptions pertaining to the seminar topic can be elicited, which is vital when negotiating philosophical paradigms. Furthermore, their application and relevance to the student, practitioner or teacher can be questioned and/or strengthened during a seminar. We agreed with Curzon (1990, p. 292) that it is the 'critical examination of another's thoughts' that enables this process.

We also wanted to explore like McNiff (1993, p. 4) 'the idea that education is concerned with the process of growth of an individual whereby the individual's life is formed and informed by the values that she holds and the knowledge that she develops'.

There were certain assumptions made by us, as leaders of a 'Masters' level' seminar, which influenced its progress. For example, we assumed a certain level of knowledge and particular attitudes to feminism/s, ethnicity and race among our colleagues. This, of course, was a mistake, since when interacting with a group of people, even when we think we know them well, we should never assume anything about them and how they will react. Going through the process of having our assumptions challenged, however, led a number of us to re-acknowledge and re-examine the future focus of our educational and clinical activities. The seminar, therefore, was a living example of promoting research mindedness, since it opened our eyes and broadened our horizons in a way that reflected Polanyi's (1969) writings on development as a transformational process which in turn encourages personal enquiry. Similarly, Brause & Mayher (1991, p. x) write: 'Living necessitates learning—and most of that learning occurs through personal enquiry, another term for research'. Finally, the seminar process led us to reflect on the question posed by McNiff (1993, p. xiii): 'How do I live more fully my values in my practice?'.

We chose Molly Bloom's soliloquy from James Joyce's *Ulysses* for a number of reasons. We wanted to use a piece of literature as a way of exploring research mindedness. The use of the arts and humanities as an educative tool within nursing and midwifery has been examined by various authors (Derbyshire 1994, Evans 1990). The soliloquy refers to a miscarriage experienced by the narrator, Molly Bloom, as well as more generally to her sexual understanding of herself. Molly's soliloquy is an emotional piece of writing and it served well as the 'voice of a woman'. It could be critiqued from a number of different philosophical viewpoints, including the feminist perspective (Harding & Hintikka 1983, Harding 1987). Indeed, as stated earlier, the reason we chose Molly's story was to emphasize the importance of exploring 'the woman's voice'.

We also wanted to see if the seminar could be used as an example of how theories are developed from data that explore 'the woman's voice'. The demand that 'the woman's voice' be heard, and the search for the 'woman's voice as central to feminist methodology' reflect what Lugones & Spelman (1983) call **nascent** feminist theory. By this they mean that:

> nascent empirical theory ... presupposes that the silencing of women is systematic, shows up in regular patterned ways and that there are discoverable causes of this widespread observable phenomenon; the demand reflects nascent political theory in so far as it presupposes that the silencing of women reveals a systematic pattern of power and authority; and it reveals nascent moral theory insofar as it presupposes that the silencing is unjust and that there are particular ways of remedying this injustice.
>
> *(Lugones & Spelman 1983, p. 574)*

For us, 'nascent' seems a highly relevant term here, not only in the sense of being a (relatively) recent theoretical perspective, but because the word also conveys the sense of being unusually reactive or volatile, as in 'nascent hydrogen' (Oxford English Dictionary 1981). This sense reflects the frequently hostile reaction that much feminist theory has engendered, not only from men but amongst women ourselves, often 'just' for desiring the knowledge. Although the nursing and midwifery professions are taking on feminist theory and practice, in general this is relatively recent and slow. Many nurses and midwives do not recognize that feminism has anything to offer them because they see it as being concerned with oppressed groups. They fail to make the connection that as women's occupations, nursing and midwifery are dominated and constrained by male-oriented medicine and managers.

The notion of nascent theory and thinking spilled over into the session itself, by which we mean there was a fluidity, volatility and uncertainty apparent within the classroom. We felt this reaction reflected the nature of the participants as well as the topic and provided a powerful learning stimulus (Curzon 1990).

The use of the audio tape was a trigger for critical uncertainty. Uncertainty and ambiguity promote critical thinking, an essential ingredient for promoting research mindedness. Critical thinking is also associated with creative or lateral thinking (Thayer-Bacon 1993). We felt that using the audio tape provided opportunities for creative thinking through exposure to the creative arts as a way of developing critical thinking and promoting research mindedness.

However, as seminar leaders we felt uncomfortable during the session. On reflection, the main reason for this discomfort was the relative lack of female voices in the discussion on feminist approaches to research and research mindedness. Even though, as is typical in groups of nurses and midwives, the women in our group far outnumbered the men, the male voices predominated. We hoped that one of the participants would challenge this state of affairs but found that we, as seminar leaders, were expected to take the initiative, which suggested the 'newness' of the topic for many of the participants. Feedback indicated that they were not only pleased to have this input on feminism, but particularly valued those aspects of feminism which intersect with gender and race. Given the silence on race and racism within feminism until relatively recently, and even more so within nursing and midwifery (Ramazanoglu 1989, Smith P 1992), we concluded that in the spirit of Maxine Hong-Kingston (1975) our seminar had contributed to 'making our minds large'.

The issue of silence is an important one in considering the demand for 'the woman's voice' and can be interpreted in a number of different ways. There is white women's silence about race and racism, and the silencing of women of colour, and of women by men. Silence can be seen as a privilege and as an oppression. There is also the related issue of speaking out which is well illustrated by the cartoon caption in Martens & Frankenberg's article (1985, p. 22): 'Well, shall we go with those who speak and won't listen, or those that will listen but won't speak?'.

The discussion of issues raised through Molly Bloom's soliloquy aided communication within the classroom setting and confirmed it as one of the most important constituents of promoting research mindedness. Further-more, the arts and humanities are able to offer much to nursing and midwifery education and practice, including subjectivity and personal experience not usually encountered within the biological sciences. The link between personal experience and communication is made by Evans (1990, p. 287) who, quoting Kirkegaard a philosopher, observes that 'when everything becomes personal, the accent immediately falls on what it means to communicate'.

BEYOND DUALISM—REFLECTIONS FOR NURSING AND MIDWIFERY RESEARCH

Debates around nursing and midwifery research have for some time revolved around discussions about method. Traditionally, quantitative methods have been viewed as a scientifically superior means of data col-lection, useful for theory testing and the development of law-like general-izations. Qualitative methods have, on the other hand, been seen as suitable for theory building and as a precursor to quantitative study. Quantitative approaches have been closely associated with the positivist paradigm and are taken to represent a realist philosophy, which assumes an independent reality existing independently of perception (Powers & Knapp 1990). Qualitative approaches are believed to embody an idealist philosophy, which holds that the world is known through human percep-tions and subjectivity (Powers & Knapp 1990); this is seen to be more closely associated with the interpretive and critical paradigms.

There is a viewpoint currently being expressed in the feminist literature that approaches and methods are fundamentally distinct entities. Methods are seen to be completely value-free, simply ways of collecting informa-tion. Methodology is, however, a more philosophical issue, comprising the assumptions that drive the research endeavour and shape the choice of method and how that method is used (Campbell & Bunting 1991). This is by no means a consensus view. Most nurse and midwife researchers still tend to see methods as reflecting certain philosophical assumptions about the nature of reality, relationships and truth.

All paradigms create knowledge that can describe and explain the phe-nomenon which is being studied. What we have seen is that the principal characteristics of the knowledge created will vary. These characteristics are:

- prediction when using positivist studies
- understanding and self-knowledge with interpretive studies
- empowerment and emancipation when the critical and feminist paradigms are used.

The type of knowledge needed will be the determining factor in the choice of research approach. When research is viewed in this light, distinctions about the relative superiority of the knowledge discovered melt away. The sole arbiter of quality will be the purpose for which the knowledge is gen-erated and how effectively it achieves this.

At present, debates in the literature have moved on from the battle lines of quantitative versus qualitative methods. There is now a widespread recognition that the nature of the research endeavour, regardless of the paradigm selected, has more similarities than differences. Paradigmatic perspectives are the result of profound philosophic inquiry, thus making them trustworthy (Dzurec & Abraham 1993) and reliable guides.

Recognizing the inherent validity of each paradigm allows the researcher to focus on the nature of inquiry (Dzurec & Abraham 1993), selecting the most appropriate means to answer the research question. It is acknowledged that paradigm choice situates the researcher within a particular philosophical context; the choice itself reflecting the researcher's comfort with its assumptions. This relates to ways of knowing about the world, and preference for working within one particular paradigm is acceptable, provided we recognize the validity of other patterns of knowing which are equally important to good nursing practice.

A knowledge of philosophy ensures that phenomena for investigation can be conceptualized in a way which gives the inquiry purpose and focus. It also means that the most appropriate methods of investigation are chosen, maximizing the explanatory power of the knowledge generated. It creates the potential for setting up sequential research studies that will contribute to nursing's theoretical base and enhance our capacity to justify care. It also encourages us to value different ways of knowing about nursing and situates the knowledge of research in its appropriate context; at once recognizing its value and its limitations to inform us about our practice.

REFLECTIONS FOR PRACTICE: ENCOURAGING AND DEVELOPING CRITICAL AND CREATIVE THINKING

The importance of developing and refining our capacities to think critically and creatively in practice cannot be overstated. In order to provide sensitive and appropriate care to people with diverse backgrounds, we must constantly question and evaluate interventions, adapting them where necessary. This demands an ability to think critically and clearly in order to substantiate proposed nursing action with a well-reasoned rationale and a willingness to enter into dialogue with other nurses and members of the multidisciplinary team.

Increasingly, situations may present themselves where there may be limited theory to guide us—times when we quite literally have to 'think on our feet'. When trying to make a 600-g baby comfortable on a hard bed, or manage his temperature as it fluctuates widely, there are few rules to follow. Caring strategies in such situations require experience, creativity and a willingness to try novel solutions.

The ability to think critically is often presented in a somewhat exclusive way, as a set of higher order skills to be acquired. We felt uncomfortable with such an elitist notion and hoped to challenge extravagant claims about the rarefied nature of critical thinking. We agreed with Smith F (1992) that anyone is capable of thinking critically if he or she has enough knowledge about the subject and that the most productive way of developing critical thinking is to develop an environment which fosters critical debate. Our experiences of the group allowed us to make some assumptions about the existing knowledge base and helped to focus the level of content. Since we also knew that class participants were grounded in positivist ways of thinking, presenting interpretivism and feminism as equally valid ways of knowing set the scene for a lively exchange of views.

Stimulating creative thinking was a central goal in our teaching plan and underpinned the decision to use a piece of creative writing. Creative thinking is largely ignored in the critical thinking literature and is identified by Smith F (1992) to be an alienating notion as it has connotations of quality and originality. This, by definition, often excludes the ordinary among us who do not perceive ourselves to be particularly gifted or artistic. Yet we daily create situations which transform fearful and alienating experiences into something that patients and families can integrate, understand and perhaps even derive some positive benefit from.

We strongly believe that the skills of critical and creative thinking are deeply embedded in the practices of nurses and do not represent esoteric qualities, only given to the chosen few. Just as we can all become better research minded practitioners, we can improve our capacities to think critically and creatively. A key prerequisite is recognizing our legitimacy to do so.

Creative and critical thinking skills can be developed in education and in clinical practice but the strategies to enhance and nurture them must reflect the nature of the skills. For critical thinking you need critical debate, at all levels and in an environment that can support and contain it. For creative thinking it is necessary to be open to the creative energy we all possess and to promote this we need methods which allow us to enter other realities and encourage imagination. The arts and humanities can be a powerful source of analogues that crystallize the essence of caring experiences. These can be helpful tools to explore in safety different ways of thinking and being which may better inform our practice.

SUMMARY

Research increases and enhances nursing and midwifery knowledge, which is an integral part of nursing's and midwifery's essence and practice. Nursing and midwifery knowledge can be said to be shaped by philosophical viewpoints or paradigms. The paradigms reviewed in this chapter are positivism, interpretivism, critical theory and feminism.

Promoting research mindedness helps us as students, practitioners and teachers to view our worlds from different philosophical perspectives and help our critical thinking.

In the seminar from which this book sprang, we decided to use an example from literature as an educational device to aid critical and creative thinking.

Research mindedness illuminates valuable issues for nursing and midwifery and creates the space for us to tell stories about and reflect on our experiences from different perspectives.

We can improve our understanding by seeking understanding from a range of experiences and reflections, in order to enhance and increase our knowledge and practice.

REFERENCES

Anderson J 1991 Reflexivity in fieldwork: toward a feminist epistemology. Image, Journal of Nursing Scholarship 23(1): 115–118

Atwood J R 1984 Advancing nursing science: quantitative approaches. Western Journal of Nursing Research 6(3): 9–15

Baxter C 1988 The black nurse: an endangered species. Training in Health and Race, Cambridge (UK)

Benner P 1984 From novice to expert: excellence and power in clinical nursing practice. Addison-Wesley, Menlo Park, California

Benner P, Wrubel J 1989 The primacy of caring; stress and coping in health and illness. Addison Wesley, California

Bernard B 1973 My four revolutions: an autobiographic history of the ASA. In: Huber J (ed) Changing women in a changing society. University of Chicago Press, Chicago

Blackburn C 1993 Making poverty a practice issue. Health and Social Care 1(5): 297–305

Blaxter M 1990 Health and lifestyles. Tavistock/Routledge, London

Bond S 1993 Experimental research in nursing: necessary but not sufficient. In: Kitson A (ed) Nursing art and science. Chapman & Hall, London

Brause R, Mayher J 1991 Search and research: what the enquiring teacher needs to know. The Falmer Press, London

Campbell J C, Bunting S 1991 Voices and paradigms: perspectives on critical and feminist theory in nursing. Advances in Nursing Science 13(3): 1–15

Chinn P 1985 Feminism and nursing. Nursing Outlook 333(3): 74–77

Curzon L 1990 Teaching in further education, 4th edn. Cassell, London

Denzin N K 1989 Interpretive interactionism. Sage, Newbury Park, California

Derbyshire P 1994 Understanding caring through the arts and humanities—a medical/nursing humanities approach to promoting alternative experiences of thinking and learning. Journal of Advanced Nursing 19: 856–863

du Bois B 1983 Passionate scholarship: notes on values, knowing and method in feminist social science. In: Bowles G, Duelli-Klein R (eds) Theories of women's studies. Routledge, London

Dzurec L C, Abraham I L 1993 The nature of inquiry: linking quantitative and qualitative research. Advances in Nursing Science 16(1): 73–79

Evans C 1990 Teaching the humanities: seminars as metalogues. Studies in Higher Education 15: 3

Fawcett J 1993 From a plethora of paradigms to parsimony in worldviews. Nursing Science Quarterly 6(2): 56–57

Gadamer H G 1975 Truth and method. Sheed and Ward, London

Gordon D 1988 Tenacious assumptions in western medicine. In: Lock M, Gordon D (eds) Biomedicine examined. D Reidel, Boston

Guba E 1990 The paradigm dialog. Sage, Newbury Park, pp 17–27

Hall J, Stevens P 1991 Feminist theory and nursing. An empowerment model for research. Advances in Nursing Science 13(3): 59–67

Harding S (ed) 1987 Feminism and methodology. Open University Press, Milton Keynes

Harding S, Hintikka M (eds) 1983 Discovering reality: feminist perspectives on epistemology, metaphysics, methodology and philosophy of science. Reidel, Boston, MA

Heidegger M 1962 Being and time. Harper & Row, New York

Hong-Kingston M 1975 The woman warrior. Picador, London

hooks b 1991 Interview. Everywoman, May

Hooton T M, Winter C, Tiu F, Stamm W E 1995 Randomized controlled trial and cost analysis of 3 day antimicrobial regimens for treatment of acute cystitis in women. Journal of the American Medical Association 273: 41–45

Humm M 1995 The dictionary of feminist theory, 2nd edn. Prentice Hall/Harvester Wheatsheaf, London

JAMA 1995 Effect of corticosteroids for fetal maturation on perinatal outcomes. Journal of the American Medical Association 273: 413–418

Jayaratne T E 1983 The value of quantitative methodology for feminist research. In: Bowles G, Duelli-Klein R (eds) Theories of women's studies. Routledge and Kegan Paul, London

Joyce B, Weil M 1992 Models of teaching, 4th edn. Allyn & Bacon, Boston

Joyce J 1992 Ulysses. Flamingo Modern Classics, London

Kelly A 1978 Feminism and research. Women's Studies International Quarterly 1: 225–232

Kleffel D 1991 An ecofeminist analysis of nursing knowledge. Nursing Forum 26(4): 5–18

Kumar V 1993 Poverty and inequality in the UK – the effects on children. National Children's Bureau, London

Leddy S, Pepper J M 1993 Conceptual bases of professional nursing, 3rd edn. J B Lippincott, Philadelphia

Lowenberg J S 1993 Interpretive research methodology: Broadening the dialogue. Advances in Nursing Science 16(2): 57–59

Lugones M, Spelman E 1983 Have we got a theory for you! Feminist theory, cultural imperialism and the demand for the woman's voice. Women's Studies 6(6)

MacPherson K 1983 Feminist methods: a new paradigm for nursing research. Advances in Nursing Science 6(1): 17–25

McNiff J 1993 Teaching as learning: an action research programme. Routledge, London

Martens J, Frankenberg R 1985 White racism: more than a moral issue. Trouble and Strife 5

Meleis A I 1987 Re-visions in knowlege development. Scholarly Inquiry for Nursing Practice 1(1): 5–19

Meleis A I 1991 Theoretical nursing: development and progress. J B Lippincott, Philadelphia

Miles A 1991 Women, health and medicine. Open University Press, Milton Keynes

Moody L E 1990 Advancing nursing science through research. Sage, London, vol 1

Morgan M, Calnan M, Manning N 1985 Sociological approaches to health and medicine. Croom Helm, London

Munhall P L 1982 Nursing philosophy and nursing research: in apposition or opposition? Nursing Research 31(3): 176–177, 181

Newman M A 1992 Prevailing paradigms in nursing. Nursing Outlook 40(1): 10–12

Nielsen J M 1990 Feminist research methods: exemplary readings in the social sciences. Westview Press, Boulder, Colorado

Oakley A 1981 Interviewing women: a contradiction in terms. In: Roberts H (ed) Doing feminist research. RKP, London

Oakley A 1990 Who's afraid of the randomized controlled trial. In: Roberts H (ed) Women's health counts. Routledge, London

Parker B, MacFarlane J 1991 Feminist theory and nursing: an empowerment model for research. Advances in Nursing Science 13(3): 58–67

Polanyi M 1958 The study of man. University of Chicago Press, London

Polanyi M 1967 The tacit dimension. Routledge and Kegan Paul, London

Polanyi M 1969 Knowing and being. Routledge and Kegan Paul, London

Polit D F, Hungler B P 1989 Essentials of nursing research methods, appraisal and utilization. J B Lippincott, Philadelphia

Porter E J 1989 The qualitative–quantitative dualism. Image: Journal of Nursing Scholarship 21(2): 98–102

Powers B A, Knapp T R 1990 A dictionary of nursing theory and research. Sage, London

Radley A 1993 Worlds of illness. Biographical and cultural perspectives on health and disease. Routledge and Kegan Paul, London

Ramazanoglu C 1989 Feminism and the contradictions of oppression. Routledge, New York

Silva M C 1977 Philosophy, science, theory: interrelationships and implications for nursing research. In: Nicholl L H (ed) Perspectives on nursing theory, 2nd edn. J B Lippincott, New York

Silva M C, Rothbart D 1984 An analysis of changing trends in philosophies of science on nursing theory development and testing. In: Nicholl L H (ed) Perspectives on nursing theory, 2nd edn. J B Lippincott, New York

Smith B 1983 Home girls. Kitchen Table Press, New York

Smith F 1992 To think in language learning and education. Routledge, London

Smith P 1992 The emotional labour of nursing—how nurses care. Macmillan, Basingstoke

Speedy S 1991 The contribution of feminist research. In: Gray G, Pratt R (eds) Towards a discipline of nursing. Churchill Livingstone, Melbourne

Stanley L, Wise S 1983 Breaking out. Routledge and Kegan Paul, London

Suppe F, Jacox A K 1985 Philosophy of science and the development of nursing theory. Annual Review of Nursing Research. Sage, London, vol 2

Thayer-Bacon B J 1993 Caring or its relationship to critical thinking. Educational Theory 43(3): 323–340

Thompson J L 1990 Hermeneutic inquiry. In: Moody L E (ed) Advances in nursing science through research. Sage, London, vol 2

Tinkle M B, Beaton J L 1983 Towards a new view of science: implications for nursing research. In: Nicholl L H (ed) Perspectives on nursing theory, 2nd edn. J B Lippincott, Philadelphia

Van Manen L 1988 Linking ways of knowing with ways of being practical. Curriculum Enquiry 6(3): 205–228

Vaughan B 1992 The nature of nursing knowledge. In: Robinson K, Vaughan B (eds) Knowledge for nursing practice. Butterworth Heinemann, Oxford

Watson J 1981 Nursing's scientific quest. Nursing Outlook 29(7): 413–416

Watson J 1985 Reflections on different methodologies for the future of nursing. In: Leiniger M (ed) Qualitative research methods in nursing. Harcourt Brace, San Diego

Webb C 1984 Feminist methodology in nursing research. Journal of Advanced Nursing 9: 249–250

FURTHER READING

The philosophy of knowledge and science

Leddy S, Pepper J M 1993 Conceptual bases of professional nursing, 3rd edn. J B Lippincott, Philadelphia, ch 5

Manley K 1991 Knowledge for nursing practice. In: Perry A, Jolley M (eds) Nursing: a knowledge base for practice. Edward Arnold, London

Moody L E 1990 Advancing nursing science through research. Sage, London, vol 1

Munhall P L 1989 Philosophical ponderings on qualitative research methods in nursing. Nursing Science Quarterly 2(1): 20–28

Schultz P R, Meleis A I 1988 Nursing epistemology traditions, insights, questions. Image, Journal of Nursing Scholarship 20(4): 217–221

Philosophic inquiry in nursing

Kikuchi J F, Simmons H 1992 Philosophic inquiry in nursing. Sage, London

Feminism

Barrett M 1987 The concept of difference. Feminist Review 26

Bourne J 1983 Towards an antiracist feminism. Race and Class XXV: 1

Bryan B, Dadzie S, Scafe S 1985 The heart of the race. Virago, London

Carby H 1982 White woman listen! Black feminism and the boundaries of sisterhood. In: Centre for Contemporary Cultural Studies (ed) The empire strikes back. Hutchinson, London

Chalmers A F 1982 What is this thing called science? Open University Press, Milton Keynes

Davis A 1984 Women culture and politics. The Women's Press, London

Ettore E 1980 Lesbians women and society. Routledge and Kegan Paul, London

Frye M 1984 On being white. Trouble and Strife 4

Gray G, Pratt R 1991 (eds) Towards a discipline of nursing. Churchill Livingstone, Edinburgh

Greene M 1966 The knower and the known. Faber & Faber, London

hooks b 1984 Feminist theory from margin to center. South End Press, Boston, MA

Humm M 1986 Feminist criticism: women as contemporary critics. Harvester Press, Brighton

Jarvis P 1985 The sociology of adult and continuing education. Croom Helm, London

Knowles M 1984 (ed) Andragogy in action. Jossey Bass, San Francisco

Knowles M 1990 The adult learner: a neglected species. Gulf, Houston

Kuzwayo E 1985 Call me woman. The Women's Press, London

Lather P 1986 Research as praxis. Harvard Educational Review 56(3)

Lorde A 1984 Sister outsider. The Crossing Press, Trumansberg, NY

Moraga C, Anzaldua G (eds) 1981 This bridge called my back. Persephone Press, Watertown, MA

O'Brien M 1989 Reproducing the world: essays in feminist theory. Westview Press, Oxford

Rich A 1976 Of woman born. Virago, London

Roberts H (ed) 1981 Doing feminist research. Routledge and Kegan Paul, London

Spelman E V 1988 Inessential woman. Beacon Press, Boston

Stanley L 1990 Feminist praxis. Routledge and Kegan Paul, London

Tang Nain G 1991 Black women, sexism and racism: black or antiracist feminism. Feminist Review 37: 1–22

Webb C 1986 Feminist practices in women's health care. John Wiley, Chichester

Experimental methods

3

Jane Say   Julie Cumpper

■ KEY ISSUES

- **Quantitative approaches to research**
- **Experimental methods and research design**
- **Laboratory experiments**
- **Quantitative approaches and experimental methods: their place in practice**

PREAMBLE

A group of student nurses were learning about biological principles by conducting laboratory experiments under the guidance of a nurse teacher. The same group of students moved to a classroom to learn about nursing research with a different teacher. Months later, as a result of a chance conversation, the two teachers realized how much their sessions had in common; surely these sessions could complement each other.

What were these factors that both sessions had in common? While the research teacher was defining, describing and discussing aspects of research, the students in the laboratory were contending with these issues in practice. There was surely potential in the laboratory session for putting into practice the theory of quantitative research and experimental **methods**. Surely the students in the laboratory could learn about biological principles and increase their research mindedness at the same time.

But why just the laboratory? The discussion widened to other experiential and participatory teaching sessions, and then to procedures in the practice setting. So many activities in these areas use aspects of the experimental research process. Many skills, such as a systematic, critical and enquiring approach, are equally valid in the areas of research, education and practice. Would it not be possible to help students and practitioners to take a fresh look at activities which they are already taking part in, as a means of increasing their research skills and enhancing research mindedness?

And so, what began as a conversation between colleagues, developed into a challenge to investigate the usefulness of activities in both educational and practice settings for exploring quantitative research and promoting research mindedness. This chapter is all about promoting research mindedness by utilizing the strong link between quantitative research methods, practical teaching sessions and the practice setting.

INTRODUCTION

In this chapter, we explore in some detail what we mean by quantitative research, showing how some of the components of this type of research may be related to clinical practice. But first let us consider what we mean by the term 'research mindedness'.

As was discussed in Chapter 1, there is no universally accepted definition for this term, and you may already have devised a working definition. The concept is rather ambiguous and probably conjures up different associations for different people. It is important, then, to clarify how 'research mindedness' will be used in this chapter. Perhaps you would like to compare your own definition with the one we have used:

> *We understand the term 'research mindedness' to imply a critical questioning approach to one's work, the desire and ability to find out about the latest research in that area, and the ability to assess its value to that situation and apply it as appropriate. It also implies a recognition of the importance of research to the profession and to patient care, and a willingness to support nurse researchers in their work. All qualified nurses should be research minded ... .*

(RCN 1982)

This definition is interesting because it addresses the importance of both the results of research and the process of researching. Let us look at these two aspects.

First, an intelligent and informed approach toward the results of formal research projects is seen as an integral characteristic of research mindedness. Much of the research that health care professionals encounter is produced using quantitative approaches. Familiarity with this type of research and its different components, as well as its limitations, will promote research mindedness by equipping health care professionals with the confidence and skills to assess the relevance of research and to apply it appropriately to their practice setting.

The second characteristic of research mindedness, according to our definition, is linked with the processes and skills involved in researching. Many of the skills required by the health care professional and the researcher are very similar. Researchers are required to approach their work systematically, using a thoughtful, critical, and enquiring approach. But many health care professionals would also recognize these skills and attitudes as being essential to areas of their work. Thus, the development of skills used within clinical practice that are pertinent to research offer a means of promoting research mindedness.

Using this definition of research mindedness means that research-based practice includes, but is not confined to, formal research projects, and research mindedness becomes an attitude, not an activity, a process, not simply a product.

We have been referring to the quantitative approach to research; perhaps it is now time to explore exactly what we mean by this term.

QUANTITATIVE APPROACHES

A **quantitative** approach to research is a way of trying to explain what is happening in the real world using numerical data or quantities. Health care professionals will be familiar with the use of numerical data in their practice; for example, height, weight and temperature are all quantities that are regularly measured. This contrasts with **qualitative** approaches to research that gather information without using numbers; qualitative approaches are dealt with in Chapters 5 and 6. For example, a study reported by Smith (1994) researching into treatment of venous ulcers used a quantitative approach that measured the performance, convenience and cost-effectiveness of two different wound care products. In contrast, researchers using a qualitative approach might, for example, examine how it feels to suffer with a venous ulcer. (The article by Smith (1994), from which we draw examples to illustrate the quantitative approach, is reproduced in Appendix 1.)

Quantitative approaches require researchers to be **objective** in their approach to the research. Objectivity means that they must be impartial and unbiased when carrying out the research and avoid including their own personal views and interpretation of what is occurring. This type of research is also viewed as being **reductionist**. This is because it is often necessary to 'reduce' a system to its component parts for the purposes of the study. For example, Smith's study into venous ulcers 'reduced' the patients' assessment of their experience of wound dressings in terms of pain, quality of life, comfort and convenience to measures on a scale for each of these abstract concepts.

Stages of the quantitative approach

Let us look at the stages undertaken by someone who is using a quantitative approach to their research. These are shown in Figure 3.1.

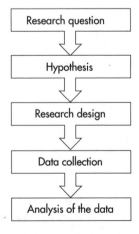

Figure 3.1 The stages of quantitative research.

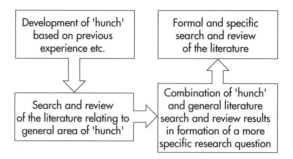

Figure 3.2 Relationship between research question and literature search and review. (Reproduced from Cormack D F S (ed) 1984 Introduction to the research process in nursing, by permission of Blackwell Scientific, Oxford.)

The research question

Often a research project begins with a question that has arisen in practice, such as: 'Is our method of treating leg ulcers really the most effective?'. This starting point is known as the research question. The relationship between the research topic, emerging question and the literature search is demonstrated in a diagram devised by Cormack (1984) (Fig. 3.2). We found this diagram helpful because it shows how the research question is partly shaped by general and unstructured reading around the chosen topic in order to give structure and focus to a more systematic literature search and review.

In quantitative research the literature review precedes data collection so that researchers can inform themselves of the material available on the topic. Janet Moir discusses this process in much more detail in Chapter 8.

Hypothesis

Although the research question expresses the overall aim of the study, it often has to be narrowed down to ensure that the study performed will be meaningful. In fact, the researchers have to make a prediction about the relationship between the factors they are studying. This is called the **hypothesis**. For example, one hypothesis for our venous ulcer study could be: 'Venous ulcers treated with product X heal more rapidly than venous ulcers treated with product Y'. Thus, the hypothesis aims to describe or test relationships and examine cause and effect. In the venous ulcer study the relationship was between the type of venous ulcer treatment and healing time.

Researchers also use a statement called the **null hypothesis**. This states that there is no difference between the factors being studied. At the start of a piece of research, the null hypothesis is assumed to be true. Only by doing the research and collecting the appropriate data can a researcher disprove the null hypothesis and therefore support the hypothesis. Can you think of a null hypothesis for the venous ulcer study? One possibility is: 'There is no difference in healing time between ulcers treated with product X and ulcers treated with product Y'.

The factors that are being investigated are known as the **variables**; in this study the variables were, of course, the healing time and the types of dressings used. Because the healing time was predicted to be dependent on the types of dressing used, it is called the **dependent variable**. The type of dressing used, which is the variable 'manipulated' by the researcher, is known as the **independent variable**. In other words, in a 'cause–effect' relationship, the independent variable (dressing) represents the cause and the dependent variable (healing time) represents the effect. One word of caution about the idea of cause–effect relationships should be introduced here. Cause–effect relationships can only really be established in carefully controlled experiments. This may not be possible in some situations such as clinical practice where many independent variables may have an impact upon the dependent variable. In the venous ulcer study, for example, the researcher noted a difference between product X and product Y in relation to a number of dependent variables, such as pain, sleep disturbance, comfort and healing time. But the technical skill of the nurse or the patient's own state of emotional well-being may also have contributed to the overall 'effect'.

The term '**correlation**' is used when variables appear to be related to each other. It is important that the researcher does not immediately assume that a 'correlation' is the same as 'cause' because, as we have just noted, it is very difficult in the clinical situation to control all the independent variables that may have an effect on the dependent variables.

Research design

In order to ensure that research is carried out in a systematic and effective way, the study must be carefully designed. One method or design that is commonly used is known as the experimental method. What exactly do we mean by experiment? Clearly, a scientific test or trial carried out in a laboratory is an experiment, but experiments can be carried out in many different areas including clinical practice, since an experiment is simply a means of testing a **theory**. Indeed, whenever anyone measures a person's blood pressure, for example, this is a very simple form of experiment. When measuring a blood pressure, a certain procedure must be followed if an accurate result is to be obtained. Similarly, research using the experimental method has certain standard conditions that aim to ensure valid results. By valid we mean that the results measure what they say they do, i.e. they are an accurate measure of blood pressure. We shall return to a discussion of the term 'valid' and its companion term 'reliable' in the section on data collection below. Sometimes when experiments are carried out outside the laboratory, such as in the clinical setting, they are referred to as 'field experiments'.

The standard conditions used in experimental method are particularly important in order to ensure that incidental factors do not affect the result of the experiment. These incidental factors are called '**extraneous variables**'. If you think back to the venous ulcer study, it may have occurred to you that many other factors in addition to the ones we identified (nurse's skill, patient's well-being) could have affected the outcome of this research. Factors such as the age or sex of the individual could have influenced the rate of wound healing. These factors are referred to as extraneous variables. As a health care professional, you will be familiar with the way that many extraneous variables can affect the measurements we make in practice, such as an elevated pulse rate when a baby cries or even diurnal changes in weight. Thus, a new-born baby's normal pulse rate is 130–140 beats per minute but when it cries vigorously (the extraneous variable) this may increase to 160 beats per minute. In terms of diurnal weight changes, it is quite likely that the weight of normal healthy people will vary. In the evening they are likely to be heavier than when they got on the scales in the morning, especially if they have eaten three full meals during the day. Body weight also depends on the amount of fluid loss through perspiration during excessive exercise or hot weather. Here we have a number of extraneous variables affecting weight, including number of meals, exercise and climate.

Any extraneous variables must be taken into consideration when undertaking research. Ideally, extraneous variables are eliminated or an attempt is made to minimize their effects on the dependent variable. This is achieved by the researcher exerting **control** over the experimental conditions. Controlling experimental research is an important aspect of the research design. As you can imagine, it is often easier to control the conditions within a laboratory experiment and eliminate extraneous variables, which in the weight example would include number of meals, exercise and external temperature. However, when research is carried out 'in the field', dealing with real people in practice settings, this can be very difficult.

In order to exert control on the conditions within 'field' experiments, there are a number of ways that a researcher can design the research to minimize the effects of extraneous variables. One means of control may be achieved by using a treatment or experimental group and comparing the results with another group, appropriately termed the 'control group'. The latter group does not undergo any manipulation of the independent variable, i.e. receives no treatment, and, because of this, the group acts as a baseline for the measurements and changes seen in the experimental group. Owing to ethical considerations, which are discussed further in Chapter 10, this can be difficult to achieve.

Consider the venous ulcer study. Here, a true control group was not used because this would have meant that the clients would not have received any treatment for their ulcers whatsoever. This would obviously be quite unacceptable. Instead, both groups of patients were treated and the dressings compared for their efficacy. Probably the best-known example of using control groups is in drug trials where a **placebo** drug that looks identical but has no therapeutic effects is given to a control group while the experimental group receives the genuine treatment. The groups are not told whether they are receiving the placebo or the drug. Using a placebo in this way ensures that the clients feel that they are being treated in the same way. There may well be considerable ethical implications for this kind of study also, and, as with any study, clients must give informed consent.

Another means of exerting control and minimizing extraneous variables is through **sampling**. When carrying out research involving subjects, for example patients or clients, the subjects or the sample involved in the study must be representative or typical of the target population.

To examine this further let us return to the trial on the treatment of venous ulcers. Within this piece of research, 40 patients with venous ulcers of greater than 2.5 cm in diameter were selected from those patients attending the Department of Dermatology in a hospital in the North of England. To minimize certain extraneous variables, patients were not included in the study if they had conditions that could affect wound healing, for example infection, immune deficiency, treatment with steroids, or malignant disease. However, as we previously stated, there are other factors such as age and sex that could affect the healing time. To overcome these types of extraneous variables, the patients were randomly allocated to two groups. One group would receive treatment with dressing X while the other would be treated with dressing Y. **Randomization** ensured that the two groups had similar characteristics and were therefore not significantly different in factors such as age, sex, mobility, work or smoking status. When using true control groups and comparing them with an experimental group, it is still important that the groups are randomized.

This approach in the design of an experiment allows the results to be generalized to the wider target population. **Generalizability** of research results is important if the findings are going to be applied to a target population. However, results from studies where small groups of clients have been used in a limited number of clinical areas may not be generalizable, owing to the small sample size and lack of practice settings. The results of the venous ulcer study would be more generalizable if a greater number of clients had been used and the study had been performed in a wider variety of clinical settings. Ideally, the results of experimental research undertaken within practice should be equally relevant to anyone with similar characteristics to the study group in any clinical setting.

The overall design of the research is important to enable other researchers to replicate the experiment. **Replication** allows the results of the original study to be verified and it also allows results to be obtained from different settings. This, as you would expect, further ensures generalizability.

Many researchers in health care consider replication and generalizability of research findings to be essential if these findings are to be used in the treatment of large populations of people in a wide range of clinical areas. **Randomized controlled trials** (RCTs) offer a means of replication and generalizability and, because of this, are a type of experimental research that has become increasingly popular within clinical practice. As with any 'true' experiment this method must demonstrate a means of exerting control over the research situation, manipulation of independent variable(s) and random allocation of clients between the control and experimental groups (Distance Learning Centre 1988).

Currently, experts from a range of health care disciplines are reviewing the results from the many RCTs that are published each week in order to offer professionals the most reliable and up-to-date evidence for their practice (Vines 1995). Databases, journals and regional health authority publications are being used to report these systematic reviews along with recommendations for practice. A critical review of nursing management of leg ulcers in the community has been published by Nicky Cullum (1994a, b), a nurse researcher. This review was one of the first to be undertaken which specifically looked at nursing interventions. Cullum considered a number of issues, including wound debridement and cleansing; types of bandages and bandaging techniques; and different types of dressings available for the treatment of leg ulcers. Overall, she concluded that there was a need for further studies to achieve more conclusive evidence about the benefits and limitations of both products and techniques.

Data collection

In order to collect data in experimental research, a means of obtaining, recording and quantifying the data is needed. This is achieved through **observation** and **measurement**. Careful observation using one's senses is required to allow accurate measurements to be performed. At the same time, the researcher must also develop some kind of tool that measures the changes that occur in the dependent variable as a consequence of manipulating the independent variable. Consider the taking of a patient's pulse. The pulse may be measured manually and timed using any watch with a second hand. This information is then recorded and documented appropriately. Other more sophisticated electronic tools such as an electrocardiograph (ECG) machine or pulse oximeter can also be used to measure pulse rate. Measurements within experimental research can be performed with a wide variety of tools from a sensitive piece of electronic equipment to a carefully designed interview schedule, scale or questionnaire.

In the venous ulcer study referred to above, Smith used visual analogue scales to measure pain. Patients were asked to mark where on a line they experienced pain from 0 = 'no pain' to 10 = 'worst pain'. She could also have designed a questionnaire or carried out an interview with patients to investigate their pain. If she had done this, she would have needed to follow careful procedures such as those recommended by Bell (1993) to ensure her questionnaire or interview contained questions that were sound (in terms of type, wording and order) and avoided such 'traps' as double questions, and leading or presumptive ones. Florence Nightingale in her *Notes on Nursing* observed that the leading question always elicited inaccurate information. She gave the following example:

> *There is no more silly or universal question scarcely asked than this, 'Is he better?' Who can have any opinion of any value as to whether the patient is better or worse, except the constant medical attendant, or the really observing nurse?*

> (Nightingale 1859)

Thus, Nightingale emphasized the key role of observation in obtaining accurate information about patients.

Various aspects of data collection are shown in parts A, B, C, D and E of Figure 3.3. It is important to remember that whichever tool is being used there is a 'human element' to the process of observation and measurement. Some aspects of the human senses, such as touch and sight, are always involved. Consider a researcher who was collecting information on patient dependency. She asked elderly patients to rate their daily living activities, on a scoring system of 0 'good/independent' to 3 'poor/dependent' devised by Hunt (1982). Activities included mobility, continence and communication. The researcher told us that she frequently rated patients as more dependent than they rated themselves. Thus, the researcher's observational skills, such as her sight and clinical expertise, influenced how she rated the patients' dependency.

Whatever the tool or equipment being used, it is important that the measurement or observation made during the research is reliable and valid. What do these terms mean? For the measurement or observation to be **reliable** 'the question to ask is whether the same observation would have been obtained by a different researcher or if collected at a different time' (Avis 1994). For example: 'two nurses taking a patient's temperature under similar conditions, and using the same thermometers and procedure, should obtain similar results' (Tierney et al 1988).

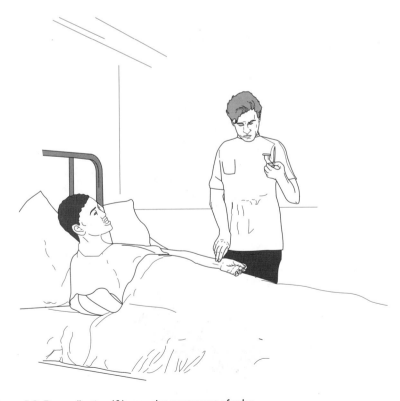

A

Figure 3.3 Data collection (**A**) manual measurement of pulse.

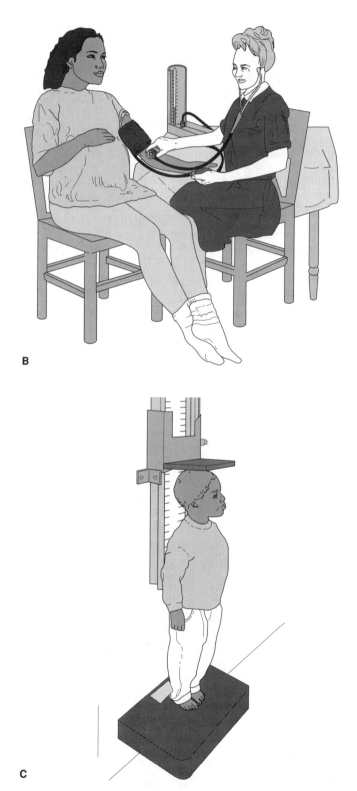

B

C

Figure 3.3 Data collection (**B**) blood pressure measurement; (**C**) height measurement.

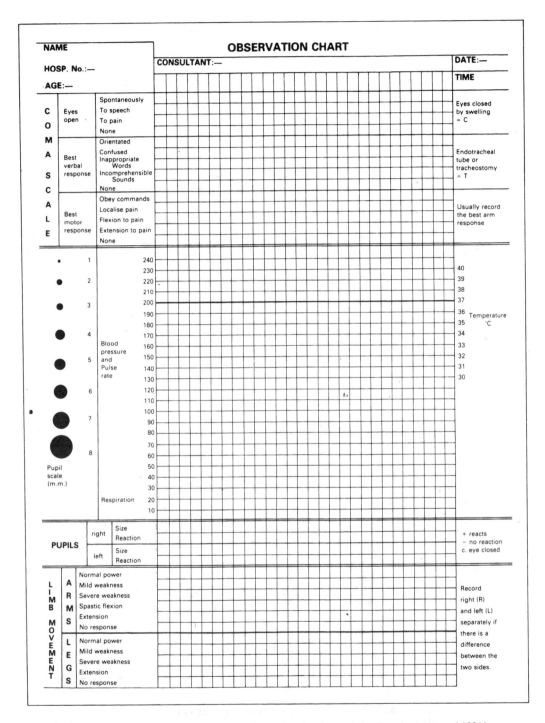

Figure 3.3 Data collection (**D**) Glasgow coma scale. (Reproduced with permission from Jamieson et al 1996.)

McGill Pain Questionnaire

Patient's Name _____ Date _____ Time_____ am/pm

PRI: S_____ A _____ E_____ M_____ PRI(T)_____ PPI ___
    (1–10)   (11–15)   (16)   (17–20)   (1–20)

1 FLICKERING QUIVERING PULSING THROBBING BEATING POUNDING	11 TIRING EXHAUSTING
2 JUMPING FLASHING SHOOTING	12 SICKENING SUFFOCATING
3 PRICKING BORING DRILLING STABBING LANCINATING	13 FEARFUL FRIGHTFUL TERRIFYING
4 SHARP CUTTING LACERATING	14 PUNISHING GRUELLING CRUEL VICIOUS KILLING
5 PINCHING PRESSING GNAWING CRAMPING CRUSHING	15 WRETCHED BLINDING
6 TUGGING PULLING WRENCHING	16 ANNOYING TROUBLESOME MISERABLE INTENSE UNBEARABLE
7 HOT BURNING SCALDING SEARING	17 SPREADING RADIATING PENETRATING PIERCING
8 TINGLING ITCHY SMARTING STINGING	18 TIGHT NUMB DRAWING SQUEEZING TEARING
9 DULL SORE HURTING ACHING HEAVY	19 COOL COLD FREEZING
10 TENDER TAUT RASPING SPLITTING	20 NAGGING NAUSEATING AGONIZING DREADFUL TORTURING

BRIEF ___	RHYTHMIC ___ CONTINUOUS ___
MOMENTARY ___	PERIODIC ___ STEADY ___
TRANSIENT ___	INTERMITTENT ___ CONSTANT ___

E = EXTERNAL
I = INTERNAL

PPI
0 NO PAIN ___
1 MILD ___
2 DISCOMFORTING ___
3 DISTRESSING ___
4 HORRIBLE ___
5 EXCRUCIATING ___

COMMENTS:

Figure 3.3 Data collection (**E**) McGill–Melzack pain questionnaire. (Reproduced with permission from Wall & Melzack 1994.)

In order to be **valid**, the measurement or observation must be a convincing and accurate means of quantifying the variable. In other words, does it actually measure what it says it does? Using a thermometer is widely accepted as a valid and reliable means of quantifying a patient's body temperature. Although we have explored reliability and validity in relation to the taking of a temperature, the same principles apply when using tools such as questionnaires, interview schedules or rating scales. For example, how valid and reliable were the scales used to measure patient dependency and pain in the studies mentioned above?

One way to demonstrate and distinguish between validity and reliability is to take the example of a clock that is consistently 5 minutes fast. The clock is said to be reliable. However, it is not valid since the time it shows is 5 minutes ahead of Greenwich Mean Time, which is valid.

When conducting research, one way to ensure validity and reliability of research tools is to conduct a pilot study to develop and try them out prior to the main study.

Analysis of the data

An appropriate method of analysis has to be chosen to deal with the data that are collected. The analysis of the data aims to demonstrate that the changes observed and measured in relation to the dependent variable are in fact due to the influence of the independent variable and are not due to chance or random occurrence. In fact, by using statistics, researchers try to prove or test that the null hypothesis is incorrect. Data analysis and the use of statistics are further explored in Chapter 4.

CASE STUDY

Although we have noted that a laboratory experiment is not the only way of conducting a quantitative research study, it is a method which can demonstrate aspects of the **methodology** quite clearly. Also, as is argued throughout the chapter, it offers a means of gaining practical research skills which may be transferable to the clinical setting. For these reasons, we are going to explore one particular experiment. We have included sufficient detail for the reader who would like to reproduce the experiment as an educational exercise.

The experiment detailed below (see Box 3.1) was chosen because it generated the original interest in the connection between teaching biology and research and it was the one we chose to present to our peers in a session on promoting research mindedness. The majority of them were more familiar with social science in natural settings than biological science and laboratory experiments. We needed therefore to check their understanding of some of the concepts being used.

■ **BOX 3.1**

Introduction

Experiments and various types of laboratory work are often used as a means of exploring biological concepts. The experiment outlined below can be used to demonstrate the importance of enzymes and enzymic reactions in body metabolism. You might like to check your understanding of these concepts in order to see how the experiment is used to present them.

Enzymic reactions

Enzymes are proteins that act as catalysts of chemical reactions, i.e. they speed up the rate of all metabolic reactions that occur within the body. Each enzyme is specific for a particular substrate or chemical. The activity of an enzyme and how effectively it increases the rate of a chemical reaction can be influenced by a number of factors including temperature. Digestion of food is facilitated by the production of enzymes in the alimentary canal. Enzymes are produced by various organs and released into the alimentary canal to break down the complex nutrient molecules into smaller molecules. These can then be absorbed by the lining of the intestine into the bloodstream.

Rennin is an enzyme produced in the stomach of new-born infants. It causes milk to clot by catalysing the conversion of the milk protein caseinogen into insoluble casein. The purpose of this experiment is to study the rate of activity of the enzyme at varying temperatures set at 0°C, 20°C, 37°C (normal body temperature) and 70°C.

The following materials are required to conduct the experiment.

Materials

- 4 test tubes
- Rennet (containing rennin)
- Pipettes
- Thermometer
- Water-bath
- Stop-clock
- Ice

Methods

As previously stated, the temperatures under study are: 0°C, 20°C, 37°C, 70°C. The class divides into four groups. Each group performs one experiment at one of the test temperatures following the procedures outlined below.

Experimental procedures

1. The water bath is prepared at the temperature specified for the group.
2. 10 ml of milk is delivered into each of three test tubes.
3. 1 ml of rennet is delivered into a fourth test tube.
4. All four tubes are placed in the water-bath for 5 minutes.
5. 0.5 ml of rennet is added to two of the tubes containing milk. The tubes are inverted once to mix and replaced in the water-bath. The stop-clock is started.
6. The clock is stopped on observing that clotting has occurred in the tubes.
7. The time taken for clotting to occur is noted and recorded.
8. The results of each group are pooled, compared and interpreted.

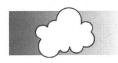

Although it may be impractical for some readers to perform this experiment, you may like to consider each stage and answer the following questions.

Could the following components of experimental research be identified:

1. *variables—dependent and independent*
2. *hypothesis*
3. *control*
4. *observation and measurement*
5. *validity and reliability*
6. *generalizability?*

To help you to explore these issues further, we describe some of the discussion that took place with our peers when they performed this experiment, with a view to highlighting experimental methodology and research mindedness. Compare your answers with our discussion.

The variables

The group had little difficulty in identifying the variables. It was quickly decided that the variables were temperature and rate of activity. However, there was some discussion about which was the independent variable and which was the dependent variable. It was eventually decided that the rate of activity was the dependent variable since the rate of activity depended upon the temperature. The variable being manipulated by the group was the temperature and thus it was agreed that this was the independent variable.

Hypothesis

The group suggested that the hypothesis could be: 'the rate of activity (as measured by the time taken for a reaction to occur) of the enzyme rennin is altered by varying the temperature at which the reaction is occurring'. Of course, the null hypothesis would have stated that the temperature made no difference to the rate of activity of the rennin.

Control

When we conducted the experiment, the group noted that the temperature was carefully controlled within the experiment. However, there was no true control group since, strictly speaking, a control should have been carried out at 'no temperature', which of course does not exist. As a compromise, we took normal body temperature to be our control (i.e. 37°C).

Observation and measurement

Direct observation was used to assess when clotting had occurred and stop-clocks were used to measure the amount of time taken for the enzyme to clot the milk.

Many of the group found the direct observation of the tubes, especially those that took some time to clot, quite boring. In fact, one group actually missed the precise moment, since they were deep in discussion and were not being particularly observant. Hence, even from this very simple experiment, it was highlighted how difficult observation can be. This was further commented upon by a member of the group, who had studied for and been awarded a PhD. She told us that at times she had found the data collection for her study (which included observation) to be difficult and laborious. She noted the importance of pacing oneself during observation in order not to become overloaded and miss valuable insights.

Validity and reliability

It was agreed that the use of a stop-clock to measure time was ostensibly a valid means of measurement, but, as one of the groups demonstrated by missing their clotting time, its reliability depended on the operators' competency. This incident showed that relying on human observation skills can lead to error. It also demonstrates the importance of ensuring reliability since, without it, misleading or incorrect results could be obtained.

Generalizability

This experiment can not be used to generalize about all enzymes in the body since rennin may not be typical of all enzymes. Also, as mentioned by the group, experiments performed in vitro (within a test tube) do not necessarily represent what happens in vivo (in the human body).

REFLECTIONS FOR PRACTICE

Having considered the quantitative research approach in the laboratory, let us now apply this approach to the practice setting.

Applying research to practice

Earlier on we looked at two aspects of research mindedness; let us revisit these now, referring specifically to the quantitative approach and applying it to the practice setting.

First, there is the idea that research mindedness involves 'the ability to find out about the latest research ... and assess its value to that situation and apply it as appropriate....' (RCN 1982).

During the last 20 years, there have been extensive developments in relation to the role of research in nursing and the means by which nursing can become a 'research-based profession' (DHSS 1972). The inclusion of research in nursing curricula is a reflection of these developments.

Health care professionals can be viewed as 'consumers' of research (Thomas & Price 1980). If this is the case, then practitioners should be able to decide whether and how to implement research findings as they become aware of them. A working knowledge of research methods and terminology will help them to do this. They can also use research to make informed choices about the delivery of patient care and argue with purchasers the need for buying proven products and processes. Smith (1994) was in a position to do this following completion of her comparative study of wound dressings, in which she showed that because the more expensive product was better all round than the other, it was also more cost-effective.

Look through some professional journals that carry research-based articles and reports. You will probably find that a substantial number of research projects are based on quantitative approaches. Familiarity with aspects of this method and the terminology used should make these reports more inviting to read, and easier to make sense of. Although it requires some experience, skill and practice to make a detailed critique of a piece of research, even beginners can ask some useful questions and can make some informed judgement about its relevance to their area of practice. Chapter 9 gives a detailed account of how to make a critical assessment of quantitative research.

Health care involves a multidisciplinary approach, and so it is useful for practitioners to have access to research from many different disciplines. Much of the research that affects patient care is based on quantitative approaches, and the 'demystifying' of these research projects may offer practitioners a better opportunity to work together in the interests of the patient.

Aspects of research in practice

The second aspect of research mindedness that we highlighted earlier was the use of the skills and processes involved in research. Several aspects of experimental research design and the process of obtaining data can actually be applied to the everyday activities that occur within practice.

Observation and measurement

Let us explore the use of observation and measurement within the practice setting.

Briefly consider and write down aspects of practice that require observation and/or measurement.

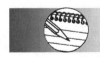

We asked a number of students and practitioners to consider this statement. Their ideas are shown in Box 3.2.

When thinking about this question you may have thought that much of direct patient care involves the concept of observation and measurement. Each day in practice, clinicians are quantifying and collecting data about individuals in their care. Consider how this compares with the researcher collecting data as part of a research project. In both instances there is the need for an orderly, efficient and accurate approach that requires a number of cognitive and psychomotor skills such as decision making, analysis, appropriate use of the equipment and a sound knowledge base. Although observations

■ **BOX 3.2**

Observations and measurements in practice

- Temperature
- Pulse
- Blood pressure
- Respirations
- Pupil size and reaction
- Fluid balance
- Wound assessment
- Pain

- Weight
- Height
- Blood glucose
- Pressure sore risk
- Head circumference
- Quality measurement
- Pulse oximetry
- Central venous pressure measurements

are performed very frequently, often by junior members of staff, they are highly complex and their importance should not be underestimated.

How do these activities and skills contribute to the overall care given to the patient? Observation and measurement are, in fact, integral to the assessment of the patient. Assessment can be viewed as 'a systematic and orderly collection and analysis of data pertaining to and about the health status of the client/patient for the purpose of making a nursing diagnosis' (Stanton et al 1990). This is a crucial issue for nurses because assessment is a fundamental feature of nursing practice and is recognized in the four stages of the nursing process, i.e. assessment, care planning, implementation and evaluation. The process is dynamic, and assessment occurs not only on the initial contact with the patient, but throughout the entire period of care. So, for example, the nurse plans care on the basis of the assessment in order to decide on the best way to implement care and then evaluate it.

Reflect briefly on a situation you have encountered where observations/measurements formed a critical part of the ongoing assessment of patient care in order to evaluate and monitor the effect of clinical interventions.

One example might be the measurement of blood glucose levels in a newly diagnosed insulin-dependent diabetic. Initially, a baseline blood glucose reading would be recorded and ongoing readings would determine the amount of insulin to be prescribed. This would also help to evaluate the patient's progress.

The assessment of risk factors associated with pressure sore development is another example requiring observation and measurement on initial contact and throughout a period of care. Well-known measurement tools for pressure sore assessment include scales developed by Waterlow (1985) and Norton et al (1975). These scales have also been subject to scrutiny. In a research-based literature review to examine the rationale for pressure sore risk assessment tools, Edwards (1994) highlighted a number of deficiencies. One problem associated with the tools was that they were used with a variety of patient populations without taking into account the different factors associated with risk, such as age and medical condition. There was also a lack of consistency among researchers as to how pressure sores were defined. All the studies had been undertaken in hospitals rather than with patients who were being nursed in their own homes. Given future trends to care for more people at home, Edwards recommends the need to redress this situation. However, her key recommendation lay in the need for a more systematic approach by researchers and practitioners to the application of the scales.

Walsh & Ford (1989) argue that 'observation is synonymous with assessment and without assessment there can be no rational individualized patient care'. This could also be said for measurement since this is inextricably linked to observation. So, the skills needed to make accurate observations and measurements should not be underestimated, since they are central to nursing practice.

Reliability and validity

As we previously discussed, any means of measurement must offer reliability and validity. Why are reliability and validity important in clinical practice?

When we perform various measurements and observations within everyday practice it is important that these observations are reliable and valid, since decisions related to the diagnosis and planning of care may be based on the observations and measurements that have been performed.

Let us consider blood pressure measurement. A throbbing headache or dizziness, which a patient complains of, may indicate that there has been a change in the blood pressure of that individual. These subjective observations may alert a clinician to this possibility but they would not be a valid assessment of the patient's blood pressure, since they would be based on impressions rather than measurement. A sphygmomanometer, however, offers a valid and objective means of measuring blood pressure. In order to maintain the reliability of the measurement, a number of factors need to be considered. Research has shown that sphygmomanometers are often defective owing to lack of maintenance (Concceicao et al 1976, Bell & Siklos 1984, Jolly 1991) and a number of other variables can also affect the blood pressure readings that are obtained. These include the time of day, the level of anxiety experienced by the patient and the technique used by the person taking the measurement. Therefore, to ensure that the series of readings obtained is a reliable measure of the patient's blood pressure, these factors must be taken into account by the various professionals performing the measurement. This is achieved by every clinician using equipment that is kept in good working order and performing the procedure and recording the observation in exactly the same manner.

Can you suggest methods that are employed within practice to ensure reliability and validity of the observations and measurements that are made?

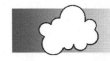

Within clinical and practice areas there are procedure and policy documents that serve as guidelines to everyday practice. To ensure that the information given in these documents is reliable and valid, they should be regularly updated and based on current research evidence. The Royal Marsden Hospital (1993) *Manual of Clinical Nursing Policies and Procedures* is probably one of the best-known documents that aims to give research-based information on carrying out procedures and facilitates practitioners to carry out procedures in a systematic way.

However, unlike a research laboratory, the clinical situation is not controlled, and sometimes reliability and validity can be hard to achieve. You may be aware of certain areas in your own practice that present particular challenges. However, the task of a research-minded practitioner is to strive to overcome these difficulties by employing the researcher's skills, such as analysis and critical thinking, and applying current research-based knowledge.

Care: the independent variable

Every intervention that is carried out within practice has a potential effect on the outcome of patient care. If we consider this from an experimental perspective, clinical interventions and patient outcome could be thought of as two correlated or related variables. There are a number of studies that have examined the effects of a nursing intervention on patient outcomes. Haywood (1975) set up an experiment to look at the effects of nurses' information giving on patients' postoperative experience of pain. Webb & Wilson-Barnett (1983) used an experimental design to find out whether postoperative counselling sessions helped women undergoing hysterectomy to recover more quickly. The researchers in these studies wanted to find out whether the independent variable (information giving, counselling as part of nursing care) was correlated with patients' better pain management or postoperative recovery.

The challenge then to the research-minded practitioner is to perform all care with the same considered approach as the researcher manipulating an independent variable. This emphasizes the importance of our practice; we may well agree with Bond (1993), who argues that interventions should have 'a reasonable chance of being effective and a minimal chance of doing harm'. So, if we accept that our practice has a direct influence upon the outcomes of care, then our approach to practice must be systematic and critical. Research mindedness is therefore not an optional extra, but must be an integral part of practice.

Quantitative approaches and holistic practice

Having said all this, there is more to health care than the experimental quantitative approach. The practice setting clearly has many significant differences from an experimental setting. The reductionist approach within this type of research has sometimes been criticized as inadequate in a holistic activity like health care. This criticism would certainly be justified if it were the only approach used. We are aware that we have emphasized repeatedly the importance of being as objective as possible when making certain observations in order to ensure accuracy. Perhaps we have made this point at the expense of the subjective side of human interaction. Quantitative measures alone will not tell us everything we need to know about a patient, and subjective observations may be equally important. Sometimes a 'hunch' or a feeling will lead on to taking a more objective observation. Sometimes the subjective experiences and feelings of the patient, which are difficult to express in words, let alone numbers, may initiate a particular type of intervention.

Take the following exemplar selected by Benner (1984) in *From Novice to Expert* to demonstrate the expert nurse's ability to pick up 'subtle changes in the patient's behavior or appearance'. Following the patient's return from the X-ray department where she had undergone an oesophageal dilatation the nurse observed that 'Later she started getting nauseated and she had streaks of very light pink drainage which I could account for by dilatation procedures, but I just had this feeling that something else was going on ... her vital signs were still stable but I indicated that I wanted the house officer to check her'.

The patient referred to in this exemplar was later found to have an oesophageal rupture. Prompt treatment was instigated because the nurse followed her feeling 'that something else was going on'.

Hence, these two aspects, the objective and the subjective, must complement each other. Thus care as illustrated by the exemplar can be described as both an 'imaginative and critical process' (Medawar 1969).

SUMMARY

The connection between skills used in experimental research and skills used in clinical practice has been an important theme of this chapter. There has been emphasis laid on the suggestion that awareness of, and participating in, experimental research activities could enhance practice and that, conversely, many nursing interventions are using aspects of the experimental research methodology. Furthermore, this gives an emphasis to the importance of research skills generally, rather than just the results of specific research projects, important though these are. This may make a significant contribution to the wider discussion on research-based practice in health care. We can improve our understanding by seeking understanding from a range of experiences and reflections, in order to enhance and increase our knowledge and practice.

REFERENCES

Avis M 1994 Reading research critically. II. An introduction to appraisal: assessing the evidence. Journal of Clinical Nursing 3: 271–277

Bell M, Siklos P 1984 Accuracy of staff and equipment. Nursing Times 80(26): 32–34

Bell J 1993 Doing your research project. Open University Press, Buckingham

Benner P 1984 From novice to expert. Addison Wesley, Menlo Park, California

Bond S 1993 Experimental research in nursing: necessary but not sufficient. In: Kitson A (ed) Nursing: art and science. Chapman & Hall, London

Concceicao S, Ward M, Kerr D 1976 Defects in sphygmomanometers: an important source of blood pressure recording. British Medical Journal 1: 886–888

Cormack D F S (ed) 1984 Introduction to the research process in nursing. Blackwell Scientific Publications, Oxford

Cullum N 1994a Leg ulcer treatments: a critical review (Part 1). Nursing Standard 9(1): 29–33

Cullum N 1994b Leg ulcer treatments: a critical review (Part 2). Nursing Standard 9(2): 32–36

Department of Health and Social Security 1972 Report on the Committee on Nursing (Chair: Professor A Briggs). Cmnd 5115, HMSO, London

Distance Learning Centre 1988 Research awareness. Module 3: the experimental perspective. DLC Research Awareness Series, London

Edwards M 1994 The rationale for the use of risk calculators in pressure sore prevention, and the evidence of the reliability and validity of published scales. Journal of Advanced Nursing 20: 288–296

Haywood J 1975 Information: a prescription against pain. RCN, London

Hunt M 1982 Patients' capacity to cope with daily living activities: assessment scale. Proceedings of the Royal College of Nursing Annual Nursing Research Conference

Jolly A 1991 Taking a blood pressure. Nursing Times 87(15): 40–43

Medawar P B 1969 Induction and intuition in scientific thought. Methuen, London

Nightingale F 1859/1990 Notes on nursing. Churchill Livingstone, Edinburgh

Norton D, Mclaren R, Exton-Smith A N 1975 An investigation of geriatric nursing problems in hospital. Churchill Livingstone, Edinburgh

Royal College of Nursing 1982 Research mindedness and nurse education: a RCN research society report. RCN, London

Royal Marsden Hospital 1993 Manual of clinical nursing policies and procedures. Harper & Row, London

Smith B 1994 The dressing makes the difference: trial of two modern dressings on venous ulcers. Professional Nurse 9(5): 348–352

Stanton M, Paul C, Reeves J S 1990 An overview of the nursing process. In: George J B (ed) Nursing theories: the base for professional nursing practice, 3rd edn. Prentice Hall, London

Thomas B, Price M M 1980 Research preparations in baccalaureate nursing education. Nursing Research 29: 259–261

Tierney A, Closs J, Atkinson I, Anderson J, Murphy-Black T, Macmillan M 1988 On measurement and nursing research. Nursing Times 84(12): 55–58

Vines G 1995 Is there a database in the house? New Scientist (21 January): 14–15

Wall P, Melzack R 1994 Textbook of pain. Churchill Livingstone, Edinburgh

Walsh M, Ford P 1989 Nursing rituals. Butterworth Heinemann, Oxford

Waterlow J 1985 A risk assessment card. Nursing Times 27(49): 51–55

Webb C, Wilson-Barnett J 1983 Hysterectomy: dispelling the myths—1. Nursing Times Occasional Paper 79(3): 52–54

FURTHER READING

Abbott P, Sapsford R 1992 Research into practice. Open University Press, Buckingham

Cormack D F S (ed) 1993 The research process in nursing. Blackwell Scientific Publishing, Oxford

Sapsford R, Abbott P 1992 Research methods for nurses and the caring professions. Open University Press, Buckingham

Wilson-Barnett J 1991 The experiment: is it worthwhile? International Journal of Nursing Studies 28(1): 77–87

Data analysis

4

Teresa Smart

■ **KEY ISSUES**

- **Making sense of data**
- **Data analysis as part of critical thinking**
- **Statistical techniques and tools of data analysis**
- **The presentation of data**
- **Pitfalls to avoid**
- **Data analysis in practice**

PREAMBLE

When we were planning our research mindedness seminars the session on data analysis came close to the end of the course. John Gordon, who chose the topic, had been a researcher involved in clinical trials and so was very familiar with experimental design and statistics. Data analysis as a topic commonly occupies a late slot in research teaching. This is hardly surprising when you consider that data analysis is traditionally represented as coming at the end of the research process (see Ch. 1). Similarly in Chapter 3 Jane Say and Julie Cumpper took us through each stage of the experimental method, finally arriving at analysis of the data. Rather than take you through the details of data analysis they referred you to this chapter. We decided therefore that it made more sense to introduce you to the techniques and tools of data analysis early rather than later in the book. Furthermore, we want to emphasize that data analysis is not the end stage or 'afterthought' of research, as is so often implied by its late appearance in teaching programmes or in representations of the research process, but part of an integrated whole. Worsley (1991), a sociology professor, illustrates this point when he writes: 'The collection of data is always undertaken in the light of the theoretical and conceptual interests of the researcher, *with analysis in mind*' (our emphasis).

INTRODUCTION

In Chapter 2, Margaret Harper and Nina Hartman introduced us to some of the issues surrounding qualitative/quantitative research debates. Nursing and health care research is caught in the crossfire of that debate.

On the one hand there has been a reaction to medical dominance in early nursing research because of the belief that sensitive topics such as quality and care are not amenable to **quantitative methods**. This reaction led to an increase in the number of studies using **qualitative** research **approaches** like phenomenology and ethnomethodology, which we discuss later in this book. On the other, the mood within the current NHS research and development strategy emphasizes the need for evidence-based practice using **randomized controlled trials**. Statistical techniques are an integral component of those trials. We want to draw your attention therefore to the importance of familiarizing yourself with statistical techniques and tools, not only to allow you to critically use current research but also as a means of getting 'sideline' topics such as care and gender on to the agenda.

It is important for nurses to acknowledge their history and to see the role statistical techniques have played in the development of nursing practice. We present two examples in the boxes below. In Box 4.1, Nuttall (1983) describes the work of Florence Nightingale whom she refers to as 'The Passionate Statistician'. Box 4.2 summarizes nine studies published by the Royal College of Nursing between 1970 and 1980. These studies used quantitative methods and their key characteristics were summarized by Spencer (1983, p27).

■ **BOX 4.1**

Throughout her long life Florence Nightingale used figures. She collected them, she sifted them and above all she analysed them. She knew that without hard facts she could achieve nothing. Even with her statistical tables she had to note 'I lost' in the margin. Without her figures and tables she knew she had no chance (p. 27).

■ **BOX 4.2**

All nine books (in which the studies were published) seemed to be concerned with quantitative methods; the key words were measurement, hypothesis testing, statistics, tables and data. On tables Anderson (1973) had 34; Wright (1974) 35; Jones (1975) 44; Roberts (1975) 45; Birch (1975) 24; Ashworth (1980) nine plus eight figures; and Crow (1980) 17. Bendall had none, although she mentioned in her introduction that she had to sacrifice 'much of the raw data and almost all of the details of the statistical analysis'.

The first four publications were part of a larger project entitled 'The Proper Study of the Nurse'. Quantification, reflected in the objective 'to develop techniques for measuring the quality of nursing care' (McFarlane 1970, p 29), was an important, though not exclusive, aspect of that project.

In his article, Spencer concluded: 'It is difficult to advocate a research method other than quantification and science, particularly as nurses have to deal with doctors who are impressive supporters of medical science, and scientific evidence may be the only kind acceptable in the world in which they work' (p. 27).

Nurses and health workers are not the only ones to feel that they have no alternative but to employ traditional scientific methods in order to gain acceptance by the Establishment. For example, Elizabeth Fennema, one of the first, and the best-known, educational researchers studying gender issues associated with the teaching and learning of mathematics, used traditional scientific methods as a way of gaining acceptability for the research in the academic world. On reflecting over 20 years of research in this area, Fennema stated: 'These studies have had a major impact. ... partly because they employed fairly traditional methodology, their findings have been accepted by the community at large'. However, she went on to say: 'but I do not believe that we shall understand gender and mathematics until scholarly efforts conducted in a positivist framework are complemented with scholarly efforts that utilize other perspectives.' (Fennema 1995).

On the basis of Elizabeth Fennema's findings, subsequent researchers were able to put the study of gender on to the educational research agenda and employ alternative approaches to future studies drawing on feminism and critical theory (Walkerdine 1989).

We have given you these examples in order to show you the importance of understanding statistical principles as part of becoming research minded. Familiarity with these tools and techniques will increase your confidence in reading research reports and prepare you to critically evaluate evidence before incorporating it into practice.

APPROACHES TO DATA ANALYSIS

Before going any further we would like to consider what relevance the notion of data analysis has to the practitioner. Writing for social workers, Everitt and colleagues (1992) state: 'Practitioners are engaged in the process of data analysis all the time. They interpret and assign meaning to all kinds of data from a wide range of sources: what they read, what they see, what they hear, what they are told, what they themselves think and feel' (p. 101). Learning about the techniques and tools of data analysis will help us to be more aware of these processes in our daily lives and practice and promote research mindedness. Statistical evidence can also assist us to present arguments and analyse situations.

For example, Martin (1990) describes a survey initiated by a Scottish pressure group who were concerned about the development of maternity services in their area and wanted to avert the potential threat of hospital closure. University researchers were commissioned to undertake the survey. The subsequent findings were used to show the local Health Board that despite some shortcomings such as staff shortage and hospital food, women were generally very satisfied with their care. Using the numerical evidence, the case was made for putting more resources into the hospitals rather than closing them. Martin writes: 'In order for the findings to be respected by the policy makers it was felt by all parties that our independence (the researchers) and "scientific objectivity" were both necessary and important' (p. 165). Although the findings of the survey did not reverse the decision to close one of the hospitals, issues such as staff shortages and their effects on quality of care were raised with the Health Board for further consideration.

As you will have gathered by now, we consider quantitative data analysis in this chapter; but data can also be analysed qualitatively. The different approaches to data analysis and presentation are described by Everitt et al (1992) as a process:

> *to do with detecting patterns in the data. In the course of analysing quantitative data, these patterns will emerge as tables, percentages, bar diagrams, pie charts and tests of significance. The exercise will be different in drawing out patterns in qualitative data. Patterns emerge through the researcher or practitioner becoming familiar with the data and yet, at the same time, being in the position of a stranger. 'Making the familiar strange' (Jeffs and Smith 1990) is crucial to the process of data analysis. It ensures that what might seem obvious questions are put to data whose meaning can so easily be taken for granted (p. 105).*

Figure 4.1 gives an overview of data analysis.

Large amounts of raw data collected by researchers are cumbersome, giving very little information to either themselves or their potential audience. They need to find ways, therefore, of organizing and presenting them in a meaningful way.

Quantitative researchers employ two types of statistical activity depending on their final aim for the study. **Descriptive statistics** are used to organize, describe, summarize and display data, so that you and other interested people can gain a sense of their main features. **Inferential statistics** are used to take data drawn from a sample of the population to infer or predict information for the population as a whole.

Qualitative researchers use accounts and narratives to seek understanding and explanation. In Chapter 5 you will look in more detail at how phenomenologists, for example, analyse and interpret data and the procedures they use to do this.

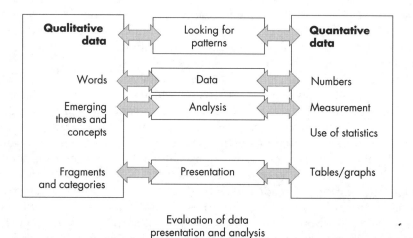

Evaluation of data
presentation and analysis

Figure 4.1 Overview of data analysis.

We shall now proceed to look in detail at the steps involved in quantitative data analysis. In doing this, I shall use some of the data and the findings from a set of research papers, two of which are discussed in other parts of this book and reproduced in Appendices 1 and 2. These are: the venous ulcers trial of Smith (1994) (discussed in Ch. 3); and the study by Macleod Clark et al (1990) of helping people to stop smoking (discussed in Ch. 9). Other studies will be referenced at the end of the chapter.

Steps in quantitative data analysis

Like Smith & Bland (unpublished work, 1976) in the study described in Box 4.3, you may have collected a large amount of raw data. As such they are cumbersome, giving very little information to either you or your potential audience. To analyse data quantitatively, we employ two types of statistical activity depending on our final aim.

The first step of the activity is to organize, describe, summarize and display data as described above using descriptive statistics so that you and other interested people can gain a sense of their main features.

Techniques used to summarize and display quantitative data include the many different ways identified by Everitt and colleagues (1992) such as: diagrams, pie charts, bar charts, histograms and box plots. The second step is to describe the data in compact form by means of some simple statistical calculations such as the average: **mean**, **median** and **mode**. We shall also consider **variance** including standard deviation.

■ **BOX 4.3**

Pam Smith, when working as a community nurse teacher in Tanzania, organized a survey of the nutritional status of children aged 0 to 5 years old. No children who had passed their fifth birthday were included in the study. The data were collected by two groups of student nurses in their fourth and final year of training at the Muhimbili School of Nursing in Dar es Salaam, Tanzania. The data were collected by the students during community health field practice.

The data collected for each child were: height, weight, sex, age, arm circumference, chest/head ratio. Descriptive statistics could be used to make sense of these data—first to display them in tables, histograms, pie charts, box plots, then to describe them in compact form by calculation of the mean and standard deviation of a set of data, e.g. the mean arm circumference of a 3- to 4-year-old girl is 15.8 cm with a standard deviation of 1.3.

The data as collected do not allow the researcher to use inferential statistics, i.e. to make predictions about the wider population of children in Tanzania or to test any theories.

However, the descriptive statistics presented the nurses with a sense that the rate of growth of the children declined as the children grew older. A hypothesis could be made that there was a link between the growth of the children and the period of time they were nourished by their mother's milk.

In order to answer this question the nurses would need to collect the data and apply inferential statistics in terms of statistical tests in order to infer information and make predictions from the correlated data.

The second step of the activity is to apply **inferential statistics**. Inferential statistics are used to take data drawn from a sample of the population to infer or predict information for the population as a whole. To do this, correlations are calculated between variables, and tests applied to measure their statistical significance.

Before I introduce you to the different techniques in descriptive and inferential statistics, however, you need to consider what type of measurements you have used to collect your data.

SCALES OR LEVELS OF MEASUREMENT

The prelude to data analysis actually concerns how we collect and categorize our data at the outset. In order to apply statistical manipulations to our data we need to be confident that they are sound in the first place. In Chapter 3 we saw that a number of different measures could be used to collect data, such as the pain analogue scale. Different tools have different scales of measurement which must be clarified as a prelude to statistical analysis.

Whilst reading this book and in your future research and practice, you will be looking at and collecting many different types of data as the following list demonstrates:

- severity of pain
- level of care
- the number of admissions to a ward
- the primary diagnosis for each admission
- different types of dressing
- milligrams of a drug
- parts per million
- area of ulcer
- ease of removal of dressing
- age, weight, height of child
- number of cigarettes smoked a day
- commitment to giving up smoking.

These types of data are collected using many different scales of measurement such as: milligrams, days, categories of illness, numerical points on a scale. The number of different types of data is immensely large but four categories or **levels of measurement** can be defined such that all types of data belong to one of them. The four categories or levels of measurement are defined as: **nominal/categorical**; **ordinal**; **interval** and **ratio** levels. They are also known as scales of measurement.

Before you analyse your data you need to work out to which scale, level or category of measurement your data belong. This is important because the amount of information you can infer from your data depends on the level of measure used, which in turn determines the type of statistical test you can apply.

Nominal or categorical level of measurement

Using this level of measurement means that you acquire the least information (from a statistical point of view) from your data. Using the nominal level of measure allows you to allocate your measure into a named category only. The data are in no particular order and you cannot make any implications about size or comparison of value of your data.

In the study *Helping people to stop smoking* (Macleod Clark et al 1990), the data collected included several examples of nominal data. Demographic data were collected from the patients according to which health authorities they came from and which social class they belonged to. The data collected were allocated to the following mutually exclusive categories:

- health authority A, B or C
- social class 2, 3, 4 (as defined by the Registrar General's Classification of Occupations).

The study will have included a question about the sex of the respondent. The investigator would then allocate the data collected into two mutually exclusive categories: male or female.

Health authority, social class and sex, are all examples of nominal measures. So also are the data obtained as a result of the question asked about the respondents' major concern about the effects of smoking. As you see below the different categories of concern are each allocated a number:

1 Effects on health of baby
2 Breathlessness
3 Lung cancer
4 Heart disease
5 Effects on health of family.

Similarly with the other examples of nominal data you can attribute numbers to the different levels or categories of data. In the following example, the investigator can ascribe an arbitrary number (or code) to the category male or female: 1 Male, 2 Female; or 7 Male, 956 Female. These numbers are markers only and represent discrete categories. They have nothing to do with ordering or imputing a value for your data. They cannot be used to make statistical statements such as: 'the mean sex of the children in the classroom is 1.7'; or 'the value of the female is twice the value of the male'.

Ordinal level of measurement

In the case of ordinal measurement, as with nominal measurement, your data can be put into discrete categories. For example, the level of pain experienced by postoperative patients can be measured according to the following categories:

- excruciating
- very severe
- severe
- moderate
- mild pain
- no pain.

These categories can then be meaningfully ordered and ranked from 'no pain' to 'excruciating pain'. Although you can say that excruciating pain is more severe than very severe pain, you cannot compare two levels of pain by saying that very severe pain is twice as great as moderate pain or even that the difference between no pain and mild pain is equivalent to that between severe pain and very severe pain.

For the study on helping people to stop smoking, referred to above, data were collected on the participants' previous smoking history. Here the data could fall into the categories of:

1	2	3	4	5
Do not smoke	Light smoker	Moderate smoker	Fairly heavy smoker	Very heavy smoker

After the educational intervention to help them stop smoking, their smoking behaviour could be measured in the following way:

1	2	3	4
Stopped smoking	Cut down substantially	Made at least one attempt to give up	No change in behaviour

In the case of ordinal data, the data can be ordered and ranked *but* we cannot say that the intervals between points of measurement have the same value. In other words, we cannot say that the interval between stopping smoking and cutting down substantially has the same value as the interval between cutting down substantially and making at least one attempt to give up.

The interval and ratio levels of measurement

The interval level of measurement allows the researcher to measure data along a scale on which the intervals between points of measurement are assumed to be exactly the same. The measurement of temperature provides us with an example of interval measurement in that we can say that the temperature differences between consecutive gradations on the thermometer are the same.

The temperature is measured in degrees Celsius or Fahrenheit. These degrees represent equal intervals, so the temperature difference between 20°F and 40°F is the same as between −20°F and 0°F. However, we cannot say that a temperature of 40°F is twice as warm as a temperature of 20°F, as a temperature reading of 0 does not mean an absence of temperature. 0 degrees F or C is arbitrarily chosen.

Taking another example, the pay structure of some school teachers is a basic salary scale plus up to five incentive allowances as follows:

Number of incentive points

0	1	2	3	4	5
Main grade	With some responsibility	2nd in charge	Year head	Head of department	Senior teacher

This tells us that the salary goes up in equal intervals; the increase is the same when a teacher moves from main grade to become a teacher with some responsibility as when he or she moves from head of department to senior teacher. In other words, it tells us that the value between 2 and 3 is

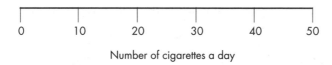

Figure 4.2 Interval scale of measurement of smoking level.

the same as the value between 3 and 4 or 5 and 6. However, it does not tell us that the senior teacher earns five times what the teacher with responsibility earns. Rather it tells us that the difference between each of the salary scales is the same. The zero is not absolute. The main grade teacher still earns a salary (even if low).

Where the zero has an absolute value, the interval level of measurement is defined as the ratio level of measurement.

For example, in the 'Helping people to stop smoking' study, expired carbon monoxide measurements were taken. The measurements of the participants' respiratory expirations were taken and recorded in the form of parts per million, i.e. 'all were smokers with readings ranging from 12 to 56 parts per million'. These measurements of parts per million represent measurements on the ratio scale of measure and we can say that a measurement of 40 is twice as high as a measurement of 20.

The difference between interval and ratio levels of measurement therefore is the presence of the value of zero. However, you do not need to be concerned about the difference. For the purpose of statistical work the interval and ratio levels of measurement can be put together in one category and treated the same.

To summarize, the 'Helping people to stop smoking' study provides examples of the different levels of measurement as follows:

- Patients can be defined as smokers or non-smokers which are examples of nominal data.
- The level of patients' smoking can be measured on the ordinal scale of measure:

1	2	3	4	5
Do not smoke	Light smoker	Moderate smoker	Fairly heavy smoker	Very heavy smoker

- The level of a patient's smoking can also be measured in the interval/ratio category on a scale such as that shown in Figure 4.2.

DESCRIPTIVE STATISTICS

A major reason for calculating statistics is to describe and summarize a set of data. A collection of numbers—the raw data—is not very informative so we need to find ways of picking out and presenting the key information in a clear, concise and comprehensible format. In this section you will be introduced to a variety of methods used to present data and to summarize data. It is difficult to cover everything in one chapter but I hope to familiarize you with statistical terms and techniques in order to give you the courage to pick up a statistics book when you need to know more.

Data presentation

Example: The work level of a general medical ward

The ward keeps a daily record of admissions, keeping note of the primary diagnosis of every patient admitted. The raw data in the ward report has the following format:

Ward: ....
Patient name: ....
Date of admission: ....
Primary diagnosis: Heart disease.

Over a 6-month period the ward has gathered a large amount of data which are not easily accessible. The nurse manager cannot easily extract information about the proportion of the different entry diagnoses, the needs for specialized nursing, the busiest times, etc.

The data can be extracted from the ward records and put into a table as shown in Table 4.1.

Here the data are more accessible and provide information on entry diagnosis and the frequency at different times of the year. For example, the table shows that the greatest number of admissions to the ward is for heart disease and that the number of admissions for bronchitis decreased from January to June. The reader is still distracted by too many numbers, however. To prevent this happening, the data in the table can be presented in the form of a bar chart (Fig. 4.3). In a bar chart the heights of the bars represent the frequency of occurrence of the data. In the case of Table 4.1, the frequency of occurrence is the number of admissions.

The chart helps the reader to gain key information for each diagnosis showing how the admissions vary over the 6 months, although how diagnoses compare with each other is not directly accessible.

Figure 4.4 presents the total number of admissions for each diagnosis. In it, we lose the information on the variation over the 6 months but gain a clear comparison between the different diagnoses.

Table 4.1 Number of admissions to a general medical ward by primary diagnosis for first 6 months of year

Primary diagnosis	Jan.	Feb.	March	April	May	June	Total
Heart disease	14	13	12	11	17	12	67
Stroke	7	10	5	7	6	4	35
Pneumonia	4	3	6	2	5	2	20
Bronchitis	12	9	10	5	2	1	38
Diabetes mellitus	7	5	6	2	2	3	22
Renal disease	1	0	2	3	3	2	9
GI haemorrhage	1	1	0	2	4	4	8
Attempted suicide	3	1	3	2	2	2	11
Others not listed	8	3	7	4	6	8	28
Total	57	45	51	38	47	38	276

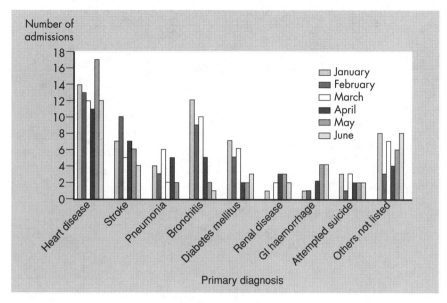

Figure 4.3 Bar chart of number of admissions by primary diagnosis.

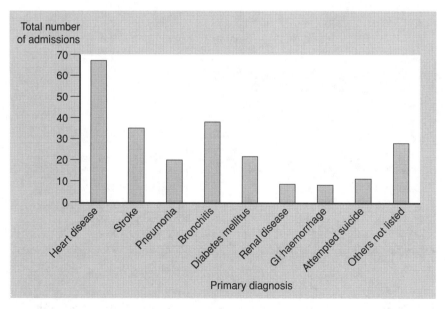

Figure 4.4 Bar chart of total admissions by primary diagnosis.

We use a **bar chart** to give a visual presentation of data when the scale of measurement is nominal, as in this case. When the scale of measurement is interval or ratio, then the data are presented by means of a **histogram**.

In Table 4.2, the data are from a ratio scale of measurement. The data are discrete (i.e. they can only represent discrete or separate values, such as 14, 16 or 24 beds—the quantity 15.4 beds does not exist). The histogram in

Table 4.2 Number of beds in the 20 wards of a district health authority

Ward	Number of beds (raw data)
A	20
B	17
C	28
D	21
E	14
F	24
G	21
H	25
I	15
J	20
K	20
L	25
M	23
N	19
O	21
P	22
Q	19
R	26
S	18
T	22
Total	420

A

Number of beds	Frequency
14–17	2
17–20	4
20–23	8
23–26	4
26–29	2

B

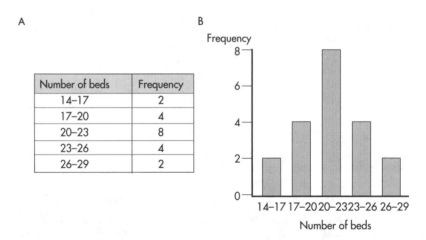

Figure 4.5 Numbers of beds in 20 wards: (**A**) frequency table; (**B**) frequency distribution (histogram).

Figure 4.5, however, shows the data as apparently continuous; the interval 14–16 contains data for the number of beds from 14 to 16 inclusive.

The definition of a histogram is that the area of the bar (rather than its height) represents the value of the frequency, although it is quite natural when drawing histograms to make the height of each bar in proportion to the value of the frequency. However, when representing frequency distributions where there is one or more unequal class interval, the method of relating the height of the bar to the frequency gives a false picture of the distribution. For example, in Table 4.3, which gives the frequency distribution of the number of girls of different ages in Bungu Village (data

Table 4.3 Number of girls by age group (based on data from a study by Smith & Bland 1976)

Age	Number of girls	To draw a histogram		
		Width of bar in months	Height of bar	Area of bar
1–2 months	8	2	4.00	8
3–6 months	16	3	5.33	16
7–11 months	10	4	2.50	10
1 year	30	12	2.50	30
2 years	6	12	0.50	6
3–4 years	18	24	0.75	18

taken from Tanzanian study summarized in Box 4.3), the frequency distribution of girls is over different units of time (i.e. months and years). The data would be misrepresented by a diagram representing the frequency of occurrence by the height of each bar since the width of the bars is not consistent.

You need therefore to present the data in two separate diagrams. In the first (Fig. 4.6A) you can plot the number of girls against age; in the second (Fig. 4.6B) you can plot the height of the bar against the width of the bar.

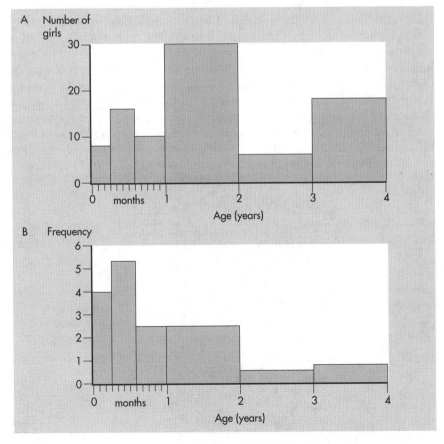

Figure 4.6 Age distribution of girls in Bungu Village: (**A**) the height of the bar represents the number in each age group; (**B**) the area of the bar represents the number in each age group.

The first diagram looks like a histogram but because the age is given over different time intervals, it does not meet the requirements. The second diagram, however, does meet the requirements to be a histogram.

Another way of giving a pictorial presentation of data is by means of a **pie chart**.

Table 4.4 gives the distribution of the nursing staff at a hospital by grade.

The pie chart (Fig. 4.7) gives an excellent visual image of how the grades are distributed.

In a pie chart the 'pie' is divided into slices. The size of each slice represents the frequency distribution. The two bits of information you need to know when drawing your pie chart are:

- the size of a slice is proportional to the middle angle of the slice
- the total angle for the complete pie is 360°.

Table 4.4 shows that there are 90 enrolled (Level 2) nurses out of a total 450 nursing staff working in Hospital O.

The 90 enrolled nurses need a slice that is 90/450 of the whole pie. The 450 nursing staff take up the angle of 360°, i.e. they represent the whole of the pie. The 90 enrolled nurses are represented by a slice with a middle angle of $360° \times 90/450$.

You have now seen how to present your data by means of pie charts, bar charts and histograms. The next question therefore is how can you summarize your data even further by one *single result*? The best way to summarize the data is by its *central* or *average* mark. In statistical terms you try to find a **measure of central tendency**. So what is the central position of a frequency distribution such as in our examples of number of hospital admissions by month or disease represented in Table 4.1 (p. 86)? How do you calculate the measure of central tendency? But also, as you will see later, it is not sufficient to summarize your data by only one central measure. You also need to summarize the **variability** of the data, i.e. the way in which the data spread out from the central measure, known as the **measure of variance**.

Table 4.4 Nursing staff from hospital O by grade	
Grade	**Number of nurses**
Registered nurses	150
Enrolled nurses	90
Students	135
Health care assistants	75
Total	450

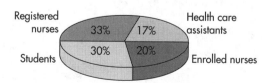

Figure 4.7 Pie chart of nursing staff by grade.

Measures of central tendency

Psychiatric nurses were given a questionnaire to gain data on their level of job satisfaction (see Table 4.5). The maximum score was 20 (high satisfaction) and the minimum was 0 (low satisfaction).

There are three ways in which we can calculate an average or central mark. These are:

The mean. The mean is the most familiar and useful measure used to describe the central tendency or average of a distribution of scores for any set of data. The mean is computed by dividing the sum of the scores by the total number of scores.

$$\text{Mean} = \frac{\text{Sum of all scores}}{\text{Total number of scores}} = \frac{\Sigma X}{N}$$

where X is each score and N is the total number of scores. The symbol Σ (the Greek letter sigma) means the sum of.

The mean job satisfaction score for the nurses represented in Table 4.5 is 10.24.

Table 4.5 Survey of job satisfaction felt by 25 psychiatric nurses

Raw scores		Scores in order	
Nurse	Satisfaction score	Nurse	Satisfaction score
A	10	N	7
B	8	R	7
C	14	I	8
D	9	B	9
E	7	F	9
F	12	H	9
G	10	K	9
H	12	M	9
I	11	T	10
J	10	A	10
K	10	C	10
L	11	D	10
M	11	E	10
N	9	O	10
O	10	S	11
P	11	G	11
Q	9	J	11
R	13	L	11
S	9	V	11
T	11	W	11
U	9	Y	11
V	9	Q	12
W	11	U	12
X	7	P	14
Y	10	X	14

Total number of nurses = 25
Sum of all scores = 256
Mean score = 10.24

The median. Another useful measure of central tendency is the median or middle score. To find the median you need to (1) put the data in order and (2) find the middle score, or rather the score that has exactly the same number of scores above it as below.

The median job satisfaction score for the nurses in Table 4.5 is 10 (the score of the 13th nurse in order).

If there is an even number of scores, i.e. there is no middle point, then you calculate the median by taking the two middle scores and finding the score halfway between them.

For example, for the following data:

5   7   7   8   8   11   11   11   13   16

There are 10 scores. The median lies halfway between the 5th and 6th score, which is 9.5.

The mode. The mode is the score that occurs most frequently in a set of data. For the data presented above this is 11.

Choosing a measure of central tendency

It is sometimes a problem for researchers to decide on whether they should choose a mean, median or mode as the most appropriate measure of central tendency for their data. I give a few examples below:

Mean. This is the most common measure of central tendency and is used when:

- the data are more or less symmetrically grouped around the central point
- this measure is needed to estimate a corresponding mean for a larger population of which you have taken a sample.

Example. The Accident and Emergency nurse manager orders sterilized dressings from the store every day. She needs to order enough but not too many dressings as there is insufficient cool storage space and the dressing has a limited shelf-life. She decides therefore to keep records of the amount of dressings she uses each day over a period of 20 days. She finds she uses a mean of 14.8 packets a day and the data are symmetrically grouped around this mean. For future ordering the mean serves as a good measure of the data.

However, if during one of these weeks there was a fire in a local factory during which a number of workers sustained lacerations and burns, there would be a huge demand for sterilized dressings. On that day alone 100 packets could be used which, if included in calculating a mean of 20 packets, would lead to a distorted measure of central tendency. In this case the median serves as a better measure, although the nurse manager will need to know she has a back-up store for such an emergency.

Median. This is not as common as the mean as a measure of central tendency but is used when:

- an extreme score distorts the data as in the case above
- there is a need to know the exact middle of the distribution.

Example. A college of higher education is only able to take half the applicants for a popular course in sociology. An entrance test is set for all the candidates and the median mark calculated. This then becomes the pass mark ensuring that half the candidates can enter the course.

Mode. This is a quick method of calculating the measure of central tendency when appropriate.

Example. A hospital pharmacy can buy a certain medication in packets of 8, 12, 24, 48 and 96 tablets. If the pharmacist has collected data on the number of different packets sold, then the best average to help her decide on an ordering policy will be the mode. She is not interested in the mean number of tablets sold per customer because this is unlikely to represent one of her stock sizes; neither is it useful to know the size of the packet that sells with median frequency. The mode, however, will tell her which packet size is sold most frequently.

You should now have an idea of how you can best represent your data by a single measure. However, often this is not enough as the example below will show.

Measures of variance

In a small research project to evaluate different methods of trying to alleviate insomnia, 18 people are divided into three groups of six and given one of three different forms of treatment:

- hypnosis tape
- sleeping pills
- drops of lavender oil on the pillow.

The treatments are randomly assigned as treatment A, B or C.
The results as a result of treatment are given in Table 4.6.
For all the treatments it is found that the mean average number of hours of sleep per night as a result of the treatment is 6. Can you say that this means that the three different forms of treatment have the same effect (i.e. each treatment gives an average of 6 hours sleep per night)? In order to answer that question you need to calculate a measure of variability or **spread**. If you look at treatment A, everybody sleeps for 6 hours a night, whereas treatment B works very well for some patients but not for others. Treatment C has a much more mixed effect. All the treatments have the same mean but very different effects.
In order to examine the data above in more detail look at Table 4.7.

Table 4.6 Results of three different treatments to relieve insomnia

Treatment	Average number of hours of sleep per night per patient						Mean average
A	6	6	6	6	6	6	6
B	3	3	3	9	9	9	6
C	4	5	6	6	7	8	6

Table 4.7 Data on three different treatments to treat insomnia: calculation of variance and standard deviation

Treatment A		Treatment B				Treatment C			
1	2	3	4	5	6	7	8	9	10
Hours of sleep X	Range, deviation, etc.	Hours of sleep X	Deviation X − μ	Absolute deviation |X − μ|	Square deviation (X − μ)²	Hours of sleep X	Deviation X − μ	Absolute deviation |X − μ|	Square deviation (X − μ)²
6	0	3	−3	3	9	4	−2	2	4.00
6	0	3	−3	3	9	5	−1	1	1.00
6	0	3	−3	3	9	6	0	0	0.00
6	0	9	3	3	9	6	0	0	0.00
6	0	9	3	3	9	7	1	1	1.00
6		9	3	3	9	8	2	2	4.00

Mean = 6 (Treatment A)

Standard deviation = 0 (Treatment A)

Mean = 6 (Treatment B) — Mean abs. dev. = 3 — Variance = 9

Standard deviation = 3 (Treatment B)

Mean = 6 (Treatment C) — Mean abs. dev. = 1 — Variance = 1.67

Standard deviation = 1.29 (Treatment C)

The simplest measure of spread is the **range**. The range is the difference between the highest and lowest scores. The range is not a very sophisticated measure, so the next stage is to calculate the **variation**. To calculate the variation you take the mean 6 (or μ) as the central score and calculate how much your scores vary or deviate from the central score $(X - \mu)$ and then add up all the values of $X - \mu$ (see columns 4 and 8 in Table 4.7). However, as you see, values of $X - \mu$ above and below the mean will cancel each other out. So a new measure called **absolute variation** is needed to overcome the problem. In the calculation of absolute variation we avoid the problem of negative and positive deviations cancelling each other out by the process of ignoring the minus sign and treating all deviations as positive. In mathematical terms we calculate $|X - \mu|$ (see Table 4.7, columns 5 and 9). Now all you have to do is calculate the mean of all these absolute deviations (add up all the absolute deviations and divide by the total number of patients).

Mean absolute deviation is the mean of all the absolute deviations.

$$\text{Mean absolute deviation} = \frac{\text{sum } |X - \mu|}{N} = \frac{\Sigma |X - \mu|}{N}$$

Variance

You had to calculate the absolute value of $X - \mu$ to overcome the problem of minus or plus deviations. Mathematicians have a way of overcoming this problem by squaring the deviations. (Remember: -4 squared is 16, which is positive, as is the square of every other negative number.)

So a new formula is suggested:

$$\text{Variance} = \frac{\text{sum } (X - \mu)^2}{N} = \frac{\Sigma (X - \mu)^2}{N}$$

To calculate the **variance**, you calculate the deviation of each value from the mean, then find the mean of the sum of the squares of the deviations.

Finally, because you need your variance to be in the same units as the original data—hours of sleep instead of hours of sleep squared—you need to find the square root. This final measure is called **standard deviation** (SD). I give the formula below and have shown how it is developed; it is worthwhile trying out some examples to check that you understand the method. However, in most cases you will use a button on your calculator or a command on a computer to calculate the mean and the standard deviation of any set of data.

Standard deviation, σ

$$\sigma = \frac{\Sigma (X - \mu)^2}{N}$$

In summary, treatment A gives a mean sleep of 6 hours and a standard deviation of 0, whereas treatment B gives the same mean sleep of 6 hours with a standard deviation of 3 (this means there is a large variation among patients in the amount of sleep each patient enjoys). Treatment C gives a mean sleep of 6 hours and a standard deviation of 1.3; therefore there is less variation in the number of hours slept by patients than with treatment B but more than with treatment A.

Normal distribution

Trendy teaching of reading methods fail—over 40% of the 7-year-olds have reading scores less than average.

This is a typical headline showing an ignorance of basic statistical understanding. If you drew a frequency graph of the reading scores of all 7-year-olds you would expect it to look like Figure 4.8.

The distribution of reading scores follows a so-called 'normal distribution', that is a distribution with a bell-shaped form and the following properties:

- symmetrical
- bell-shaped
- its mean, median and mode fall in the same place on the curve
- the two tails never actually touch the horizontal axis.

In a normal distribution, then, you should expect 50% of the scores to lie below the mean and 50% above it; so you would certainly expect 40% of the 7-year-olds to have reading scores less than average. Also, it is expected that a further 34.13% of the scores will lie within 1 standard deviation above the mean and 34.13% within 1 standard deviation below the mean. A remaining 15.87% of the population gain very high scores and a similar percentage gain low scores.

It is important to note that many of the things we study and measure in our research can be assumed to come from populations that are normally distributed. When you apply many of the statistical tests that are discussed in this chapter you will assume that the population you are **sampling** from has this typical normal distribution. What is more interesting is that even if the population does not have a normal distribution, if you take a large enough number of samples of the same size (e.g. 100 samples of 10 people) and calculate the mean score of each sample, then these sample means will form a normal distribution.

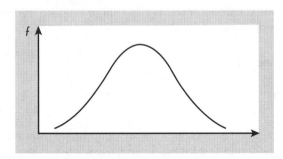

Figure 4.8 A normal distribution.

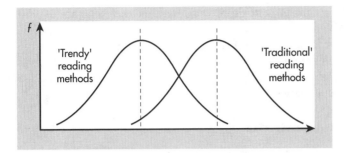

Figure 4.9 Normal distributions of data with different means.

The normality of most population distributions allow us to test whether a treatment has the effect of producing a new population with a higher mean or whether these new 'high' results are high by chance because each normal distribution has a proportion of high results.

For example, the next headline could be:

Traditional methods are best. Pupils from a school employing 'traditional' methods of reading were tested and found to have reading scores above average.

In statistical terms this headline is saying that the pupils from the 'traditional' school belong to a new improved normal distribution (see Fig. 4.9) with a higher mean. There is, however, a chance that these pupils belong to the same population distribution as those attending the school with 'trendy teaching methods', but lie in the top of the right tail; approximately 5% of the 'trendy' population have scores at least 2 SD above the mean so you are only 95% confident that the improved grade is due to the application of 'traditional' methods. When giving the results of a statistical test you must also state your level of confidence that the improved scores are due to the treatment and not due to the chance that they lie in this high area of the untreated population. This will be dealt with in the next section.

HYPOTHESIS TESTING AND THE
APPLICATION OF STATISTICAL TESTS

In Chapter 3 we considered hypothesis testing. Here we shall look at the application of basic statistical tests involving rules and formulae. You can think of these tests as a 'black box', i.e. we have no idea what is in the box. We put data into the 'box' in order to ensure that a 'result' comes out. Sometimes we have to use formulae based on mathematical principles as if they were a 'black box' without worrying too much about why the formula is structured in a particular way. What is more important is to take the output from the formula (your 'black box') and develop confidence to explain what it (the output or result) means. For example, you may be studying family size in North Wales and obtain a mean for the number of children under 5 years old in these families. You may be led to say on the basis of this mean that there is something different about family size in North Wales compared with other regions in Britain. A formula or test will tell you whether this difference is 'significant' or not. You will not stop there, however, since you will want to interpret your finding and ask further questions of the data. In order to do this you will need to draw on inferential statistics.

Inferential statistics

The need for inferential statistics

When you have collected, displayed and described your data you may feel that it provides you with what looks like strong evidence for the performance of a treatment.

For example, in Chapter 3 you were referred to the trial of two different types of dressing on venous ulcers. In this study the changes found as a result of the application of two different types of dressing are presented as a table (see Appendix 1, Table 3, p. 311). The table shows that the dressing Granuflex appears to be superior to the dressing Alginate in all areas except cost, which is higher. So decisions about whether to pay more for a more effective treatment have to be made. However, when statistical tests appropriate to the type of data were applied, it was found that although disturbance of sleep as a result of ulcer pain improved more for Granuflex, this difference between the treatment groups was not statistically significant, although it approached significance. The only aspect of the treatment where the difference was statistically significant was the ease of removal of the dressing. What does the statistical significance mean and how do you find out if your data show significance or not? You may collect data that seem to show that an improvement results from a particular treatment but in fact the application of a statistical test shows that the difference is not significant. You will find that this is often the case in your research.

First, I am going to refer you to some data collected as part of a small research project in clinical practice (Reid & Boore 1987).

Using the pain scale:

Excruciating	5
Very severe	4
Severe	3
Moderate	2
Just noticeable	1
No pain	0

10 patients who had just undergone major abdominal surgery were monitored eight times over a 2-day period for the severity of their pain. For each patient the total pain score for the eight periods was found.

During the next 3–4 weeks, the health workers in the ward—nurses and doctors—took part in the study and their subsequent discussion led to a raised awareness of the issue of pain management. The study was then repeated with 10 new patients matched for similar age and operation. The data collected are given in Table 4.8.

Table 4.8 Patients' pain scores before and after increasing staff awareness of pain management

Before reading and discussion		After reading and discussion	
Patient	Total pain score	Patient	Total pain score
A	19	Q	10
B	18	R	8
C	20	S	11
D	10	T	7
E	17	U	15
F	12	V	8
G	22	W	9
H	14	X	12
I	14	Y	10
J	15	Z	9
Total	**161**	**Total**	**99**

The 'Before' data give a mean pain score of 16.1 per patient over the 2-day period of eight readings yielding an average of 2.01—this is *moderate* level of pain.

The 'After' data show a mean of 9.9 per patient and hence an average pain score of 1.24 per occasion which is just more than *just noticeable* pain. The research report notes that all involved in the project were pleased at what they saw was a marked reduction in the pain as a result of their raised awareness of the issues. There was no statistical test applied. Hence, the research is not transferable and there is no defined level of confidence that the reduction in pain was a result of the action and not the result of random fluctuation. In other words, it is quite likely that the changes in the patients' pain scores were due to the reading and discussions taking place amongst the staff resulting in better pain management. Statistically, however, we are not able to define how confident we are that the results did not occur by chance. Irrespective of the staff's increased awareness there is no guarantee that the changes in the patients' pain scores might not have occurred anyway. In order to be sure that the changes were statistically significant and had not occurred by chance you would need to apply statistical tests to your data.

Applying statistical tests to your data

Experimental design

In this section you will look at the application of statistical techniques to data collected from experiments. In a later section you will be introduced to testing data using a correlation design.

What are statistical tests and how do they work?

First, a cheerful note. Now computers and statistical software will do most of the work in applying the tests. Added to this there are professional statisticians who are available to advise you on which test and why. What you need to do is gain confidence in:

- choosing an appropriate test
- learning to interpret the results.

The basis of a statistical test is posing a question that you want to be answered. Examples of such questions are:

- Does an awareness of pain management techniques by nursing staff lead to a reduction in pain experienced by postoperative patients?
- Does the application of dressing B to a venous ulcer lead to a reduction in the pain suffered compared with dressing A?
- Is there a link between the access elderly diabetic patients have to a nutritionist and the stability of their sugar levels?

These questions can each be posed as a **hypothesis** that we will try to show the truth of by means of a statistical test.

- *Hypothesis 1:* Awareness of pain management by nursing staff leads to a reduced level of pain experienced by postoperative patients.
- *Hypothesis 2:* The application of dressing B to a venous ulcer leads to a reduction in the pain suffered compared with dressing A.
- *Hypothesis 3:* The more contact an elderly diabetic has with the nutritionist the greater the stability of his or her sugar levels.

To investigate these hypotheses a statistical test is applied. This test tells us if there is an improvement as a result of the treatment. However, even if there is an improvement we are still left with the question of whether the improvement is due to the treatment (greater pain awareness, different dressing, more time) or is just the result of chance and the fact that in any normal distribution there is a small proportion with scores at least 2 standard deviations above the mean.

To deal with this problem, you need from the start to state how **confident** you wish to be that the change is due to the treatment and not due to chance.

Levels of confidence

You can apply a test that states that statistically you are 99% confident or 95% confident that the treatment worked. In other words, there is only a 1% or a 5% possibility that the results of the treatment are due to chance.

P is the symbol for the **level of confidence** or the probability that the results have not occurred by chance, i.e. the treatment did make a difference.

$P < 0.01$ means that the P (probability) that the difference occurred by chance rather than as a result of the treatment is < (less than) 1 in 100.

In Smith's trial of the two modern ulcer dressings, dressing B was found to be statistically significantly superior in terms of a decrease in ulcer area ($P < 0.01$). This means that dressing B led to a greater decrease in ulcer area than dressing A. A test showed that this was statistically significant at $P < 0.01$. That is, there is less than a 1 in 100 chance that the improvement was due to random chance and so we can be 99% confident that dressing B is superior in this aspect of treatment.

If the P value is < (less than) 0.05, this means that the level of confidence is 95%; $P < 0.1$ means that there is a 1 in 10 chance of the effect being random and hence we are only 90% confident the results did not occur by chance. Normally, the highest acceptable value of P is 0.05, which means we need to be 95% confident that our results have not occurred by chance.

Null hypothesis, H_0

Mathematicians believe, however, that it is far better to state the hypothesis in terms of 'there is *no chance*', 'there is *no relationship*', 'there is *no improvement*' and then to prove that this hypothesis, now called a **null hypothesis**, falls down. A null hypothesis is also known as a statistical hypothesis of no difference. You need to rewrite your hypothesis, called H_1, as a null hypothesis, known as H_0. The hypotheses stated above would be stated as null hypotheses in the following way:

- *Null hypothesis 1:* There is no relationship between the awareness nursing staff have of pain management and the level of pain experienced by postoperative patients.
- *Null hypothesis 2:* There is no difference between dressings A and B in terms of pain suffered.
- *Null hypothesis 3:* There is no relationship between the amount of nutritional information received by an elderly diabetic and the stability of his or her sugar levels.

Choosing a statistical test

You are now ready to apply a statistical test based on a hypothesis, a null hypothesis and a chosen level of confidence (say $P < 0.01$). What test would you use?

The types of statistical analysis used on data depend on the design of the experiment and the type of data. Figure 4.10 sets out which hypothesis test you can apply for which type of data and experimental design.

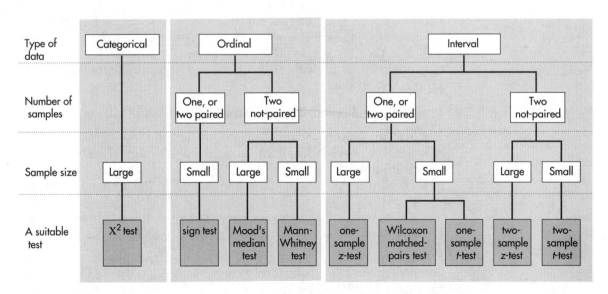

Figure 4.10 Which test to use? All the tests given for use with ordinal data can also be applied to interval data. The χ^2 test can also be applied to ordinal or interval data if suitable categories are defined. (Reproduced from Open University 1983.)

I will illustrate my point by means of some examples. Beforehand, however, I need to introduce you to the concept of **parametric** and **non-parametric** tests.

Many statistical tests are heavily dependent on the normal distribution curve. These tests assume therefore that samples are drawn from normally distributed populations which allow us to estimate the parameters of such populations. Data drawn from such populations are assumed to yield parametric data on which parametric tests can be applied.

But there are many cases where it would be wrong to assume a population has a normal distribution, such as the distribution of unemployment amongst a group of school leavers. It is possible to test differences amongst this population by using a non-parametric test. Such tests do not assume the normality of a distribution and are used for analysing nominal or ordinal data.

A parametric test is more sensitive than a non-parametric test and will show more easily whether your hypothesis stands. On the other hand, a non-parametric test is much more simple to apply. An example of this difference is as follows.

You wish to test a patient for anaemia. You can look at the colour of the inside of the lower eyelids or you can take blood to make a haemoglobin count. This latter way gives you a more accurate reading and is the equivalent of a parametric test. The first approach is quick and easy and will allow you to register some changes after a treatment. It is easier and less invasive to apply but is less accurate and is the equivalent of a non-parametric test. Which test you can use depends on the way in which the data were collected.

As previously stated, a parametric test is a more sensitive tool but there are fairly rigid assumptions as to when it can be applied. If these conditions are not met, then a non-parametric test must be used. Statisticians have developed a set of non-parametric tests equivalent to most of the well-used parametric tests. These tests are not the poor relation but can be very powerful for applying statistical tests to large samples of ordinal data for example.

Conditions under which a parametric test can be applied:

- The data must be measured on an interval/ratio scale of measurement.
- The data should come from a sample that is (roughly) normally distributed.
- The sample subjects should be randomly selected from the target population.
- If data from two samples are being compared, the way in which the results of both sets of data vary should be roughly similar.

For example, if you are comparing the birth weight of babies of smoking and non-smoking mothers, then if the range (i.e. the difference) between the smallest baby and heaviest baby is broadly similar for both groups of mothers, you can apply a parametric test. If the range of weights for babies of smoking mothers is 4 lb 3 oz compared with 6 lb 4 oz for non-smoking mothers, then you will need to apply a non-parametric test.

A non-parametric test should be applied when the data are ordinal or when the conditions listed above are not met.

You will find in some of the examples quoted in this chapter and in your reading of research that, at times, the assumptions on which the selection of a particular type of test is based seem to be violated. However, Christine Hicks (1990) says:

> *as long as the data are interval/ratio and there are* no major *violations of the other three criteria, a parametric test may be used. So when choosing between a parametric test and a non-parametric test concentrate primarily on the type of data you have. Second, while parametric tests require stringency as to the type of measurement used, non-parametric tests are less fussy. They can normally be used with* any *level of data. If you are not sure whether you can use a parametric test on your results, always choose the non-parametric equivalent since this is an error to caution (p. 79).*

The worked examples below will give you a view of how a decision is made about which test to apply. It is not within the scope of this chapter to go through each test. When you have collected data you may seek the help of a statistician to help you analyse the data. Having some understanding means that you will not feel disempowered by contact with the expert. Statisticians are there to help and they do that by going through a set of logical decision steps.

Example I

A drug company wished to test the efficiency of a new oral contraceptive by trying it out on volunteers. 2000 volunteers were allocated randomly to two groups: the experimental group of 1000 women took the new contraceptive whilst the control group of 1000 women took an existing contraceptive. At the end of the 1-year period, each woman taking part in the test was recorded as either having conceived or not. Suppose that only one of the 1000 women taking the new contraceptive had conceived by the end of the year, whereas 15 out of the 1000 women taking the existing contraceptive had conceived (Table 4.9). How would you go about testing and interpreting these results?

The scale of measures for 'Conceived' or 'Not conceived' is nominal or categorical.

Since the data are nominal, if you consult Figure 4.10, the only test possible is the χ^2 (chi-squared) test.

Table 4.9 Testing a new oral contraceptive: conception rates in experimental and control groups (data from Open University 1983, Unit C1, *Testing New Drugs*, pp. 24–25)

	Experimental group	Control group	Total
Conceived	1	15	16
Not conceived	999	985	984
Total	1000	1000	1000

The drug companies are interested in determining whether there is a relationship between the *type of contraceptive* and the *number of women who conceive*. Now the two variables are defined (*type of contraceptive* and *number of women who conceive*) and you can set up the hypotheses showing the link between them.

Hypothesis H_1: There is a relationship between the number of women who conceive and the type of contraceptive they use.

Null hypothesis H_0: The type of contraceptive used and the number of women who conceived is totally independent.

As a result of applying the chi-squared test, the researchers show that you can reject the null hypothesis H_0 in favour of H_1 at the 5% significance level ($P < 0.05$) and conclude that there does seem to be a relationship between the type of contraceptive used and the number of women who conceived in the 1-year period.

Example 2

Pain management awareness by nursing staff and level of pain felt by patients (Table 4.8, p. 99).

These ratings are ordinal. A rating of 19 is a higher pain rating than a rating of 10 but it is not possible to say what the difference in ratings is in terms of how much pain.

The data are not matched in pairs but rather matched as a group—the same number of patients of approximately the same ages and the same types of operations. The data set is small.

If you consult Figure 4.10, you will see that a suitable test for this type of data is the Mann–Whitney test because the data are ordinal, the two data sets are not paired and the sample is small. Here I am introducing you to the range of tests available for testing different sorts of data rather than showing you how to calculate them. This would be the job of a statistician or a computer programme.

Hypothesis H_1: The pain levels after the raised awareness of pain management are different from before.

Null hypothesis H_0: There is no difference between the pain levels before and after changing the awareness of pain management.

Correlation design

In the previous section you saw that when you design an experiment you start off with a hypothesis that states that there is a relationship between the two variables of the design. Then the hypothesis is tested by manipulating one variable and observing the effect on the other. In correlation design, as in experimental design, you start off with a hypothesis which predicts a relationship between two variables but then you do not manipulate either of the variables but make a series of measurements of the two variables in order to observe if there is a relationship between them. If there exists a relationship (called **correlation**) between the two variables then we can use the value of one variable to predict or *infer* the value of the other variable.

Consider the correlations between the following pairs of variables (Cases 1–6):

1. alcohol consumption and incidence of urinary tract infection
2. number of minutes the doctor spends with the patient and the level of anxiety felt by the patient
3. level of fears and worries about smoking and motivation to give up smoking (see Macleod Clark et al 1990, Appendix 2)
4. age of the man and his sperm count
5. the IQ of the child and the number of months the child was breast-fed
6. quality of nursing care in a ward and level of support gained by student nurses from the ward sister.

How do you measure association, pattern or correlation between two sets of variables?

A quick visual way to analyse the possibility of a relationship between the variables is to plot the two sets of data as a **scatter graph** with one variable along the horizontal axes and the other along the vertical axes (Fig. 4.11).

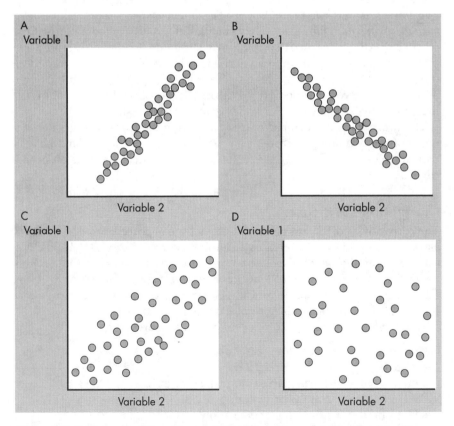

Figure 4.11 Scatter graphs: (**A**) positive correlation; (**B**) negative correlation; (**C**) relationship between variables not clearly defined; (**D**) no correlation.

Figure 4.11A shows that *high* scores on variable 1 seem to be linked with *high* scores on variable 2 and also *low* scores on 1 linked with *low* scores on 2. If this is the case, you can say that there is a **positive correlation** between the two sets of data. Examples of positive correlation could be the data in Cases 1, 3 and 6.

Figure 4.11B shows that *high* scores on variable 1 seem to be linked with *low* scores on variable 2 and also *low* scores on 1 linked with *high* scores on 2. That is, as one variable increases the other decreases. This is called a **negative correlation** and Cases 2 and 4 (above) could provide examples of such data.

Figure 4.11C shows that the relationship between the data is not clearly defined, although one could be tempted to think that there is a positive correlation. Case 3 is an example of this, as a recent study has shown that contrary to beliefs there is no significant correlation between breast-feeding and the child's IQ.

Figure 4.11D shows a zero correlation, since the points are so scattered that no sign of a straight line can be observed.

The graphical method gives you a sense of whether there is a correlation or not. However, a sense is not good enough. In the smoking study the researchers wanted to see if there was a positive correlation between the two variables: *motivation to stop smoking* and *concerns about health consequences of continuing to smoke*. They calculated what is called a correlation coefficient—the Spearman correlation coefficient—and then verified by means of statistical tables the level of significance or level of confidence. (Look back at the section on levels of confidence (p. 100) which tells you how confident you can be that the correlation observed is due to a relationship between the variables rather than random chance.)

To summarize, in correlation design, a number of measurements are made of two variables. A correlation coefficient is calculated and then statistical tables are consulted to give the level of significance of the observed correlation.

Correlation coefficient

The correlation coefficient gives you the degree of correlation—how much association—and is calculated as a number between -1 and $+1$. Positive numbers state the level of positive correlation and negative numbers the level of negative correlation. The closer the coefficient is to $+1$ or -1 then the higher is the correlation and the closer to 0 the lower the correlation (Fig. 4.12). The coefficient is normally denoted by the letter r.

Approximate guidelines for level of correlation are:

0.00 to 0.19	a very low correlation
0.20 to 0.39	a low correlation
0.40 to 0.69	a reasonable (modest) correlation
0.70 to 0.89	a high correlation
0.90 to 1.00	a very high correlation.

A value of r of 0.8 is a high correlation. However, in order to state with confidence that there is a positive association between your two sets of

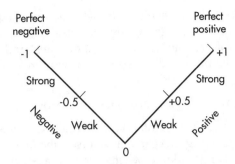

Figure 4.12 Relationship between the value of the correlation coefficient and the level of correlation.

data, you need to refer to a statistical probability table which tells you whether your correlation has statistical significance at a defined confidence level. The level of confidence will depend on the size of the sample used.

As in experimental design, there are a number of statistical techniques designed to test correlation. Which one you use depends on the type of data, the scales of measurement, etc. It is beyond the scope of this chapter to go into all the different tests in great detail. Below I list the most common tests to give you some idea of when and how they should be applied, followed by a worked example.

Statistical tests for correlation

1. The Spearman test is a non-parametric test for two sets of ordinal or interval/ratio data.
2. The Pearson test is a parametric test for two sets of interval/ratio data.
3. The Kendall coefficient of correlation test is a non-parametric test for three or more sets of data; data can belong to the ordinal or interval/ratio scales of measurement.
4. Linear regression tests: two sets of data; data are shown to be significantly correlated for prediction of a score given the value of the other score.

Worked example 1

A ward sister interviewed by Pam Smith and colleagues (Smith et al, unpublished report, 1992) noted the importance of preparing patients both psychologically and physically for their operations. She said: 'You prepare the patients psychologically and physically for their operations and after a little while you can sense it straight away whether this patient is going to do well after the operation or not. You can sense it somehow' (p. 56).

The way in which this statement could be evaluated is by collecting data from a number of randomly selected groups of patients on the length of time spent talking to the nurse about their operation and the level of anxiety they experienced prior to their operation.

Hypothesis H_1: The longer the time a nurse talks with the patient about the operation the less anxious the patient is about the operation.

Hypothesis H₀: There is no relationship between time spent talking with patients and the anxiety experienced by patients.

Time is collected in minutes (from 3 to 20 minutes) and level of anxiety is measured on a five-point ordinal scale of measurement:

1	2	3	4	5
Very calm	Calm	Slightly anxious	Anxious	Highly anxious

The length of time variable is interval/ratio and the anxiety level gives us ordinal data. You are trying to see if high values of the time variable give you low values on the anxiety scale, i.e. whether there is a negative correlation.

The results are given in Table 4.10.

For this design, because the data are ordinal we must use the Spearman test. To find the **Spearman rank order correlation coefficient** r_s you apply the following formula:

$$r_s = 1 - \frac{6\sum D^2}{(N^3 - N)}$$

where D is the difference between the values of A and B when they are both put in rank order; $\sum D^2$ is the sum of the squared values of the difference between the ranked scores; and N is the number of paired scores.

Procedure: Table 4.10 provides the following information:

- Column 1 gives the subject—each subject is defined by a number from 1 to 15.

Table 4.10 The effect on anxiety of psychological preparation of patients for their operations: data from study and calculation of the Spearman rank order corrrelation coefficient, r_s

1	2	3	4	5	6	7
Subject	Variable A length of time in minutes	Variable B anxiety score	Rank of A (a)	Rank of B (b)	D (a – b)	D² (a – b)²
1	5	4	3	12.5	–9.5	90.25
2	10	2	9.5	4.5	5	25
3	6	3	4.5	8	–3.5	12.25
4	3	5	1	15	–14	196
5	12	3	11	8	3	9
6	8	3	7.5	8	–0.5	0.25
7	15	3	13	8	5	25
8	13	2	12	4.5	7.5	56.25
9	6	4	4.5	12.5	–8	64
10	10	1	9.5	2	7.5	56.25
11	7	3	6	8	–2	4
12	20	1	15	2	13	169
13	4	4	2	12.5	–10.5	110.25
14	18	1	14	2	12	144
15	8	4	7.5	12.5	–5	25

$N = 15$

$N^3 - N = 3360$

$\sum D^2 = 986.5$

$6\sum D^2 = 5919$

$r_s = 1 - 5919/3360 = -0.76$

- Columns 2 and 3 give the data collected from the study.
- Columns 4 and 5 give the two variables 'time' and 'anxiety score' placed in rank order. (Note: When putting in rank order, give a rank of 1 to the lowest score and 2 to the next lowest score. If two or more scores have the same rank then assign each of them the mean value of the ranks they would have been assigned if they had been different. For example, two scores ranked 8 would have been 8 and 9 if they had been different from each other so both are assigned a rank of 8.5. Three scores sharing a rank of 7 would have been ranked 7, 8, 9 if they had been different, so all are assigned a rank of $(7 + 8 + 9)/3 = 8$.)
- Column 6 holds the difference between the ranks for time and anxiety.
- Column 7 is the value in column 6 squared and the sum of all the numbers in this column give the sum of D^2.

The next step is to find the value of r_s from the formula given above. The formula may look complex and you do not need to know in detail how it is derived. However, it may be helpful to recognize the following assumptions on which it is based:

- The data in a non-parametric test is ordinal and hence only the order and not the size of values of the anxiety levels 1 to 5 is relevant. We could have measured anxiety levels as 5 to 10 or any other sequence of five numbers. In the calculation of the Spearman rank order correlation you need to replace the scores for time and anxiety level by the rank scores.
- The difference column can contain positive and negative numbers and all of these must contribute to the coefficient rather than cancel each other out. Hence the need to create column 7 which is the square of the difference (squaring the difference produces all positive numbers).

The result of this test has produced a negative correlation coefficient of r_s of -0.76. This is a high negative correlation. But is the correlation significant and at what level of confidence? To find this out the figure of 0.76 must be looked up in a statistical probability table to find out whether this figure represents a significant correlation between the length of time spent talking and the level of the anxiety. The sample size is $N = 15$. For sample sizes of $N = 14$ (there is no value for $N = 15$ in the table I used) the following critical values for each level of significance are given:

N	0.05	0.025	0.01	0.005
		Level of significance		
14	0.456	0.544	0.645	0.715

The table will give you the critical value of r_s at various levels of significance. For your value of r_s to be significant at a particular level m, it should be equal to or larger than the critical value for m that is associated with the N in your study.

From this table it can be seen that this correlation (0.76) is significant at the 0.005 level, so there is less than a 0.5% chance that this result is due to random error.

This test shows that there is a high negative correlation between the time spent by the nurse talking to the patient before the operation and the patient's level of anxiety, and this correlation is significant at the 0.005 confidence level.

The other correlation coefficient test that you will see frequently used is the **Pearson product-moment correlation coefficient** test. This is a parametric test that can be applied only for interval or ratio data. Again the calculation seems complex and often produces large numbers, but if you follow the instructions step by step carefully, using a calculator or computer, you will arrive at a result—remember that your calculated value should lie between + 1 and – 1.

Worked example 2 (data from Hicks 1990, pp. 208–209)

There is a suggestion that the length of time a woman has been taking the contraceptive pill will affect the time it takes for her to conceive.

Hypothesis H_1: There is a relationship between the length of time a woman has been on oral contraceptives and the time it takes to become pregnant subsequently.

Hypothesis H_0: There is no relationship between the length of time on oral contraceptives and the time it subsequently takes to become pregnant.

The data in Table 4.11 were collected from 12 randomly selected women to test this hypothesis.

Table 4.11 Relationship between length of time on the contraceptive pill and time taken to become pregnant after ceasing to take the pill: data and calculation of the Pearson product-moment correlation coefficient, r_p

Subject	Variable A Length of time on pill	Variable B Length of time to become pregnant	$A \times B$	A^2	B^2
1	4	6	24	16	36
2	2	5	10	4	25
3	7	7	49	49	49
4	10	4	40	100	16
5	1	5	5	1	25
6	11	10	110	121	100
7	9	12	108	81	144
8	5	18	90	25	324
9	3	6	18	9	36
10	6	9	54	36	81
11	7	3	21	49	9
12	10	7	70	100	49
$N = 12$	$\Sigma A = 75$	$\Sigma B = 92$	$\Sigma(A \times B) = 599$	$\Sigma A^2 = 591$	$\Sigma B^2 = 894$
	$(\Sigma A)^2 = 5625$	$(\Sigma B)^2 = 8464$			

$$r_p = \frac{12 \times 599 - 75 \times 92}{\sqrt{(12 \times 591 - 5625)(12 \times 894 - 8464)}} = 0.16$$

Degrees of freedom $= N - 2 = 10$

These data are suitable for a parametric test (they are ratio data and satisfy the assumptions noted on p. 102). Hence, you will apply the Pearson product-moment test to calculate a correlation coefficient r_p using the following formula:

$$r_p = \frac{N\Sigma(A \times B) - \Sigma A \times \Sigma B}{\sqrt{((N\Sigma A^2 - (\Sigma A)^2)(N\Sigma B^2 - (\Sigma B)^2))}}$$

where N is the number of pairs of scores; A is the value of each score for the first variable—number of years on the pill; B is the value of each score for the second variable—length of time to become pregnant.

The calculation produces a correlation coefficient of $r_p = 0.16$. This value must then be looked up in a statistical probability table to see whether it represents a significant correlation between the length of time on oral contraceptive and the length of time taken subsequently to become pregnant. In order to do this it is also necessary to know the number of degrees of freedom associated with the sampling. In this case, the number of degrees of freedom is $N - 2 = 10$.

A value for r_p of 0.16 with 10 degrees of freedom is not significant, i.e. there is no significant relationship between the length of time on oral contraception and the length of time taken to conceive.

REFLECTIONS AND CONCLUSIONS

In this chapter we have taken you through a number of key concepts about using statistics to organize and analyse data and test ideas. We have given you a flavour of how to go about this with many examples from practice. Even experienced researchers do not make decisions about study design and statistical tests on their own. They seek the help of statisticians early on in their study in order to ensure that the data they collect are sound so that they can test hypotheses, summarize, describe and present their data visually prior to seeking inferences and explanations.

In a study undertaken by Pam Smith and colleagues, assistance was sought from a statistician in order to help them ask questions of their data. The statistician assisted them to analyse quantitative data from a questionnaire, a visual pain analogue scale and a check list of patient dependency. The variables under study were 'anxiety and depression', pain and dependence in patients undergoing hip and knee replacements. The data complemented qualitative data as part of a study of the effects of emotional care on patient outcomes (Smith et al, unpublished report, 1992). I want to emphasize to you that in analysing such complex data you cannot be expected to undertake it alone. The statistician has the expertise in the techniques but you have the expertise in the topic which informs your questions, understanding and explanation, which in turn shape the hypotheses and findings. The statistician advised Pam Smith and her colleagues on the tests to use in order to assist them to make assertions about their data with confidence that they had not occurred by chance. They found, for example, that significance tests allowed them to say that there was a positive relationship between the emotional style on a ward and pain management. They also found that patient dependency was related to whether the patients had had the same professional looking after them throughout their hospital stay. The levels of significance were such that they were able to have confidence that their results had not occurred by chance. Talking to patients and continuity of care did seem to make a statistical difference to the patients' recovery. The qualitative findings of Smith et al, in which they described through narratives and accounts what their patients told them about emotional care, as presented in the box below, were supported statistically. By using statistics to support their qualitative findings they were able to convince their medical colleagues that narratives and accounts were just as important as numbers.

■ BOX 4.4

The nurses were very very sympathetic and they picked me up when I was feeling low (p. 25).

I hadn't slept for a couple of nights and I suddenly felt so fed up with pain. The nurse came to me and she said 'Don't worry. Why don't you lie on your side rather than your back'. And she sorted out the bed so nicely and got me comfortable. It was her skill in that. But at the same time she could see I was worked up and yet her whole manner took that in. She was very very good (p. 29).

As Say and Cumpper demonstrate in Chapter 3, we use numerical skills and intuition every day in practice. Learning how to formalize those skills through learning about quantitative data analysis, is part of becoming research minded. Furthermore, knowledge and understanding of quantitative data analysis is very important in the present climate of an NHS research and development strategy committed to randomized controlled trials as part of evidence-based health care. As the examples from Nightingale (Box 4.1) and Martin (1990) have shown, evidence based on numbers and 'hard facts' is important for constructing arguments and influencing policy. Our knowledge of statistics also helps us to critically and constructively read articles (such as those reproduced in Appendices 1 and 2) and to decide whether the evidence being presented is sound.

Often statistical evidence is taken as the ultimate proof of the **validity** and **reliability** of research findings. We want to leave you with some concluding thoughts. Statisticians, like researchers, are not all the same. There are no right and wrong ways to treat data. Statisticians use judgements about the data when they apply statistical tests according to the largeness or smallness of a data set; the type of data being collected and the questions being asked of the data.

We shall give the final word to John Gordon, who was the original instigator of this chapter. He wrote in a conclusion to an early draft that: 'The crux to the statistical approach is the need to know the basics to enable you to solve the complex or at least be able to ask the right questions of others who might advise you on the type of analysis that best suits your data'. Research-minded people are those who not only look ahead to aid their research but also look back and learn from their experiences for next time.

Statistical manipulations are tools and like any tool you have to learn to use them effectively. This chapter, and indeed this book, show that the way in which we teach and learn is a crucial element of success.

We hope that working through this chapter has been fun and that you will feel able to return to the worked examples again and again as part of your equipment for being research minded.

REFERENCES

Department of Health (Research and Development Division) 1991 Research for health. HMSO, London

Everitt A, Hardiker P, Littlewood J, Mullender A 1992 Applied research for better practice. Macmillan, Basingstoke

Fennema E 1996 Mathematics, gender and research. In: Gila H (ed) Towards gender equity in mathematics education: an ICMI study. Kluwer Academic Publishers, Dordrecht

Hicks C 1990 Research and statistics: a practical introduction for nurses. Prentice Hall, New York

Jeffs T, Smith M 1990 Using informal education. Open University Press, Buckingham

McFarlane JK 1970 The proper study of the nurse. RCN, London

Macleod Clark J, Haverty S, Kendall S 1990 Helping people to stop smoking: a study of the nurse's role. Journal of Advanced Nursing 16: 357–363

Martin C 1990 How do you count maternal satisfaction—a user-commissioned survey. In: Roberts H (ed) Women's health counts. Routledge, London, pp 147–166

Nuttall P 1983 The passionate statistician. Nursing Times 79 (Sept 28): 25–27

Open University 1983 Unit C1. Testing new drugs. In: Statistics in society. MDST 242. Open University Press, Milton Keynes, pp 24–25

Open University 1983 Unit C5. Review. In: Statistics in society. MDST 242. Open University Press, Milton Keynes, p 6

Reid N, Boore J 1987 Research methods and statistics in health care. Edward Arnold, London, pp 114–117

Smith B 1994 The dressing makes the difference: trial of two modern dressings on venous ulcers. Professional Nurse 9(5): 348–352

Spencer J 1983 Research with a human touch. Nursing Times 79(12): 24–27

Walkerdine V 1989 Counting girls out. Girls and Mathematics Unit, Institute of Education. Virago, London

Worsley P (ed) The new modern sociology readings. Penguin, Harmondsworth

Phenomenology

5

Nina Stephenson   Veronica Corben

KEY ISSUES

- The contribution of phenomenology to research mindedness
- Phenomenology as philosophy, approach and method
- Phenomenology as an alternative to positivist science
- The use of art and literature in the study of phenomenology
- Experiential learning: a case study of phenomenology in action
- The use of phenomenology to interpret practice

PREAMBLE

Phenomenology is a **qualitative** inductive research approach that is accessible to all, whether students, practitioners, mentors or teachers. It is particularly suited to the study of complex and nebulous **concepts** such as care, love and happiness, which are difficult to quantify. We see phenomenology as a way of looking closely at seemingly ordinary, everyday experiences in order to 'taste' and 'feel' another person's frame of reference and to see the world through that person's eyes.

Phenomenology is a complex research approach, which uses rigorous and effective research methods to collect and analyse rich data to illustrate another person's world. Despite its complexity, phenomenology can be communicated in a novel and simple way without losing the richness or uniqueness of the approach.

As we describe in our case study, we used works of art to present and demystify phenomenology in an easily understood way as a means of promoting research mindedness. We chose phenomenology for our topic because we had learnt so much from undertaking phenomenological research for undergraduate degrees. We learnt not only about the research process but also gained insights into other people's worlds which enhanced our teaching and practice as nurses. We refer to our two studies in the chapter. Nina sought to understand the experiences of spouses living with an elderly functionally mentally ill partner; Veronica explored the experience of being a bank nurse.

INTRODUCTION

Phenomenology is a research approach that is firmly based in practice. It is a way of seeing the world through another person's eyes. By losing ourselves in the experience, we can produce valuable, rich data. Phenomenology bridges the theory–practice gap and goes a long way towards demystifying research and dispelling the myth that research is only for the enlightened minority.

By exploring phenomenology and its application to the practice of nursing, we emphasize the need to prepare knowledgeable doers to break down the barriers and fears surrounding the researcher role and encourage critical thinking.

We hope that as the complexity of phenomenology unfolds, and a need for and awareness of the skills of research becomes clearer, the value of research mindedness in relation to phenomenology will also become clearer to you. We are not suggesting that you necessarily need to undertake phenomenological research; but that you need to be aware of, and understand more fully, the approach and the value of existing studies to your practice.

How do we define research mindedness and what is phenomenology's contribution to its promotion? Research mindedness is a way of interpreting and thinking that helps health care students, teachers, mentors and practitioners to feel confident about various research approaches, question and seek information about their own clinical practice and value existing research. Research mindedness is not necessarily about doing research but being aware of the availability and content of research studies and what it means to use them in practice. The Briggs' report (DHSS 1972) did not ask all nurses to be researchers, only that they seek the value of research. Sometimes the interpretation of the report has served to alienate health professionals, who may see research as the domain of the few not the ownership of the whole.

By using novel ways of promoting research mindedness we highlight the value of research in practice. We want to avert the danger that the word research may serve to compartmentalize theory and practice into separate units. We hope to promote a new mentality about research which will enable you to incorporate it into your daily experiences.

PHENOMENOLOGY AS PHILOSOPHY, APPROACH AND METHOD

The aim in nursing and other health care professions has been to use research to predict and control care using traditional scientific methods (Oiler 1981). We see these methods as reducing human beings into small **quantitative** units which give no clue to how they fit into the dynamic living whole.

Phenomenology provides a different philosophical basis from the traditional scientific approach to research. For nursing, which is regarded as an art as well as a science, a philosophical perspective that is not rooted in traditional science ensures that experiences are not reduced to quantitative measures.

Phenomenology was developed by German philosophers Husserl (1859–1938) and Heidegger (1889–1976). Heidegger's writings have influenced the work of American nurse theorist Patricia Benner. Heidegger's approach to phenomenology falls within the interpretive research tradition, which is summarized in Chapter 2 (p. 24). It is underpinned by the **philosophy** known as existentialism. By existentialism we mean the way one views the world, stressing the personal 'here and now' experience and responsibility and the demands they place on the individual as a free agent in a deterministic and seemingly meaningless universe. We can therefore understand that phenomenology by its very nature is a descriptive and inductive research method. Omery (1983) states that 'the task of this method is to investigate and describe all the phenomena, including human experience, in the way these phenomena appear'.

The phenomenological research approach serves the caring goal of understanding the 'lived experience' of every individual and the world these individuals live in.

The word '**phenomenon**' is used to describe the human lived experience of a particular aspect of life. We see the nature of a 'phenomenon' as an experience, maybe an everyday one such as being tired, or a more unique one such as seeing a child walk for the first time. The purpose of phenomenology is to attempt to describe and understand the essence of these experiences in a qualitative way.

The main features of phenomenology as we refer to it throughout this chapter are summarized in Box 5.1. The concern of phenomenology is with the nature of being, the here and now, 'as it is'. This shows that the approach is rooted in experience. As noted above, the idea of 'here and now' is part of the philosophical notion of existentialism.

■ BOX 5.1

Main features of phenomenology
- It is anchored in experience, not theory.
- Its concern is to understand:
  - —the way people exist in the world
  - —the significance of everyday things and events
  - —the phenomenon 'as it is', the 'lived experience'.

Phenomenology means looking at the experience as you see it at this moment in time, a sense of 'existing' or living now. The phenomenologist's viewpoint is based on the premise that any experience is a valid and fruitful source of knowledge. Phenomenologists also maintain that intuition (developing one's consciousness through looking and listening) is important in the development of knowledge. However, human meaning should not be inferred from a sense of impression alone.

At this juncture, you may wonder why phenomenology is useful to you? In your practice, for example, there may be rich experiences which you would like to examine more deeply. If nursing research is to be rooted in practice, using the phenomenological approach to looking at these experiences may enable you to promote and develop your nursing knowledge by providing meaning and richness to everyday experiences.

The value of such individual experiences is highlighted in the practice-based works of Beck (1992), Forrest (1989) and Morse et al (1994). Morse and colleagues used patients' narratives to elicit and understand the essence of 'lived comfort', illustrating how each patient was the source of unique experience. Beck (1992) described how it feels to be a mother suffering from post-partum depression, whilst Forrest (1989) looked at the experience of caring. Other examples include what it feels like to be a novice nurse (Benner 1984) and the lived experience of being a bank nurse (Corben 1992). All of these studies are illustrations of unique experiences with commonality of meanings.

Phenomenologists endeavour to make their research participants actively involved as 'co-researchers' rather than 'subjects'. This approach can be compared with the relationships nurses develop with their patients as partners in care. We all need to accept that patients and 'co-researchers' are more skilled at highlighting their own feelings than we who are outside the experience. This issue has been recognized and highlighted in Benner's (1984) eloquent exemplars of expert psychiatric nursing practice such as the one presented in Box 5.2 below.

■ BOX 5.2

I was making my rounds and I walked in. And I said, 'Hi, I'm Sue, you must be Ann'. And she said 'What the hell is it to you? I'm so goddamned mad'. I was just amused by it and said 'Well, why don't you tell me about it?'. I knew from the beginning that there was such pain under her vile language—such intensity, almost agony … (Benner 1984, p. 68).

This exemplar illustrates how the patient, Ann, like a co-researcher, had let the nurse, Sue, feel what it was like to be in her shoes. The nurse has participated in the patient's 'lived experience' of psychiatric illness.

We see reflective practice as a possible application of the phenomenological research approach. Schon (1987) describes reflection in action as tantamount to the 'lived experience', the way the individual perceives the phenomena at that point in time, the unique experience. However, we would add that in order to ensure the phenomenon being investigated is as it truly appears or is experienced, a necessary criterion is that the investigator must approach the phenomenon to be explored with no preconceived **operational definitions**, an open mind, as a sponge waiting to absorb the experience and describe the phenomenon as it appears.

Do you do this in your practice? We see health care professionals reflecting on their practice every day, even though they may be unaware of doing so. Making us aware of the unaware is for us the true value of the phenomenological approach. As nurses, teachers, students and mentors, we all absorb the experience of caring for others. We use this method daily (during the handover report, in the coffee room) by describing to each other the richness of our patient–nurse interaction. However, we do not acknowledge our **bias** and are not always explicit in our motives, which if one is 'research minded' can be recognized.

Everybody coming to any experience brings biases, life experiences, ways of seeing and doing, which are ingrained and an integral part of their personalities and social context. Our beliefs and values colour the way we perceive the world.

Phenomenologists suggest that we should **'bracket'** feelings, temporarily suspend our own preconceived beliefs and look at the phenomenon with wide-open eyes, with knowledge, facts and theories held at bay, and concentrate on and absorb the phenomenon. In practice, we are led to believe that we should, as nurses, be bias-free. However, in reality, we inevitably carry around preconceived ideas, which can sometimes lead to a self-fulfilling prophecy.

Reed's (1994) study of nursing expertise in the care of long-term elderly clients serves to highlight this issue. Reed was left in a quandary about the selection criteria for her interviewees since they appeared not to demonstrate expertise in the nursing care of elderly clients (see Box 5.3).

■ BOX 5.3

'Did this mean that the nurses I had interviewed had no expertise? They had all been on the ward for several years, in the care of the elderly for even longer. Were they perhaps nurses who simply had not developed expertise, or was there no expertise in the care of the elderly to develop? I had avoided selecting nurses on the strength of managers' evaluation of them, because I felt that these evaluations would be suspect; sometimes nurses are valued by managers for the expertise they present, rather than the expertise they have. Perhaps I needed to re-think this ... (Reed 1994).

In re-thinking her selection criteria of expert nurses, Reed demonstrated insight and research mindedness by questioning her original bias in not selecting nurses (for interview) on the strength of their managers' evaluation of them.

Phenomenology's usefulness lies not only in the rich uniqueness of its findings, but also its possible generalizability. Field & Morse (1985) suggest that generalization may be based on similar meaning rather than exact duplication of essence. By 'clustering' data into themes we can ascribe similar meaning to phenomena without exact duplication. Exact duplication is not possible in unique living beings. Clustering themes, therefore, is a way of articulating the essential structure of the phenomenon. Colaizzi's framework (Fig. 5.1) is commonly used by phenomenologists to do this. Colaizzi is just one of several theorists whose techniques can be drawn on to conduct phenomenological research (see Omery 1983 for others).

Box 5.4 demonstrates Beck's (1992) use of Colaizzi's framework to identify themes from clients' perspectives about the structure of the phenomenon 'post-partum depression'.

By using a phenomenological approach we can highlight and access the unquantifiable experiences of daily life and can enable people to empathize with one another by noting that 'it's like that for me too' (Morse 1991).

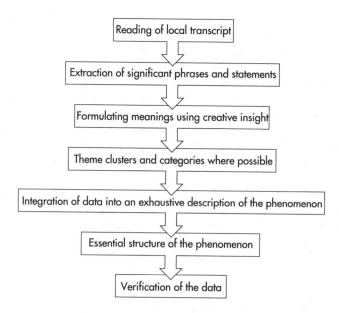

Figure 5.1 Phenomenological data analysis (adapted from Colaizzi 1978).

■ **BOX 5.4**

Sample of the 11 theme clusters that constituted the fundamental structure of post-partum depression (Beck 1992)

Theme 1

Mothers were enveloped in unbearable loneliness owing to discomfort with others and a belief that no-one else understood what they were experiencing.

Theme 2

Contemplating death provided a glimmer of hope to end their living nightmare.

Theme 3

Obsessive thoughts of being a bad mother and of questioning what was happening to them consumed the mothers' waking hours.

Theme 11

Besieged with insecurities, the mothers needed to be mothered themselves.

From then on we can, if we choose, infer wider generalizations (Beck 1992). These wider inferences can then become the first step in **theory** development.

However, it is essential that the philosophical approach underpinning phenomenology is understood from the outset, since it represents a major departure from the traditional empirical research tradition. Looking at the phenomenon in detail enables you to provide meaning to an experience which is often not quantifiable. What are some of the methods available to us to collect this rich data about the essence of lived experiences?

Methods of collecting data in phenomenological research

Phenomenological information can be collected by three methods, all of which are used regularly by practitioners in the course of their work. We shall refer to these methods again in our case study. They are:

- observation
- unstructured interviews
- diaries/journals.

Observation

Skilled **observation** is an everyday tool of the practitioner, who checks the nonverbal cues given by patients, clients, their family and friends. For example, you could use this method to observe and describe concepts such as client dependency or pain.

Unstructured interviews

Unstructured interviews are conversations with a purpose, which enable us to extract rich and often unquantifiable information about the nature of a range of feelings, such as anxiety, fear, happiness.

This is probably the most common form of data collection in phenomenology (Field & Morse 1985) and can also readily be translated to a practice setting. Research rooted in practice can focus on client perceptions of their experiences, for example researching the anxiety arising from admission to hospital by using informal conversations with clients as the equivalent of unstructured interviews.

As we describe below, we both used this method in our own research studies, Veronica to examine the role of the bank nurse (Corben 1992) and Nina to understand spouses' experience of living with an elderly mentally ill partner (Stephenson 1993). Veronica had actually been a bank nurse and therefore understood deeply the experience which she was asking others to describe. Nina, on the other hand, had not had direct experience of being an elderly spouse caring for a mentally dependent partner but had worked with such clients as a nurse.

Diaries/journals

Though this method is used least in phenomenology, as nurses we are increasingly being encouraged to keep reflective diaries or journals to document specific experiences or to monitor our professional development. Information collected in this way could be used to examine different approaches to care, such as primary or team nursing, or document the development of a new role such as that of a clinical nurse specialist or lecturer/practitioner.

Uses of phenomenology

Let us consider the following examples of when we might use the phenomenological approach to research:

• To study under-researched areas where little or no literature is available, such as in Veronica's bank nurse study (Corben 1992).

• To study areas of practice which are difficult to quantify, for example in areas of mental health as described in Nina's study (Stephenson 1993).

• As part of triangulation, to complement quantitative methods to research a complex topic. Triangulation in phenomenology may provide the extra perspective to a previously quantified phenomenon such as empathy.

Triangulation means combining more than one approach to research by using a variety of approaches and/or methods to provide different perspectives on the same phenomenon. The term is geographical in origin, meaning to ascertain one's position by comparing it to more than one other known location.

• As a method of examining daily phenomena in practice (such as client communication), in order to look at them in a rich and living way.

Van Manen (1990) suggests that phenomenology makes teachers and practitioners more sensitive and competent in understanding experiences in practice as well as making them better researchers.

Van Manen also suggests that phenomenology distinguishes itself by its courage and resolve to stand up for the uniqueness and significance of the experience described, a task not often attempted by other research approaches. It enables one to 'borrow' others' experiences and reflect on their deeper meaning to come to a better understanding (Van Manen 1990). This approach can be seen in classic studies by well-known authors who demonstrated real, lived experiences in a truly phenomenological way. Examples of this are Albert Camus' (1960) description of a doctor's experience of chronic life-threatening illness in *The Plague* and Florence Nightingale's experience of being a nurse in *Notes on Nursing* (1859). You can read these descriptions in Boxes 5.5 and 5.6.

Camus provides a description of being totally immersed in the real experience described at a particular moment, i.e. the real nature of the influence of plague on people. Nightingale demonstrates the intuitive understanding of the interpretation of a patient's colour by an experienced nurse.

The value of research mindedness is demonstrated here through the valuing of these well-known works. Research mindedness becomes a way of life: we see others through their writings trying to provide meaning to ordinary but complex experiences.

Works of art can also provide a medium for looking at the essence of a phenomenon. In our case study we used works of art to generate ideas from a number of pictures which we asked our colleagues to examine as if for the first time.

We had been drawn independently to the link between art and phenomenology by browsing through Van Manen's (1990) literature. Van Manen speaks of art as a lived experience, and reminds us that art transforms the

■ **BOX 5.5**

It was by such lapses that Rieux could gauge his exhaustion. His sensibility was getting out of hand. Kept under all the time, it had grown hard and brittle and seemed to snap completely now and then, leaving him the prey of his emotions. No resource was left him but to tighten the stranglehold on his feelings and harden his heart protectively. For he knew this was the only way of carrying on. In any case, he had few illusions left, and fatigue was robbing him of even these remaining few. He knew that, over a period whose end he could not glimpse, his task was no longer to cure but to diagnose. To detect, to see, to describe, to register, and then condemn—that was his present function. Sometimes a woman would clutch his sleeve, crying shrilly, 'doctor, you'll save him, won't you?' but he wasn't there for saving life; he was there to order a sick man's evacuation. How futile was the hatred he saw on faces then! 'You haven't a heart!' a woman told him on one occasion. She was wrong; he had one. It saw him through his twenty-hours day, when he hourly watched men dying who were meant to live. It enabled him to start anew each morning. He had just enough heart for that, as things were now. How could that heart have sufficed for saving life?

(Camus 1960)

■ **BOX 5.6**

The experienced nurse can always tell that a person has taken narcotic the night before by the patchiness of the colour about the face when the re-action of depression has set in; that very colour which the inexperienced will point to as a proof of health.

There is, again, a faintness, which does not betray itself by the colour at all, or in which the patient becomes brown instead of white. There is a faintness of another kind which, it is true, can always be seen by the paleness.

But the nurse seldom distinguishes. She will talk to the patient who is too faint to move, without the least scruple, unless he is pale and unless, luckily for him, the muscles of the throat are affected and he loses his voice.

Yet these two faintnesses are perfectly distinguishable, by the mere countenance of the patient.

(Nightingale 1859)

lived experience into 'transcended configurations'. This means that art enables ideas at a particular point in time and space to be transmitted to others as a truly 'lived experience'.

The notion is not new since Heidegger uses Van Gogh's painting *Shoes of the Peasant* in his *Reflections on Truth* (1977) to provide powerful examples of the lived experience. The use of literature, as we saw in Chapter 2, can similarly help us make more interpretive sense of lived experiences.

We now present a summary of our own research projects to show you how we were able to use phenomenology even though we were both new to research and new to the approach.

OUR OWN EXPERIENCES OF DOING PHENOMENOLOGICAL RESEARCH

Nina's research

In my research I sought to understand the experience of spouses living with an elderly functionally mentally ill partner (Stephenson 1993). It enabled me to put myself into the other person's shoes: to taste, touch, smell and feel as they must taste, touch, smell and feel.

As noted above, Field & Morse (1985) suggest that generalization may be based on similar meaning rather than exact duplication of essence; this was illustrated in my own work (Stephenson 1993). I discovered that all the spouses whilst having similar experiences also had unique ones, as shown by their expression of anger, presented in Box 5.7 below.

■ **BOX 5.7**

Mrs D: 'I get very, very angry, I'll tell you.'
'Years ago, I could cope, as you get older you can't … I lose my patience.'
'He gets frustrated, so do I, but I just close my mind.'
'I am one of 13 so I have learnt to close my mind. I used to be able to read a book with anyone around me. You close your mind.'

Mrs C: 'I get very, very angry—I'll tell you I swore at him … keeps me sane!'
'I admit I hate his guts, I'll admit to you, but you can't suddenly think he's not my husband any more. It's what I took on, you can't give up.'

Both these statements are unique expressions of anger. Both spouses are living and coping with their experience in individual but also similar ways.

We have already discussed how as nurses we are led to believe that we should be bias-free. However, in reality, we inevitably carry around preconceived ideas with us. In order to avoid this tendency, phenomenologists suggest that we 'bracket' feelings, as a means of temporarily suspending our preconceptions so that we can concentrate on and absorb the phenomenon. In my own work (Stephenson 1993) I attempted to approach the participants without any preconceived ideas, but owing to my own life experiences I inevitably had some biases and notions about why spouses continued living with their mentally ill partners. I accepted all data as given and tried to understand them from the perspective of the participants who were going through the experience of living with the elderly mentally ill sufferer. During data analysis, I identified 'guilt' as a recurring theme. Was this coincidental or a self-fulfilling prophecy? For example, had I expected spouses to be motivated by guilt to care for their relatives?

In the spirit of phenomenological research I also wanted the spouses to participate actively and be involved in the project as 'co-researchers' rather than 'subjects'. It also highlights that they are more skilled than we are in highlighting their own feelings about their unique experience.

Veronica's research

My study of the lived experience of being a bank nurse (Corben 1992) is an illustration of how I was able to describe a unique experience that has a commonality of meanings.

As noted above, unstructured interviews are conversations with a purpose which assist us to extract rich information about the nature of feelings such as anxiety. I used this method in my own study to examine the role of the bank nurse. I had actually been a bank nurse and therefore understood deeply the experience that I was asking others to describe to me through unstructured meaningful conversation.

My study illustrates the development of the phenomenological process (Box 5.8). Relating issues to one's own experience may add more value, accessibility and clarity to the issues raised because of one's own direct involvement. The role of the researcher in listening to difficult or otherwise inaccessible data, enabling the participant to examine the phenomenon as it is for them here and now, and then analysing the data and returning them to the participant for verification was powerfully reconstructed through the experience of examining the bank nurse's role.

I had been privileged to enter the world of the bank nurse through phenomenology, to begin to understand what uncertainty and fear their role produced, and what it really felt like to not really belong anywhere. As researcher, I enabled the participants to cast aside the agenda with which they came to the interview, and to look with 'wide open eyes' (Oiler 1981) at what emerged from their role as they viewed it, here and now. I was enabled to explain how vulnerable participants may feel (Box 5.8) and

---

■ BOX 5.8

The lived experience of being a bank nurse: meanings and themes

Formulated meanings:

- Not knowing an individual bank nurse professionally means being unaware of his or her potential and not daring to take risks.
- Being moved around produces extra stress and ignorance of the current workload. This can be transmitted as a lack of knowing to clients and their families.
- Being a bank nurse means having to find another method of showing others one's professional skills and knowledge without appearing over-confident. It means being treated as someone who knows very little.
- The bank system has no support network for the nurse. It means keeping quiet and struggling on.

Recurrent theme: 'need'.

Theme clusters:

a. the need to be recognized for what I am
b. the need to be recognized for what I know
c. the need to develop my knowledge further.

also how important the need for skilled support is. The study also showed the need for sensitivity and skill in handling the uncovering of the many deep-seated frustrations and fears in relation to the bank nurse's role.

CASE STUDY

In our case study, which is based on the seminar we presented for the 'Promoting research mindedness' module, we had to be mindful of creating a safe environment for our colleagues to understand the complexity and sensitivity of phenomenology without fear, intimidation or humiliation. We developed a fun, innovative method to relay information about phenomenology. We wanted to be sensitive to the needs of our colleagues, but also to convey how to use phenomenology to access the 'lived experience'.

Four main principles guided our approach to our session:

- the creation of a safe environment
- the use of an inductive teaching and learning method
- the use of the group facilitator as a role model for the phenomenological researcher
- the value of phenomenology to promoting research mindedness.

The use of poetry and art

The use of poetry or art provides a safe but meaningful experience that can be used by all health care practitioners, students and teachers to experience the phenomenological approach to research. We chose to use works of art because much of the literature we had read linked art and phenomenology to each other. The paintings we chose are: Constable's rural scene of *Salisbury Cathedral* (Fig. 5.2), Van Gogh's still life of *Sunflowers* (Fig. 5.3) and Botticelli's *Primavera* (Spring) (Fig. 5.4). These paintings represent different eras in art history. Their creators came from different countries and cultures. Botticelli, for example, was a Renaissance painter and used imagery from Greek and Roman mythology. He was Italian and lived from 1446–1510. Constable was a British painter and lived from 1776–1837. He is well known for his realistic representations of rural life. Van Gogh's paintings are also very familiar. Born in 1853 in the Netherlands, Van Gogh suffered from recurrent episodes of mental ill health which sadly ended in suicide in 1890.

In Chapter 2 reference is also made to the use of literary works to demonstrate the richness of experience that can be used to teach about approaches to and methods of research.

Paintings and literature may enable you to appreciate the subjective nature of phenomenology. The lack of firm conclusions presented in novels and poetry allows the reader to share and learn through the writer's experience. The unquantifiable and often inaccessible data gained from examining art or literature may be for you, like our colleagues, a reflection of your own personal experiences as a professional carer. For example, facial expressions in a picture may remind an oncology nurse of a patient's moment of anguish, or a description of joy may remind a midwife of the safe delivery of a child.

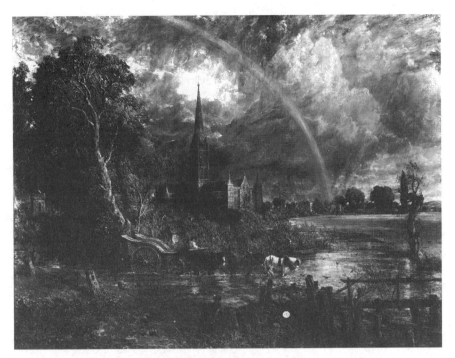

Figure 5.2 John Constable, *Salisbury Cathedral*. (Reproduced by courtesy of the Trustees, The National Gallery, London.)

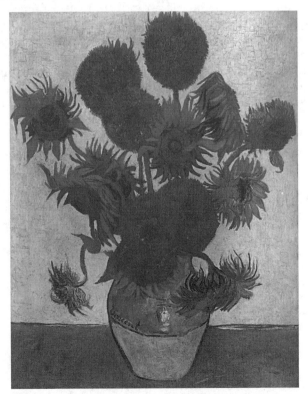

Figure 5.3 Vincent Van Gogh, *Sunflowers*. (Reproduced by courtesy of the Trustees, The National Gallery, London.)

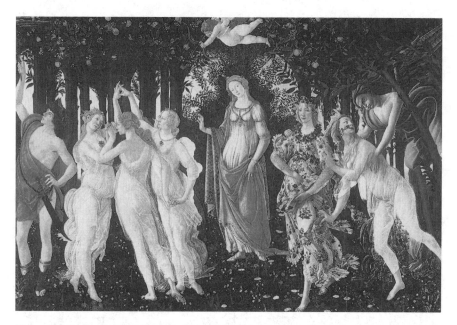

Figure 5.4 Sandro Botticelli, *Primavera*. (Reproduced by permission of the Uffizi Gallery, Florence.)

Inductive teaching and learning

The phenomenological method is an inductive one. Induction involves developing knowledge from the specific, i.e. the phenomenon being observed, to a general premise. The phenomenologist comes with an open mind, waiting to describe the experience as it appears, here and now, and from which conclusions and descriptions may be developed. In a similar way you may look at the care of a wound for a particular client without being influenced by what others have said about it, but evaluate it as you see it in the here and now.

In our seminar we chose to follow an inductive approach to teaching and learning about phenomenology by drawing on the 'data' gathered from the individual experience of looking at the pictures.

After the 'data gathering', we developed the theoretical underpinnings of the approach by teasing them out from issues arising during group discussion (Fig. 5.5). In this way, the principles of the phenomenological approach

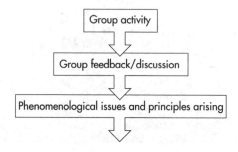

Figure 5.5 Inductive reasoning in action.

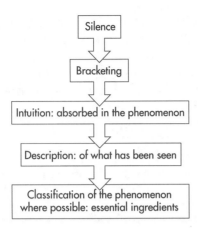

Figure 5.6 Systematic phenomenological method (adapted from Oiler 1981).

could be demonstrated as summarized in Figure 5.6. Phenomenological findings are usually presented as text that contains detailed descriptions and interpretations of the phenomena under study.

Using the facilitator to demonstrate the researcher's role

We used our role as facilitators in our session as a means of demonstrating the importance of the researcher's role in phenomenology. The development of the role highlights the need for a skilled, sensitive person to encourage accurate and appropriate data collection from the participant and also to provide help and support during the process (Parse et al 1985). You as teacher or practitioner can essentially emulate the researcher's role as you listen, observe and gather information about your students or clients. Our own research studies, summarized above, both demonstrated the need for sensitivity and skill in handling feelings such as anger and anxiety during data collection.

You may like to follow the instructions for the following activities, feedback and learning points we presented to our colleagues.

Activity 1: Individual observation of the picture—'the lived experience': gathering the 'data'

Spend about 15 minutes in silence looking at, thinking about and immersing yourself in the picture you have chosen to be the phenomenon you wish to experience.

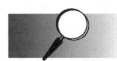

Whilst looking at the picture of your choice:

- *Attempt to put everything else out of your mind, including any previous experiences which might be aroused by looking at the picture.*

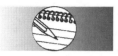

- *Look at the phenomenon with 'wide open eyes' (Oiler 1981), i.e. only focus on the experience of looking at the picture and on nothing else at all.*
- *Describe in writing everything you can about the picture as you see and feel about it, in a way that you could share with others. This is to enable you to grasp the essential meaning of the experience by entering into it (Van Manen 1990).*

Compare this activity with Beck's clear but highly meaningful instructions to participants in her study of post-partum depression presented in Box 5.9.

■ BOX 5.9

Please describe a situation in which you experienced post-partum depression. Share all your thoughts, perceptions and feelings that you can recall until you have no more to say about the situation.

(Beck 1992, p. 167)

For meaningful interpretation of the essence of an experience the need for silence is vital (Oiler 1981).

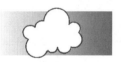

Stop for a moment and consider the value of silence in other situations, say in your role as a practitioner or teacher.

The moments of silence in conversation with clients or students allow time for information to sink in or for them to put their feelings into words. Silence also enables the practitioner to consider how to plan and implement excellence in care, or the teacher or mentor to assist students to think meaningfully about their actions. The use of silence in this way can be linked to the principle of bracketing (Oiler 1981). Bracketing as referred to earlier is a phenomenological concept involving suspending all other ideas from one's mind whilst focusing on the experience itself, a discipline that the practitioner or teacher may find invaluable. The systematic phenomenological approach, summarized in Figure 5.6, becomes a way of thinking, developing and living.

We would now like to give you feedback in the same way as we did to our colleagues.

Feedback from Activity 1

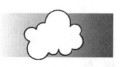

- *Reflect on your experience—how difficult was the exercise?*
- *Were there problems with setting aside all previous relevant experiences?*
- *Was the 'here and now' difficult to identify?*
- *Were there difficulties putting thoughts into words?*
- *How comfortable were you with living and feeling the experience meaningfully?*

- *What influence did the cultural beliefs and values mirrored through the pictures have on your ability to interpret the experience of looking at them?*

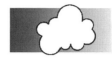

Key learning points. Refer back to the section on 'Phenomenology as philosophy, approach and method' (pp. 116–123).

Can you make links with this section and Activity 1 in relation to:

- *Phenomenology's main features (Box 5.1): the understanding of the existential approach: no preconceptions; here and now; the nature of being; how does the picture actually appear to me today?*
- *Its philosophical basis: rooted in existentialism; anchored in experience, not theory; its concern is to understand the way things or people exist 'in the world'?*
- *Research mindedness: valuing what others have already seen and described and painted and applying it to practice?*

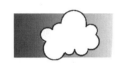

Activity 2: Reflecting on, talking and writing about, interpreting the 'data'

As noted above, our colleagues' knowledge was developed inductively by allowing them to recall their observations during group work (Fig. 5.5). We helped them to identify issues, then related them to phenomenological principles. A mentor may work in this way by using student examples to encourage them to think more meaningfully about their practice and enabling them to relate practice back to theoretical principles.

You too could share your 'observations' from your chosen picture in discussion with others who looked at a similar picture.

- *Identify the different methods of gathering and recording data during this experiential learning exercise.*
- *Discuss the data collected in terms of the substantial difference or similarity of reflections and interpretations among yourselves.*
- *Emphasize and respect the differences and uniqueness of your individual reflections and interpretations.*

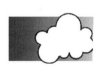

- *Consider ways of writing about your reflections and interpretations in a way that you feel comfortable with and yet is understandable to others.*
- *Did there appear to be an overriding theme to the experience which everyone identified?*
- *Did a particular aspect seem especially significant?*
- *What type of feelings were generated by the experience?*

Feedback from Activity 2

If you have undertaken this activity for yourself, compare whether other people came up with different or similar interpretations of the same pictures. During our session, for example, Constable's rural scene produced an overriding theme of peacefulness. Van Gogh's *Sunflowers* produced a similar feeling of peacefulness but also one of beauty and spirituality. Botticelli's *Primavera* produced a wide variety of interpretations of both the environment and the individuals in the scene, including a notion of purity. We were, however, least at home with Botticelli's mythical imagery. However, his picture provided fresh perceptions and stimulated the development of new ideas about what constituted the phenomenon of *Primavera*, i.e. Spring. The style and topics of Constable and van Gogh's paintings were culturally closer to our own experiences.

You may be able to attribute the differences in interpretation to the beliefs and values that influence the different ways in which we interpret things. Similarly, beliefs and values influence how individual clients are perceived by nurses.

Key learning points. The data gathering and recording methods used in our case study illustrate the need for a phenomenon that is difficult to access, to be seen and felt in context (Field & Morse 1985). For example:

• Observation of a patient, student or client, can be compared to the process of observing and experiencing the pictures.

• Journals or diaries can be used to capture the essence of the phenomenon in the written form.

• Unstructured interviews are a means by which the research participant can relive an experience verbally. This was demonstrated during discussion of how our colleagues interpreted the pictures and sought clarification from each other about their observations.

• The process is **inductive** rather than **deductive**—developing knowledge from the experience of observing the pictures rather than using existing knowledge to develop and test **hypotheses** about them.

• The very uniqueness of personal and individual data might provide clues and meaning for others.

• The role of participants as collaborators ensured that our colleagues, like research participants, invested more than a passing interest in the project and became emotionally involved as a result (Ford & Reutter 1989).

• The role of researcher can be likened to our role as facilitators within the group, where we become more than **objective** researchers by living the experience too.

• Consider the notion of prereflectivity, i.e. how we experience the 'here and now' rather than as a reflection afterwards. Prereflectivity enables us to understand the 'lived experience' in the here and now but also its changing nature as it is translated into 'data'.

• Phenomenological interpretation: look at the richness and variety of the data collected but also its personal or subjective nature. Many of our colleagues described individual and unique experiences in relation to the pictures but also common themes about the pictures began to emerge, such as fear, peace, purity.

Activity 3: Organizing and analysing the data; developing 'findings'

Once recurrent themes for each picture were identified, we took our colleagues through the procedural steps of organizing and analysing phenomenological data in order to generate findings. We outline those procedures below.

- From your observation and subsequent understanding of the picture you selected, you will begin to see themes emerging. Compare this process with the development of themes in Veronica's study (Box 5.8).

- Attempt to cluster and categorize your interpretations and feelings into themes. Themes involve the search for common threads which frequently appear and help to describe the experience (Van Manen 1990).

- You can also try to write a description of the experience, looking at it from all angles and using all the available information by developing themes that characterize the phenomenon. Van Manen (1984) suggests that one way of accessing experiences is by writing about them. He says 'responsive-reflective writing is the very activity of doing phenomenology. Writing and re-writing is the thing' (p. 68). In other words we experience the phenomenon by writing about it.

- See what happens when you compare your observations with those of others to see whether they come up with the same interpretations and reactions to the pictures as you.

Feedback from Activity 3

During our session, the pictures by Van Gogh and Constable produced several common themes whereas Botticelli's, which was much less familiar, did not. Art is a powerful medium and is open to wide interpretation in the same way as our own opinions and experience colour our living, practice and teaching.

Key learning points:

- As teachers or practitioners, we need to use creative insight to understand the meaning of the phenomenon being transmitted either through a visual image or a person's words. Colaizzi (1978) calls these formulated meanings (Fig. 5.1).

- Look at the emerging themes and clusters and/or try to produce an exhaustive written description of the phenomenon, as prescribed in Figure 5.1.

- This process could be used to develop a clear picture of what a phenomenon like breathlessness means to an asthmatic patient or a person with chronic bronchitis.

Morse & Field (1995) give the following example from Clarke's (1992) study entitled *Memories of Breathing: A Phenomenological Dialogue: Asthma as a Way of Becoming*: 'the reader can identify with the mother's and daughter's experience of managing asthma. The reader does not have to be an asthmatic to sense the essence of breathlessness, the mother's concern, and the daughter's attempts to "not panic" (to appear normal) and devise ways to take her breathalyzer inconspicuously in the presence of her peers' (p. 152).

• Consider the role of the researcher in handling difficult and inaccessible data and yet remaining true to it. In our session each individual had exchanged observations and interpretations with other colleagues. We used this activity to draw attention to the responsibility researchers have in phenomenological research when making interpretations about participants' experiences. The researcher's formulated meanings about a phenomenon (in this case a picture) should not decontextualize those of the participants.

Activity 4: Confirming the truth: validity (credibility) and generalizability (transferability)

If you have been carrying out this exercise as we did, now see what happens when you give your categorized or descriptive data to people who have not seen the picture. Find out whether they come up with the same interpretations or have the same reactions to it as you. You may want to consider the problems of interpreting other people's experience. Think about factors that affect the accuracy of your interpretation and analysis and the **validity (credibility)** and **generalizability (transferability)** of your findings to other people and places.

Morse & Field (1995) write: 'Validity (in phenomenological research) rests in the richness of the discussion. Does the description of essence make sense to anyone else?' or, citing Ray (1994), 'Does it make sense within the context of nursing practice?' (p. 23).

The re-interpretations of the categorized or descriptive data are then returned to the original 'owners' for scrutiny and confirmation of their truth and accuracy. In this way we were following Oiler's (1981) recommendation for testing validity by checking whether 'findings are recognized by those who had the experience'.

We were conscious of the need to be sensitive and supportive when returning 'findings' to the original participants. We wanted to be sure that nobody got upset on seeing them, since we can never know what associations a particular phenomenon has for others. In phenomenological research, the researcher needs to be particularly aware of this when exposing participants to 'findings' in order to confirm their validity (credibility), since a participant may thereby relive an upsetting experience.

Key learning points:

• Validity (credibility): we achieve validity by examining the lived experience as the participant sees it. In phenomenology the validity of the findings may be confirmed by the individual participant. Similarly in our practice, our interpretation of an experience, say the sudden collapse of a patient, may be unique to us but our account may also have resonances for others who witnessed the same event. They will also bring their own unique perceptions of the experience.

Validity or credibility of phenomenological research may also be confirmed by readers who subsequently recognize an experience in the clinical setting, which they had previously only read about, such as Field's (1981) description of the experience of giving an injection.

• Generalizability (transferability): if an experience is so unique to an individual it may be impossible to transfer it to other situations. On the other hand, the description of a phenomenon may provoke the response that 'it's like that for me too' (Morse 1991) allowing you to apply the findings to your own situation. Beck (1992) shows how the development of themes and concepts about post-partum depression (presented in Box 5.4) may be used to generate findings that are transferable to other women outside the **sample** who are also suffering from post-partum depression.

Generalizability or transferability of phenomenological research may also be confirmed when the findings concur with those of existing studies.

• Research mindedness is promoted by encouraging practitioners and teachers to make links between the process and findings of phenomenological research in order to build on and develop their existing knowledge about sensitive and hidden experiences and encourage students to do the same.

Case study summary

The case study demonstrates the experience of using art to reflect on the process and value of the phenomenological research approach. You may still be left with the question of whether art is appropriate to demonstrate and interpret the approach. In our session, a variety of interpretations arose from the same pictures, which demonstrated how different the same phenomenon may appear to different individuals. We need therefore to ask in what way our upbringing, beliefs and values affect our interpretation of events.

Art was felt by most of our colleagues to provide an experience that was safe in which to explore feelings in a meaningful and in-depth way. The session reaffirmed that phenomenology provides a systematic approach with which to uncover and describe the essence of a variety of phenomena and give richness and meaning to our care. It also demonstrated the relevance of phenomenology to reflection on practice.

Being able to build on your existing knowledge and experience may enable you to develop concepts about phenomena at your own pace and for them to contribute to your practice. We, for example, utilized our own experiences of undertaking phenomenological research as well as art to demonstrate the approach. Similarly, practitioners and teachers can use their clinical and pedagogic experience as the basis for developing phenomenological insights.

The complexity and rigour of the approach was demonstrated as a way of justifying and valuing existing phenomenological research as part of promoting research mindedness. Two very distinctive approaches were developed in the session to encourage an appreciation of phenomenology: (1) the everyday phenomenological view of the world through the use of art and experience; and (2) the appreciation of its rigour through reviewing contemporary research studies, such as those of Field (1981), Benner (1984) and Beck (1992).

REFLECTIONS FOR PRACTICE

The practitioner or teacher is able to use phenomenology as an ongoing way of life to examine daily experiences as lived phenomena, without necessarily conducting research. Rather, phenomenology can be built into our practice to give us a unique perspective on the way we view everyday experiences as part of 'research mindedness'.

We can use it to conduct one-off case studies of situations in which we find ourselves with our clients or students, involving ourselves as we did with the pictures to 'stay right in there' in the world we share with others (Van Manen 1990). Anxiety surrounding the admission of a child to hospital might be one such example during which we try to keep close to the experience of the young patient and his or her parents.

Phenomenology as a research approach is appropriate when researching areas of health care where data are rich but difficult to document and describe and consequently under-researched. By virtue of its existential nature, phenomenology examines the 'here and now' and is not dependent on conducting a literature review first. Hence, a lack of information to provide a starting point is not the barrier it is to some research approaches.

However, the word 'phenomenology' may itself be off-putting to practitioners, teachers and students. In order to overcome this, we prefer to describe phenomenology as the 'talk–taste–live experience'. We found in our session that, by referring to phenomenology in this way, our colleagues were motivated to discover more about it as a research approach and their participation was enhanced. Difficult issues such as bracketing and data analysis need to be well illustrated to demonstrate their significance. Relating them to existing studies may therefore be of benefit, to compare with the process of describing, analysing and developing findings from a work of art or a piece of literature.

We were able to show by referring to our own studies (Corben 1992, Stephenson 1993) the systematic and rigorous methods of phenomenological research for collecting and analysing data (presented in Boxes 5.7 and 5.8) and its value to the practice of health care. The perennial complaint that qualitative research lacks rigour could be laid to rest by examining studies which demonstrate phenomenological methods in action rather than in principle.

Phenomenological research can be used by expert practitioners with clinical credibility to demonstrate the approach to others and as a means of bridging the theory–practice gap (McCaugherty 1992). Phenomenology's power as a research approach and method lies in its being rooted in practice and experience which enables the practitioner to examine care provision in a research-minded way. Used in this way, phenomenology also demonstrates that learning is a lifelong dynamic process.

CONCLUSION

Throughout the chapter, we have attempted to highlight how phenomenology can be seen as part of everyday experience and a way of looking at the world both personally and professionally. Until now, you may have viewed research as esoteric and the domain of the enlightened few. We feel that phenomenology is different. It provides a valuable philosophical perspective that is accessible to teacher, mentor, practitioner or student. An awareness of this qualitative research approach enables us to understand the richness of the lived experience and develop the quality of the care we give.

For us, the use of phenomenology to promote research mindedness has two facets. One is the adaptation to a research-led way of life, by which we continue to develop nursing knowledge through researching 'ordinary' experiences. The other is the awareness associated with using existing studies to help us to value these as a means of improving our own professional development. In either case, we do not necessarily need to conduct research ourselves. By being mindful of where others have trodden using phenomenological research, we can use it as a springboard for future action.

REFERENCES

Beck C T 1992 The lived experience of post-partum depression: a phenomenological study. Nursing Research 41(3): 166–170

Benner P 1984 From novice to expert: excellence and power in clinical nursing practice. Addison-Wesley, Menlo Park, California

Camus A 1960 The plague, 2nd edn. Penguin, Aylesbury

Clarke M 1992 Memories of breathing: a phenomenological dialogue: asthma as a way of becoming. In: Morse J M (ed) Qualitative health research. Sage, Newbury Park, California, pp 123–140

Colaizzi P 1978 Psychological research as the phenomenologist views it. In: Valle R, King M (eds) Existential phenomenological alternatives for psychology. Oxford University Press, New York, pp 48–71

Corben V C 1992 The lived experience of the bank nurse. Unpublished dissertation. Buckinghamshire College of Higher Education

Department of Health and Social Security 1972 Report of the Committee on Nursing (Chair: Professor Asa Briggs). HMSO, London

Field P A 1981 A phenomenological look at giving an injection. Journal of Advanced Nursing 6: 291–296

Field P A, Morse J M 1985 Nursing research: the application of qualitative approaches. Chapman & Hall, London

Ford J S, Reutter L J 1989 Ethical dilemmas associated with small samples. Journal of Advanced Nursing 15: 187–191

Forrest D 1989 The experience of caring. Journal of Advanced Nursing 14: 815–923

Heidegger M 1977 Reflections on truth. Harper Row, New York

McCaugherty D 1992 Integrating theory & practice. Senior Nurse 12(1): 36–39

Morse J M (ed) 1991 Qualitative nursing research: a contemporary dialogue. Sage, Newbury Park

Morse J M, Bottorff J L, Hutchinson S 1994 The phenomenology of comfort. Journal of Advanced Nursing 20: 184–195

Morse J M, Field P A 1995 Qualitative research methods for health professionals, 2nd edn. Sage, Thousand Oaks

Nightingale F 1859 Notes on nursing. In: Skretowicz V (ed) Notes on nursing. Scutari, London

Oiler C 1981 The phenomenological approach in nursing research. Nursing Research 31(3): 178–181

Omery A 1983 Phenomenology: a method for nursing research. Advances in Nursing Science 5(2): 49–63

Parse R R, Coyne A B, Smith M J 1985 Nursing research: qualitative methods. Bowie, Maryland

Ray M A 1994 The richness of phenomenology: philosophic, theoretic and methodologic concerns. In: Morse J M (ed) Critical issues in qualitative research methods. Sage, Thousand Oaks, pp 117–133

Reed J 1994 Phenomenology without phenomena, a discussion of the use of phenomenology to examine expertise in long-term care of elderly patients. Journal of Advanced Nursing 19: 330–341

Schon D A 1987 Educating the reflective practitioner. Towards a new design for teaching and learning in the professions. Jossey-Bass, San Francisco

Stephenson C N 1993 A qualitative report of a phenomenological study of the experiences of spouses living with an elderly functionally mentally ill sufferer. Unpublished dissertation. Anglia Polytechnic University

Van Manen M 1984 Practising phenomenological writing. Phenomenology + Pedagogy 2(1): 36–69

Van Manen M 1990 Researching the lived experience: human science for an action sensitive pedagogy. Althouse, Ontario

FURTHER READING

Koch T 1995 Interpretive approaches in nursing research: the influence of Husserl and Heidegger. Journal of Advanced Nursing 21: 827–836

Ethnomethodology

Benny Goodman   Frank Strange

6

■ **KEY ISSUES**

- **Everyday nursing practice is the focus of study**
- **Assumptions and taken-for-granted behaviours in nursing practice are highlighted**
- **Ethnomethodology is identified as a means of fostering a critical approach to social and nursing science**
- **What counts as sound scientific knowledge for nursing practice is questioned**

PREAMBLE

The aim of this chapter is to examine the meaning of ethnomethodology for health professionals, and more particularly, its relevance for research-based practice. We believe that the critical and alternative approach to social science adopted by ethnomethodologists can be utilized to help us understand more fully the human condition and the nature of nursing work. This chapter, like the others in this book, grew from the presentation and review of a session which took place at the Institute of Advanced Nursing Education at the Royal College of Nursing.

The session was entitled 'Ethnomethodology' and was part of the 'Promoting research mindedness' module. We conducted the session by getting the group to examine which features they thought would lead to a death being classed as suicide. We did this so as to examine how 'social facts' are constructed. This is in contrast to Durkheim (1897) and the positivists, who contend that we can treat social **phenomena** (such as suicide) as value-free social facts which are open to scientific measurement and analysis. We argued that suicide should not be studied as a measurable 'fact' but rather as something constructed by society, especially coroners. We applied a similar argument to examine how nursing concepts such as the 'bad patient' are constructed. The middle part of the session involved looking at the historical development of ethnomethodology, its current stance and relationship to the rest of social science. We concluded by looking at examples of nursing research from the perspective of ethnomethodology.

INTRODUCTION

In this chapter, we have followed a format similar to other chapters in this book. We begin by discussing why we chose ethnomethodology as a way to promote research mindedness and what that means to us. This is followed by an examination of the ethnomethodological perspective to ensure that the reader is familiar with its central concerns. The discussion involves looking at the philosophical underpinnings of both ethnomethodology and of science. The relevance of ethnomethodology to clinical practice, research and teaching is also addressed. In the final section we present some critical reflections on the understanding and use of ethnomethodology for ourselves and in practice.

ETHNOMETHODOLOGY AND RESEARCH MINDEDNESS

The contribution of ethnomethodology is to bring to light a set of important, unexamined and unarticulated background assumptions.

(Tilley 1980)

Ethnomethodology is a branch of sociology created by Howard Garfinkel (1967), and is a relatively new approach to the study of the production of knowledge in the social sciences. The term literally means 'the study of people's methods' and its aim is to understand the everyday world in which we live. It developed from the dissatisfaction that some social scientists had with the traditional scientific **method** as applied to the study and understanding of people.

Just a brief word here about ethnography, which is a related research approach but should not be confused with ethnomethodology. **Ethnography**, a subdiscipline of anthropology, is also concerned with the study of people but has traditionally taken a broader approach than ethnomethodology. Ethnography is the detailed study of small groups such as gangs, nurses, patients and their subcultures in a range of settings such as hospitals and housing estates. The ethnographer concentrates on in-depth case studies to understand local worlds at the level of group cultures rather than individual, face-to-face interactions.

Ethnomethodology, on the other hand, sees our understanding as being constructed by personal as well as social experiences. It sets itself the task, therefore, of describing the means by which we create and reproduce our social world at the level of our everyday face-to-face interactions. Normally, our interactions with one another occur quite smoothly. If an acquaintance enquires of me 'How are you?', I do not give a detailed account of my medical status. I merely reply, 'Fine, thanks'. I know without really thinking about it that the request was not for a medical history but that the acquaintance was just passing the time of day.

It is these taken-for-granted rules and assumptions that contribute to the 'commonsense view' which helps our everyday lives run more smoothly. Fairclough (1989) sees common sense as underpinning **ideologies**, which can be thought of as shared bodies of ideas that reflect the beliefs of a culture or group. The right to free speech could be considered as a widely accepted ideology in western culture. Fairclough thinks that ideological ideas, such as organizing people in hierarchies, have their origins as a doctrine. If the doctrine or ideology is accepted by the powerful, then it becomes part of everyday language. The repetition and unquestioning acceptance of the ideology mean that what started out as an idea eventually becomes accepted as the commonsense view of the world.

This commonsense view of the world that we all share is what ethnomethodology looks at in an attempt to examine how it becomes created, recreated and accepted as the unquestioned way that things are. It is the commonsense view that affects many of our perceptions of what is 'normal' or the right way of doing things.

The Royal College of Nursing (1982) considers that research mindedness 'implies a critical and questioning approach to one's work, the desire and ability to find out about the latest research in that area and apply it as appropriate'. According to this definition, research mindedness can be seen as consisting of three factors: a critical approach; the ability to appreciate the value or otherwise of some research; and the skill of using research in practice. The ethnomethodological perspective is critical in that it levels criticism mainly at the traditional methodology and assumptions of social science.

Ethnomethodology's contribution to research mindedness therefore helps us to examine background assumptions when critically questioning practice. Knowledge and reality in nursing come from socially created phenomena, which ethnomethodology then seeks to uncover. The **positivist paradigm** in nursing science gives a partial explanation at best and, at worst, distorts the nature of knowledge and therefore of practice. **Positivism** approaches the study of social phenomena in very much the same way as the natural world is studied by physicists, biologists and chemists, i.e. by **objective observation**, **measurement** and the development of **theory** on the basis of causal laws (see Ch. 2 for a fuller discussion of positivism).

This classical view of knowledge, by which only science can explain the world, strongly contests the validity of alternative perspectives. Whilst some social scientists accept that there are alternative and equally valid perspectives on knowledge and the world, many perceive knowledge as an unchanging entity, existing independently of human experience. These differences of opinion are also demonstrated by the heated debates associated with **qualitative** and **quantitative** research **methodologies**. The aim of this chapter is not to become involved in this ongoing and unresolved debate, however, since it has been discussed at some length in Chapter 2. Instead, we wish to present the benefits of examining how scientists, like the lay public, use unexamined knowledge about the world in their scientific theorizing.

At this point you may be thinking 'what has this got to do with my nursing work or understanding of research?' As practising health care workers it is valuable to understand that, like some scientists, we may also hold on tightly to particular ways of knowing. Becoming research minded means freeing ourselves, if possible, from restrictive thought processes, to engage critically in examination of ourselves and to make explicit our assumptions and values. This may well be too much to ask, but is at the heart of the search for knowledge and professional practice.

To many social scientists, the criticisms of traditional scientific method within the social sciences are justified. The application of the scientific method to surveys, questionnaires and statistical analysis has not resulted in the same 'success' as when used in the physical sciences to solve physics and engineering problems. For Kessen (1991) the failure of science to solve the social problems of the human condition leads to the need to do two things: first, to re-examine the methods scientists use to describe and explain the world; and second, to examine how knowledge is socially 'constructed' when people interact.

The social construction of knowledge leads to alternative ways of perceiving the world. For example, we could use religion to describe the world as God's creation. 'God' could be used as an explanation for anything from the origin of humanity to individual events such as the birth of babies with congenital abnormalities. Alternatively, we could follow Darwin's teachings on evolution and survival of the fittest to think about the origins of the species and the low survival rate of babies with congenital abnormalities.

Religious and scientific world-views are products of the society in which they occur. Ideas have no independent existence from the human beings who create them: they are 'constructed' and shared socially. The **social constructionist perspective**, which views the individual as the builder of perceptions that are strongly culturally influenced, fits comfortably with the view that situations are both indexical and reflexive. These concepts, referred to as '**indexicality**' and '**reflexivity**', are central to the ethnomethodological approach and we will return to them in more detail later. Because they are so important to our understanding of ethnomethodology we have provided short explanations of these concepts in Box 6.1.

The value of ethnomethodology (as a way of thinking) for promoting research mindedness is that not only is it critical but its perspective is at the level of individual interactions that take place in the everyday world. Such a perspective could be beneficial for nurses whose practice is very much focused on individual patients and their interpretations of what is happening to them. Ethnomethodology can be used to examine how we as nurses construct such concepts as 'quality of life', 'attachment' and 'good care' which we use in research as real and measurable entities. The approach can also be valuable in examining how people construct their beliefs about health, illness and disease. It has been argued (Becker & Rosenstock 1984) that the development of health beliefs has a reflexive and indexical quality. Such a perspective, involving criticism, examination and application to practice, fulfils the RCN (1982) aims of promoting research mindedness, and therefore ethnomethodology can be regarded as being a valuable and alternative perspective with some explanatory power.

Ethnomethodology is as much a way of thinking as a research tool. Bowers (1992) argues that it involves taking a philosophical position on the production of knowledge. Perhaps we need to go further and say that, as a 'critical' mode of thinking, ethnomethodology forces examination of some of our cherished assumptions and practices and an analysis of nursing's position within wider society. This position moves on from the early pioneers of ethnomethodology who focused on the everyday practices without analysing why we practice as we do or recognize the external

---

■ **BOX 6.1**

Indexicality

Indexicality is a central concept within ethnomethodology. It refers to the need to take into account the context around words and phrases to give us meaning. All words and phrases are indexical. To understand anything we have to know the context within which they are spoken. The phrase 'how are you?' means one thing when a friend asks at a casual meeting, and another when a general practitioner asks at a surgery. This is because the context of a chance encounter with a friend differs from that of meeting a professional for a consultation. If you remove the context from around the words, their precise meaning is lost.

Reflexivity

Reflexivity of accounts refers to the process whereby our knowledge of our social world explains and is explained at one and the same time. We continually engage in procedures to account for the world, i.e. to explain it. These accounts are reflexive. When we come across a 'bad' patient we know this because we use an 'account' to tell us that this particular patient is 'bad'. This account incorporates ideas about bad patients such as noncompliance, i.e. 'bad' patients do not do as they are told, do not take their medication on time or complain about the hospital food. This reflexive account both explains that the patient before us is 'bad' whilst at the same time the behaviour of this particular 'bad' patient confirms that the account is correct.

---

social constraints on behaviour. The recent example of the nurse who performed an appendicectomy, albeit on the advice of the attending surgeon, is a case in point. Her action created a huge debate around accountability and legality, about why nurses can extend their roles to perform certain functions and not others. The decisions are made by those who are more powerful in medical and nursing hierarchies.

Ethnomethodology has been seriously criticized because of its failure to address the issue that our methods for making sense of the world and our thought patterns are conducted within a system of social relationships involving differences of power. That is to say that there are external constraints upon us which may limit choice, not just in action but also in ways of thinking. The nurse who performed the appendicectomy thought that she would be protected by her medical colleague and her years of experience as an operating theatre sister during which she had performed similar procedures.

Another example is that of a child born into a society committed to a particular regime, such as Nazism during 1930s Germany. The child is restricted by the predominant ideology and culture of the society in which he or she is growing up, which may be reinforced at home and at school. This limits the child's exposure to other ideas and world-views. In any society that espouses fundamentalist ideas (e.g. women are inferior; certain races and religions are superior), open criticism of alternative world-views such as feminism and egalitarianism is unlikely, so that the child's opportunities for developing alternative perspectives are limited.

ETHNOMETHODOLOGY:
THREE PHILOSOPHICAL TRADITIONS

To understand ethnomethodology's approach, it is worth examining its historical development in relation to theories about knowledge. Habermas, a distinguished German sociologist, social philosopher and critical theorist (1984), does not consider knowledge to be a fixed and unchanging entity. Rather, it can be seen as a creation arrived at through experience and various approaches to its production. As you saw in Chapter 2, the means by which we arrive at ways of knowing about the world are traditionally classified into three types: the positivist, the interpretive hermeneutic and critical theory. The need to seek alternative perspectives to knowledge production, over and above positivism, grew from an increasing realization that science did not have the answer to all the world's problems, especially those with a social origin. This realization has been referred to as the failure of the positivist dream (Kessen 1991). We shall now briefly define each of these approaches so that you can see how they differ from each other.

Positivism

The positivist or empirical approach to knowledge is rooted in methods of science. Scientific method is based on **empiricism** (a word closely related to experiment and experience) in order to establish the factual basis of knowledge through careful, detached, objective measurement, followed by **replication** and the confirmation of recurring patterns and relationships within the data. Positivist **philosophy** perceives the universe as deterministic or lawful and the role of science is to discover the causes or determinants of particular events. This philosophy also underpins positivism in social science and is elaborated in Box 6.2 in relation to Durkheim's work on suicide.

■ **BOX 6.2**

Emile Durkheim (1897), a French sociologist, produced a major piece of work on suicide as an example of the use of a positive science of society and argued that we treat social facts as 'objects'. Therefore, we could treat social life as a topic to be used for research, using a methodology similar to that of the natural sciences. The same positivist 'way of knowing' (also referred to as epistemology) creeps into nursing research when we assume that nursing is 'out there' waiting to be discovered and analysed, or feel that knowledge is a fixed entity, awaiting discovery (Rogers 1989). The positivist approach may work for inanimate objects. However, even this has been questioned, as in the field of quantum physics, where assumptions of predictability and causal laws are being challenged (Capra 1984).

Durkheim examined suicide rates to theorize about what makes particular groups more prone to taking their own lives than other groups. This form of thinking suggests that something in the social structure (in this case religion or class) affects behaviour. The social structure, i.e. our location within it, such as our class position, has an effect on individual behaviour. Durkheim used the official statistics on suicide rates as a resource for his theories in order to make his own interpretations from the data.

However, Durkheim's research fails to address the real issue, and that is: 'How does a death get categorized as a suicide in the first place?' By failing to address this, the commonsense procedures adopted by coroners get incorporated unexamined into the research process. As Atkinson (1971, 1978) argues, suicide is 'created' by coroners who use a mixture of scientific and lay theories to classify a death as suicide. Therefore, any examination of why suicide occurs using the official statistics will incorporate unexamined lay theories.

Interpretive hermeneutics

The interpretive hermeneutic approach is both a theory of and a method for interpreting meaningful human action. Its concern is with obtaining an authentic version of actions or creations, through behaviour, books or pictures. The approach developed from the problems encountered when interpreting biblical text. These problems arose, not just in the sense of translating text from the original Greek and Hebrew into English but in understanding the meanings of the words and phrases themselves. The term 'Yahweh' in Hebrew translates into 'I am' in English, but the meaning of that phrase is not the same in the two languages. Yahweh does not merely refer to anyone's state of being but to some unfathomable aspect of God. This understanding can only be reached by unpicking the meanings held by the original authors.

Scholars who used these approaches found that they needed to consider the experiences of the author as well as the text itself. To obtain an authentic version of the text, the researcher adopts a subjective perspective which involves consideration of the lived experience of the person or group under study. As noted in Chapter 5, the consideration of the lived experience is also a concern of phenomenology.

When Jesus is referred to as the 'Lamb of God' it is necessary to grasp the understandings and meanings ascribed to that phrase by early Jewish writers to fully comprehend its meaning. It is not an insult. The writer is not describing Jesus as a little woolly animal but refers to Jesus as God's ultimate sacrifice, as in the Old Testament. This true interpretation would be lost without understanding what the original writer meant.

The hermeneutic method is twofold. First, it involves analysis of the relationship between the creator of an act and the person interpreting it. Secondly, it requires analysis of the act in relationship to the wider whole that gives it meaning. For example, a painting could be understood by reference to the political, economic or cultural context in which it was produced. You might argue that today's artistic culture, which produces buildings made of steel and glass and abstract paintings, is a reaction to older styles of past decades.

Critical theory

Critical theory is a form of social analysis which, as its name implies, entails the exercise of critical judgement. Its aims are to uncover the hidden assumptions and value judgements that underpin the dominant ideologies of a group and debunk their claim to authority. Some researchers and activists such as Brazil's Paulo Freire (1987) argue that a critical approach can be empowering as it enables people to examine the forces that shape their hierarchical and social relationships within society. Franz Boas (cited in Fairclough 1989) summarizes the empowering and releasing nature of a critical perspective in a rhetorical question and answer. He asks: 'How do we recognise the shackles that tradition has placed upon us? For if we can recognise them, we are also able to break them' (Fairclough 1989, p. 1). In nursing terms, once we realize through critical examination that ritualistic practice may be shaped by hierarchical relations, then we may be free to change.

ETHNOMETHODOLOGY: SCIENCE AS KNOWLEDGE OR IDEOLOGY

Ethnomethodology grew from humanistic and phenomenological traditions but incorporates a more critical perspective. Its methods and perspectives, therefore, share features of both interpretive hermeneutics and the critical way of knowing. Morris (1977) thinks that all ethnomethodologists share two key assumptions: first, that we are not merely acted upon by social forces, but constantly shape and create our own social world through interaction with others; second, that special methods are needed for studying the human condition. Both these assumptions arise from the traditions from which ethnomethodology developed. The **interpretive hermeneutic approach** acknowledges subjectivity and perceives the physical world of nature as different from the social world of culture. This difference is neither recognized nor acknowledged in the scientific objective approach which has traditionally dominated medicine and nursing.

In the natural sciences (physics, chemistry, biology), the elements studied are devoid of meaning for the elements concerned. Stones and atoms do not have emotions. Humans, however, assign meaning to actions. When we see a person drop a cup, we can interpret it as an accident or say that it was dropped on purpose; we attribute meaning to the action, describing it as accident or design, which in turn affects future action. However, the stance of formalized detached science is remote from this, and social scientists tend to view social settings as 'out there' and independent of people's actions at any given moment.

Alfred Schutz (1972), who combined phenomenology and sociology, suggests that social scientists employ a different type of **construct** or **concept** when practising science. Constructs are things whose existence is inferred from our observations. Their existence is as yet unproven because the evidence is not yet available. The gene is a classic example of a thing that started as a construct and was later found to have existence in the physical world. Social scientists such as Schutz often use the terms construct and concept interchangeably. A construct is a concept that has been given a more systematic definition to enable scientific hypothesizing and measurement in the 'real' world. Therefore a construct has qualities that allow it to be measured.

Schutz refers to the constructs that scientists use as **second degree constructs**. Second degree constructs are theoretical terms like 'attachment' and 'quality of life', which social scientists construct to help explain the world. They then proceed to measure and analyse them in a scientific way. People usually operate in the commonsense world of **first degree constructs**; terms like 'attachment' and 'quality of life' mean something different to them.

Stress is a lay concept that has many meanings in everyday speech (Schutz's first degree construct) but the scientist needs a more precise definition, an **operational definition**, to allow investigation to proceed (Schutz's second degree construct). An example is Selye's (1956) 'general adaptation syndrome', which tries to define stress in a particular way. The use of the word construct is to point out that concepts do not have independent existence and meanings outside of human beings. We collectively and individually 'build' or construct meanings and concepts both as lay persons and scientists.

According to Garfinkel (1967), a sociologist and 'father' of ethnomethodology, we make sense of social situations as they proceed. Each of us brings our personal experiences or resources to the situation, but it is through the interaction and the context that we construct our understanding of what is going on. To ethnomethodologists, each social situation is ongoing and different, which they refer to as the 'reflexivity' and 'indexicality' of situations (see Box 6.1). Hence, in order to classify a patient as a 'good' patient, we resort to our understanding of what for us constitutes a 'good' patient. This understanding depends on context and taken-for-granted assumptions. However, researchers may use the words 'good' and 'bad' as second degree constructs to mean something different to everyday understandings.

Causality, the laws of cause and effect as applied to the social sciences, can be seen to be more than a mechanistic linear relationship between A (the cause) and B (the effect). The interpretative process is also required to understand that relationship. For example, we are not merely acted upon by social forces (e.g. our class position determining which kind of schools we go to) but we actively engage in interpreting what our education means in our everyday experiences and the bearing it has on our choice of schools. This process includes the use of human qualities such as motives, beliefs and attitudes, which many social scientists believe can be measured in a rigorous, detached and scientific manner but which ethnomethodology denies.

Schutz and the ethnomethodologists believe that the scientific analysis of concepts such as 'motivation' and 'attitude' are not possible, because of the differences that exist between everyday life and scientific theorizing. The everyday life in which we live is embedded in the here and now, it is ongoing and is the accomplishment of interaction.

As we have stated, Garfinkel (1967) considers behaviour to be 'indexical', i.e. dependent on context for its meaning. The situation or context in which we find ourselves can be a powerful influence on our behaviour and, more importantly, on our understanding of the behaviour of others. Our behaviours vary depending on whether we are in the workplace or at home. If you were to treat your relatives as though they were your patients, they would be surprised and confused, especially if you attempted to take their temperatures and pulses every 6 hours. A behaviour pattern that is acceptable in one context is not deemed appropriate in another and is governed by rules that are taken for granted and assumed.

It is these taken-for-granted rules that patients follow when they allow intimate examinations of their bodies to be undertaken by health care professionals (Lawler 1991). The nurse's uniform or the doctor's white coat, the clinical setting and the experience of sickness are the context that permits such examinations. Change the context and the rules change. A white coat elsewhere means something different. Bowers (1992) describes how this process works with community psychiatric nurses (CPNs) visiting clients at home. The home setting changes the nature of the interaction between the nurses and the client. Importantly, it changes the nature of the power relations between them, because the CPN is now the 'invited guest' in the client's home. You can read Len Bowers' ethnomethodological account of home visits made by CPNs in Box 6.3.

■ **BOX 6.3**

Bowers argues that home visits are socially constructed events in the sense that talk depends upon the setting and context. In this case the context of the home exerts pressure upon the events, i.e. being a visitor defines the CPN's visit as that of a meeting of friends. The participants draw upon the stock of knowledge that typifies the behaviour of hosts and guest to conduct the visit and to set the scene. The power relations are altered because the setting for the visit is the patient's home. The patient is firmly in charge which allows him/her to take the lead at every turn. Only in matters seen by both participants as clearly related to medicopsychiatric issues will the nurse become more assertive.

Behaviour, and our understanding of it, also vary depending on whether we are subjects in experiments or just interacting with friends. The power of context can be simply demonstrated. Look at Figure 6.1: the middle character is either the letter 'B' or the number '13', depending on whether the figure is read vertically or horizontally. Just as the home context helped to define the interaction between the CPN and the client as described by Bowers, so the context of a list of numbers or a list of letters defines the middle character as a 'B' or '13'.

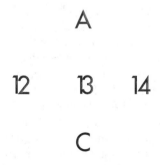

Figure 6.1 The power of context: the central symbol can be perceived as either the letter B or the number 13 depending upon whether it is read as part of a sequence of letters or numbers.

Not only do ethnomethodologists have a different perspective on the nature of knowledge and the value of science, but their level of investigation also differs. Whereas some social scientists are more concerned with things at the broader, macro- or societal level, ethnomethodologists are concerned with events at the micro- (individual) level. For health care professionals who engage with people at the individual or micro-level, the questioning and critical approach adopted by ethnomethodologists can be a useful and alternative means of shedding light on the human condition. We need to understand the individual contexts and interactions within which practice takes place. Generalized statements about patient care do not help us predict with any certainty what any one patient needs.

ETHNOMETHODOLOGY AND NURSING

We are now going to look at how the concepts of 'good' and 'bad' patients, suicide, blood pressure and physical intimacy can be looked at from an ethnomethodological viewpoint using the notions of indexicality and reflexivity. An important point to grasp is that we are dealing with the issue of historically dominant ways of thinking (i.e. the positivist) in nursing and social science. Therefore, by applying an alternative way of thinking, using what Heritage (1984) calls the 'social microscope', we may be able to see things that on the surface are hidden from us. For example, individualized care in nursing is a central concept, and it could be taken for granted that it is actually carried out in practice. An examination of practice may reveal that it exists as a guiding philosophy only.

A further example is Lawler's attempt to 'explore very deliberately what nurses know and take for granted' when dealing with the human body and to examine 'generalized social methods nurses use to manage the body' (Lawler 1991, p. 1). Lawler states a number of research questions that very clearly give the flavour of the ethnomethodological approach. For example, Question 4 asks 'how the *context* of care is *constructed* [italics added] so that it is socially permissible to touch the body to provide nursing care'. Question 1 asks 'How, in becoming nurses, they overcome what they have been socialised to believe about the body, body exposure, and body accessibility in our culture' (Lawler 1991, p. 7).

The ethnomethodological approach is also illustrated by Atkinson's (1971, 1978) work on suicide, and by Kelly & May (1984) who discuss the shortcomings of research into 'good and bad' patients which we discuss below.

Ethnomethodology seeks to uncover the **'accounting procedures'**, knowledge, and theories used by coroners when they engage in their work. An accounting procedure is the process we use to make sense of the world, drawing on everyday theories and commonsense taken-for-granted knowledge to 'socially construct' a phenomenon such as suicide. The suicide rate, therefore, is not an independent fact waiting to be discovered but a product of the accounting procedures that coroners engage in. The incidence of suicide, therefore, is dependent on how it is classified. Any research into suicide must, therefore, explain and describe the accounting procedure. In other words the researcher needs to examine the ways in which coroners take a death and classify it as suicide.

The investigation of everyday, taken-for-granted activity is explicitly addressed by Lawler (1991), who argues that there is a need to explore nurses' experiences as a 'window to the body' in order to understand 'how the body is constructed in social life' (p. 1). In the spirit of ethnomethodological enquiry, Lawler addresses the need to investigate the 'accounting procedures' she used in her study since 'the subject matter was familiar to me in the sense that I knew about these things in a way which had not yet been translated into language, that is, it was about the things I had learned *to take for granted* as a nurse, and which I wanted to be *made explicit*;' (Lawler 1991, p. 5, italics added). Put another way, Lawler was interested in the host of attitudes, assumptions, values and knowledge used during everyday nursing work that contributed to nurses' construction of the body. It is these constructs that need examining to discover more about the hidden, private and invisible parts of nurses' work. Lawler developed a theory from her data which she called 'somology'. Somology refers to the management of the body in nursing; it describes and explains the rules and taboos associated with how practitioners approach the human body.

Lawler's study shows us how the body and its meanings are constructed by nurses in the same way that suicide is constructed by coroners. To understand the way nurses interact with patients in intimate ways, the context (i.e. the indexical nature) and the accounting procedures (the reflexive nature) have to be made explicit.

We all have our taken-for-granted assumptions and commonsense knowledge on suicide and nursing on which we would agree. Why do we agree? What are our taken-for-granted assumptions and commonsense knowledge on suicide or nursing? Do we in fact share the same assumptions or would we in some instances disagree on what we define as nursing or suicide? We can explore this question further by taking another popular concept used by nurses, that of the 'good' and 'bad' patient. Kelly & May (1984), two sociologists, address our taken-for-granted assumptions in their critique of the literature on 'good' and 'bad' patients. We all know a good patient and a bad patient when we see one. But how do we go about classifying patients in this way? Kelly & May argue that in many of the studies that they looked at 'the assumption is that the readers share with the researcher a common universe of discourse in which ideas like good and bad, appreciative, wilful and manipulative, when applied to patients are unambiguous'(p. 151).

This statement presents us with a problem. If we were to list all the characteristics of a good or a bad patient, we may come up with a list that we all agree on. However, this is an assumption that requires further examination. Would we, in fact, all agree? We may agree on the words which should go on the list such as 'unappreciative' or 'noisy', but would we all totally agree on what these characteristics meant in real life? Kelly & May think not and argue for the close examination of the taken-for-granted aspects of medical and nursing interaction with patients, which they say was 'hardly examined in the nursing literature surveyed' (Kelly & May 1984, p. 151). In other words, they suggest that the quality of those interactions is affected by our unexamined assumptions about whether we see the patients we are relating to as 'good' or 'bad'.

The second difficulty about a list of characteristics is that each item is not an objective fact with an independent meaning. Rather, each characteristic derives its meanings from everyday use. In other words, the characteristics are social constructs, which could mean different things to different people and are open to change. Even apparently objective phenomena like symptoms and medical diagnosis are relative in that they are perceived differently from culture to culture and class to class (Helman 1990, Mitchell 1984, Shilts 1987), as is demonstrated in Box 6.4.

■ BOX 6.4

Randy Shilts, investigating the origins of the AIDS epidemic in the USA, clearly demonstrates how cultural values, mixed with uncertainty, muddy the waters of scientific investigation and categorization. Research was being carried out in both France (at the Institut Pasteur) and in the Center for Disease Control in the USA. Much of the American research focused on gay men, because the epidemic was first brought to notice in the gay communities in San Francisco, Los Angeles and New York. Shilts quotes Dr Jacques Leibowitch, working in Paris, who was 'curious to see that (AIDS) was promoted as a homosexual disease', putting it down to Americans' 'obsession with sex'. For the French scientists, a virus could not discern between the sexual orientation of its respective hosts (Shilts 1987, p. 103).

This example shows how scientists in the USA and France were influenced by their cultural settings and by the communities they worked with. The example also shows how even a seemingly 'objective fact' such as a disease category is open to different labels, interpretations and treatments. For a detailed discussion on culture, health and illness and how they interact we refer you to Helman (1990).

Taking another example, is blood pressure an objective fact? We can measure a patient's blood pressure and come up with a reading. But what does it mean? Pause and reflect on this question.

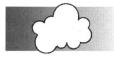

You may conclude that physiological concepts and disease categories are not necessarily facts. Helman (1990), a medical anthropologist, would certainly argue that culture and social background affects medical data and categorization. Citing the apparent predominance of chronic bronchitis in the UK and of emphysema in the USA, Helman argues that the same constellation of symptoms and signs are being diagnosed and labelled differently in the two countries. This example demonstrates that an apparently objective disease category is open to variable interpretation.

Returning to our example of blood pressure, how do we interpret the reading '150/90'? As you read this, you may be using your own stock of knowledge to give it meaning. A non-medical person in the USA may read and interpret '150/90' as a basketball score. The reading is therefore 'indexical', i.e. it depends on its context for interpretation. The context for health care professionals would be 'clinic' or 'hospital', with patient's age, medical condition, psychological status, medications and previous history all giving it further meaning. The figure is also 'reflexive' in that we make sense of it by reference to an 'underlying pattern' which would then indicate to the professional whether the patient could be diagnosed as having hypertension. This underlying pattern in nursing is created by a mixture of commonsense taken-for-granted knowledge and scientific knowledge of physiology.

We use these different forms of knowledge to create an 'underlying pattern' to make sense of the reading. If our underlying pattern includes the categories '75-year-old patient', then we adjust our interpretations of the blood pressure reading accordingly, since a reading of 150/90 is not considered high for a person of that age. We are, of course, simplifying the process that takes place, but just as a coroner categorizes a death by reference to the underlying pattern that explains suicide, so we categorize a reading by reference to the underlying pattern that explains blood pressures.

In order to understand this process it may help to detail it further. A coroner has had a case presented before him or her. Is this death a suicide or not? The underlying pattern would suggest that certain questions be asked based on the knowledge of what constitutes a suicide. For example, is there a suicide note? Was there a bottle of pills nearby? Does the deceased have a history of depression? If evidence is presented that fits this underlying pattern, then it not only suggests that a suicide has occurred but provides further confirmatory evidence that the underlying pattern is correct. The case is reflexive, because by referring to the underlying pattern, it both confirms and explains that a suicide has occurred. In other words, the coroner uses the underlying pattern associated with suicide to confirm or deny the case before him or her.

In the case of the blood pressure reading of 150/90 in the 75-year-old described above, we also used underlying patterns to make sense of the evidence. Underlying patterns by which we filled in the details, such as age, helped us to make a judgement as to whether the reading was indicative of hypertension. If a second case in which a blood pressure reading of 150/90 were obtained, and the details included '21-year-old patient with no previous medical history of hypertension', then our underlying pattern that 'young fit people do not have such high blood pressure readings' would lead us to conclude that the patient may have hypertension. If the same high reading on three separate occasions was obtained, then the truth value of the underlying pattern associated with hypertension would be confirmed.

The interest of the ethnomethodologist in all of these cases would be in how the underlying patterns to which we referred came into being. Helman (1990) suggests that one factor in the process is the cultural variability of interpretation by which practitioners actually come to make their decisions, a view shared by ethnomethodologists. We may ask 'how does this stock of knowledge used by practitioners get created and used in everyday life?' We would suggest that nurses engage in accounting procedures to make sense of a blood pressure reading and it is this accounting procedure and its cultural influences that is of interest to ethnomethodologists.

A simplified account of Durkheim's work as presented in Box 6.2 suggests that suicide rates vary for different social groups based on the official statistics. As argued, however, this is a distortion as the statistics were used as 'resource' and not as a 'topic' for research. The question should be: how does a death get categorized as suicide in the first place (as differing methods of categorizing lead to differing rates)? Similarly, the incidence of asthma in a population depends on how it is classified: what exact respiratory condition counts as an incidence of asthma? In nursing, how do we categorize anxious patients? If research states that information-giving reduces anxiety, what exactly do we mean? Ethnomethodologists would seek to uncover not only how nurses classify a patient as anxious but what they mean by information giving.

One of the few ethnomethodological studies in a health care setting is Sudnow's (1967) work on death and dying, in which he demonstrates that death as a category has social as well as physiological elements. Just as coroners construct suicide, so in a hospital setting death and dying are constructed and exist not just as physiological changes but involving a whole series of social interactions, meanings, definitions and practices carried out by health care workers. Death and dying, in this sense, are constructed by all the individuals involved.

Similarly, we may use an ethnomethodological approach to clarifying nursing practice as it actually happens rather than how it theoretically happens. Cash (1990) argues that nursing *is* what nurses *do*. Nurses themselves think they know what they do and some non-nurses think they know what nurses do (Griffin 1983), and nursing theorists create things such as a 'theory of nursing', or 'conceptual nursing models'. You will be familiar with a variety of nursing models and theories, such as Watson's theory of caring, Roper's model based on the 'activities of daily living'; Orem's self-help model or Roy's adaptation model. However, might it be a fundamental error to assume that these theories and models are fixed entities? The ethnomethodologist would suggest that it is misleading to assume that nursing is an objective category that is 'out there' waiting to be discovered and theorized about. Nursing is an ongoing social construction conceived daily by nurses as they interact and interpret everyday events in a variety of settings.

Instead of taking for granted certain categories or constructs, or imposing theoretical categories and constructs on to nursing, perhaps we should examine the everyday occurrence. Take the concept of caring which is central to nursing. Cash (1990) seems to suggest that this concept is not applicable to nursing alone but is shared among the other caring professions, such as social workers and teachers. If an activity is to be defined as nursing by the presence of caring, then any activity carried out by lay persons and professionals which also involves caring would have to be defined as nursing also. Caring as *the* defining concept of nursing is therefore not applicable. Cash's argument demonstrates the dangers in failing to examine, not just the theory but the actual practice of everyday concepts associated with nursing. Being research minded is when we seek to uncover the processes by which we all categorize and give meaning to concepts such as 'suicide', 'blood pressure', 'asthma', 'death', 'anxiety', 'information giving' and 'caring' and question their appropriateness.

CHALLENGE, CHANGE AND
THE LEARNING PROCESS

Ethnomethodology and its philosophical base can present a challenging view to some of our most cherished ideas about the world. This was certainly the case for us when we were planning our session on ethnomethodology to present to our peers. Our experience led us to reflect on how we get caught up in 'webs of our own making' (Lambert 1993) when trying to understand the world and the nature of nursing work. Do we dare venture 'out of the cave' and see the world as it might be? This analogy of a 'cave' can be found in Plato's *Republic* (Lambert 1993). We have summarized it below in Box 6.5.

■ BOX 6.5

Imagine a dark underground cave, at the mouth of which is a large fire. The light from the fire tries to penetrate the gloom inside the cave. Deep inside, there are people who are chained, unable to move around. The only thing that they can see is the cave wall which is illuminated by the fire outside. The light has the effect of throwing shadows on to the wall, and so, for those in the cave, these shadows become reality. The shadows are given characteristics and names as if they were real things. Knowledge and truth, for the cave dwellers, lie in the shadowy forms before them. They know no other world.

Suppose one of the cave dwellers were released from the chains and allowed to go outside. That person's world and reality would change dramatically. He or she would discover new things and perhaps come to see that the shadows were merely products of the light from the fire. A whole new world would open and provide the opportunity to see things in literally a different light. Things that were hidden before would now be seen and the cave dweller could begin asking a thousand different questions about this complex new world.

The cave dweller then goes back into the cave to tell the others of what has been experienced. Would they or could they listen? Their reality lives in the shadowy forms before them; they have no way of understanding what is being explained; they do not have the knowledge to help them gain real meaning from the new stories.

Lambert (1993) uses the analogy of the cave to argue that nurses often trap themselves in a web of their own making and that to free themselves they need to go outside the cave. The cave represents a well-established and traditional way of thinking, such as the medical dominance of health care and the influence of positivism in social and nursing sciences. The shadows can be seen as analogous to the images of nursing and nursing work that are created by the way nurses are occupationally socialized into particular modes of thinking.

These modes of thinking are characterized by such subjects as the biological and behavioural sciences, pharmacology, medicine and surgery, which are based on the traditional scientific method. Nursing knowledge or epistemology has traditionally been founded on the natural sciences such as biology or physiology. Carper (1978) argues, however, that nursing knowledge is far more complex than is commonly understood. Nursing knowledge does not rely exclusively on the disciplines just mentioned. Carper argues that there are four forms or ways of knowing that nurses draw upon. Nurses use scientific knowledge, personal knowledge, aesthetic knowledge and ethical knowledge during practice. For example, scientific knowledge views the patient as a physiological system and helps explain disease processes, whereas ethical knowledge is used to examine the moral and ethical dimensions of care. Benner (1984) discusses intuitive knowledge used by expert practitioners, which cannot always be explained in scientific terms or even explained by practitioners themselves. Intuitive knowledge, like Carper's aesthetic and personal knowledges, involves the use of feelings and experiences rather than textbook knowledge to make skilled judgements and decisions. How does ethnomethodology contribute to the knowledge debate? For some, it will mean an examination of the personal belief systems that underpin their own ideas of what science is. For others, it will allow a consideration of the nature of taken-for-granted knowledge. The case study that follows should allow you to look more closely at issues of science, knowledge and belief systems.

CASE STUDY

In our case study we take you through some of the issues raised when presenting a seminar on the contribution of ethnomethodology to research mindedness. We also draw on much of the material we have considered in the chapter so far to look at key concepts associated with ethnomethodology that can be used in everyday practice and teaching.

Taken-for-granted knowledge

Our first aim in our seminar was to introduce our peers to the subject of taken-for-granted knowledge. We asked them to imagine that if they were coroners, what information they would need to permit them to classify a death as a suicide. You will already be familiar with the stock of knowledge they drew on to ask questions such as: How was the body found? Was there a history of ill health? Was a suicide note found? By discussing these questions with your colleagues you will be able to get at and make explicit the 'accounting procedure' that is taking place in order to make sense of the particular case being considered. You could then use a nursing example from one of the many we identified above, to make the same point. In the seminar we asked our colleagues to consider what makes a 'good' or 'bad' patient.

Try this activity for yourself. How do you categorize a patient as 'good', 'bad', 'popular', 'unpopular'? What knowledge do you use to create your category? What do you look out for in a patient?

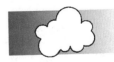

You could take another example such as 'the ward round'. How do you describe a 'typical' ward round? Your descriptions or **'typifications'** may include behaviours that are taken for granted, such as the nurse or junior doctor pushing the notes trolley behind the consultant. Ethnomethodologists define 'typifications' as 'recipes for action that exist in the culture as a whole'. On some wards it may be taken for granted that the senior nurse such as the sister or charge nurse accompanies the consultant on the ward round, regardless of whether patients have been cared for by their named nurse, primary nurse or team leader. What other taken-for-granted behaviours can you identify in your everyday work and why do they happen in that way? The taken-for-granted behaviours we identified in connection with ward rounds, for example, appear to be intimately linked with the hierarchical organization of hospital wards.

Discussing these taken-for-granted behaviours can illuminate many issues pertinent to the delivery of care. At the same time we would be engaging in ethnomethodological 'behaviour'. We then considered how research uses these 'typifications' and accounting procedures as a resource, as Durkheim did, rather than as a topic of inquiry.

Indexicality

We considered the key concept of indexicality by giving our colleagues the following piece of text to read with no explanation about what the subject matter was. We asked them to read it 'blind' to try to make sense of what was in the text. As you will see, because the text is without context, it is unlikely that you, like our colleagues, will be able to interpret what is going on. When they had finished reading the text, we put it in context. They then re-read it, this time with a different understanding.

> *The procedure is really quite simple. First you arrange things into different groups depending on their make up. Of course one pile may be sufficient depending on how much there is to do. If you have to go somewhere else due to lack of facilities that is the next step, otherwise you are pretty well set. It is important not to overdo any particular endeavour. That is, it is better to do too few things at once than too many, in the short run this may not seem important, but complications from doing too many can easily arise. A mistake can be expensive as well. The manipulation of the appropriate mechanisms should be self explanatory and we need not dwell on it here. At first, the whole procedure will seem complicated. Soon, however, it will become just another facet of life. It is difficult to foresee any end to the necessity for this task in the immediate future, but then one can never tell.*

> (Bransford & Johnson 1973, p. 722, cited by Hilgard et al 1979)

Reading the above text 'blind', it is difficult to understand what is being referred to. However, given the context 'doing the laundry' all becomes clear. Nursing talk also produces many indexical expressions, the meaning of which will be unclear to the lay person unfamiliar with health care settings. The context 'hospital' gives a very different meaning to the phrase 'you need to drink plenty tonight' from that of the context 'stag night'.

We were able to think of many other examples in the classroom and you to will be able to come up with many of your own.

Ethnomethodology as critique of positivist science

We also asked the group to identify research papers written from a positivist perspective. They were then asked to re-read them using the ethnomethodological framework to critically analyse them. Research critique is a demanding activity and surveys have shown that many students and registered nurses do not have a great deal of experience in this (Bircumshaw 1990, Webb & Mackenzie 1993). However, research critique does promote research mindedness by assisting us to evaluate the usefulness of particular pieces of research. Chapter 9 in this book will take you through the skills required to critically evaluate research with particular reference to the paper *Helping people to stop smoking*. You might like to apply an ethnomethodological approach to a critical evaluation of that paper.

Constructs

We then focused on the 'constructs' found in positivist research and asked the group how these were created by the researcher. We also created a list of common nursing concepts in order to examine their origins. This activity also addresses the issue of taken-for-granted knowledge; you might like to try it for yourself.

Consider the following concepts commonly used by nurses:

1. *nil by mouth*
2. *patient reassured*
3. *tender loving care (TLC)*
4. *individualized care*
5. *constipated*
6. *confused*
7. *off duty rota*
8. *drug round*
9. *pain*
10. *quality of life.*

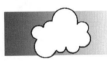

These constructs may at first glance seem to present little problem. We all know when a patient is constipated or has been reassured, or do we? How do we know and what accounting procedures do we engage in to come to such decisions? Walsh & Ford (1989) argue that many nursing practices are still based on ritual and mythology. We argue that recourse to ritual or unthinking practice has its roots in an uncritical examination of everyday practice. By examining how nurses exactly go about their business, we may be able to see what the true grounds of knowledge nurses actually use are and come to a decision as to the efficacy, appropriateness, and rationality of nursing work. Lawler's (1991) study of somology, referred to above, is an excellent example of this.

We found that engaging in a learning experience from an ethnomethodological perspective using experiential learning methods, and engaging our peers in critical thinking and analysis, rather than relying on mere exposition of the concepts, was challenging. Although as a group we had not engaged in carrying out research we were developing research mind-edness as we started to question the basis of knowledge and knowledge production (epistemology) in social and nursing science.

THOUGHTS AND REFLECTIONS:
PERSONAL CHALLENGE

As we have argued throughout this chapter, because ethnomethodology presents such a radically different approach to the world it forces us to reflect upon our own commonsense views. There was a realization for us that there was difficulty in grasping the reflexive, indexical and ongoing nature of social situations. Fish are always the last to discover water and there is a tendency to think that social situations can only be analysed in a detached and objective way and not as an ongoing interactive whole. For example, we could study how patients play the sick role based on a sick role theory (Parsons 1950) and examine how patients behave when ill from an objective standpoint, 'standing above' and observing behaviours. Alternatively we could analyse the interaction between nurses and patients, examining the context within which they find themselves and how they together negotiate roles and behaviours and the meanings they both bring to the situation.

A belief in a deterministic social universe, a universe whose laws and truths can be discovered by careful application of the scientific method, is challenged by ethnomethodology. Durkheim is persuasive when arguing a law of social forces affecting individuals. A law that links poor social integration (cause) with increased risk of suicide (effect) makes a lot of sense. However, ethnomethodology calls into question the existence of social laws and forces. This is because, unlike positivist social science, it is not primarily concerned with the linear relationship between cause and effect. Its focus is on the reflexive and indexical nature of this relationship, on people's assumptions and taken-for-granted behaviours, on how we use context in everyday social actions and on how perceptions are shaped by the context and concepts that we use.

The concern of ethnomethodology is with generating an understanding of the social world, which is considered to be radically different from the physical world. It does not compete with science as the only means of explanation, but offers an alternative and critical perspective, arrived at from a different approach by analysis of a different level.

The realization and acceptance that there can be more than one way of knowing produces a 'dissonance' or unease, and requires that we re-exam-ine some of our approaches to different types of research and their value for health professionals. In our own case the result of these reflections was a more critical approach to the positivist tradition. These points will now be described.

The dominant paradigm within nursing research has been that of the positivistic tradition, with its emphasis on objective reality and its claims to adopt a neutral approach to data which are collected in an objective manner. Whether this detached and neutral view of the world is possible remains a keenly debated subject as you saw both earlier in this chapter and in Chapter 2 of this book.

Kelly (1955) proposed that our perception of the world is to a great extent governed by our theories or concepts concerning the world. According to Kelly, we see the world through goggles that are put in position as the result of experience and culture. We cannot remove the goggles, merely alter their focus and perspective as a result of new experiences. This is what happened to us during the preparation of the seminar.

Kuhn (1962) also refers to this perceptual **bias** and describes it as the theory ladenness of perception. His examination of science reveals how many observations are conditioned by the expectancies and classificatory schemes of the observer. He notes that 'groups of scientists see different things when they look from the same point in the same direction.' (Kuhn 1962, p. 129). The claim that the theories of science born of empirical observation are value-free at both the personal and cultural levels also requires examination. The kudos which western culture attaches to science has led to the findings of researchers being widely implemented because they are regarded as having great truth value.

Kessen (1991) considers that the findings of scientists are held in such esteem that the publications of prestigious researchers are interpreted as the equivalent of natural law. The struggle between the Anglican bishops and Charles Darwin in the last century over whether life on earth had been created or evolved can be seen as a watershed when science began to overtake Christianity as the most reliable source for knowledge of the world.

Science as 'ideology' can be illustrated by Bowlby's theory of maternal deprivation. This theory, which considered that babies who were separated from their mothers were at risk of psychological problems in later life, was widely accepted. Ideology crept into Bowlby's theory when he uncritically assumed that it was separation from *mothers* that was the problem rather than separation from a caring adult. Bowlby was a product of a society that generally uncritically accepted female roles in child care. It became part of the post-war social policy and Tizard (1991) argues that it was influential in pressurizing women back into the home following the freedom which they had experienced during the Second World War. Bowlby's theory was a theory that fitted the times and so went largely unchallenged. More recently, Rutter (1979) argued that infants become attached to other caretakers such as fathers, sisters and brothers, so the effect of not being constantly with your mother is not as hazardous as Bowlby claimed. Bowlby's work also led to the belief that it was the mother who was the focus for attachment and so his theory can be seen to be biased through gender-specific spectacles.

These criticisms of science reveal that researchers are not immune to the cultural haze that clouds and gives value to all perception. They also imply that researchers need to examine the way that they create the concepts which they use in their investigations. Perhaps it is too much to expect Bowlby to examine why he used the concept of maternal deprivation rather than parental or care deprivation, given the dominant cultural context of his time which automatically linked child care with women. However, a critical and questioning approach which seeks to understand cultural expectations and assumptions, combined with an awareness of one's own values, should be the aim of all health researchers. We, too, have our own professional biases, prejudices and values sometimes camouflaged as nursing theory and practice. Is it possible to uncover our assumptions and taken-for-granted knowledge?

Positivist science has come in for some criticism, not least from ourselves. However, it is extremely valuable when it comes to understanding large populations and can help us to predict outcomes and allocate resources, factors which are extremely important in health care. Science operates in the macro-world, i.e. the world of large populations, groups or organizations. Those who deliver health care to patients and clients are situated at the interface of the organization and the individual.

Schon (1991) argues that expert practitioners operate at the micro-level which he describes as the 'swamp-like' regions of uncertainty rather than the high ground of the certain and absolute. He refers to professionals practising in the indeterminate zones where 'uncertainty, uniqueness and value conflict escape the canons of technical rationality' (Schon 1991, p. 6). For example, when a patient is critically ill and does not wish relatives to know, the nurse may be placed in a difficult position when confronted by the relatives. This ethical dilemma in care cannot be easily solved by applying a law or principle; it is not straightforward. When a car does not start, we can apply principles to find out why, such as first check to see if there is any petrol.

Nurses engage with their patients at the individual level. When operating at this level, evidence from scientific studies such as that which predicts that 20% of people who experience cardiac arrest will do so in the first hour following infarction (Chamberlain & Vincent 1984) is of limited value. What the practitioner wants to know is what this particular patient will do. Science does not inform us of certainties regarding individuals, only probabilities concerning groups. Probabilities concerning populations are vital when allocating resources at the macro-level, they are of less value when operating at the micro-level which is where the practitioner operates. Like the skilled builder, health workers need different tools to operate at different levels.

However, accepting that there is a relative quality to all perceptions and observations can lead to an 'infinite regress', wherein we accept everything as relative and nothing as real. Giddens (1976, p. 166) describes those who have become locked in to accepting nothing as real as: 'Intrepid travellers all now left swirling helplessly in the vortex of the hermeneutic whirlpool'. If ethnomethodology suggests that all scientific accounts and explanations of the world are constructed by scientists working with particular cultural values, this criticism could be levelled at ethnomethodology itself. Ethnomethodology's account is just another way of describing the world and is therefore no more or less valid than anybody else's view. This is referred to as the infinite regress of '**relativism**' by which we cannot accept anything as 'real'. If there is no absolute truth except that there is no absolute truth, then the statement that 'there is no absolute truth' is not true either.

The aim of ethnomethodology is not to spin in this whirlpool but to examine how constructs are created and how they become accepted as common sense. Paradoxically for us, an examination of the central concepts and philosophy of ethnomethodology created a whirlpool all of its own in which long-held beliefs were challenged.

CONCLUSION

Ethnomethodology has been termed a 'social microscope' (Heritage 1984). What would it reveal if focused upon nursing and nursing work? It may show us how nursing is constructed, accomplished and recreated by nurses in their everyday activity. It would seek to clarify 'the intricate web of behaviours through which nursing identity is secured' (Bowers 1992). It would clarify the host of assumptions and typifications in use. Perhaps we would examine what our theories in use were (i.e. what we do) as opposed to our espoused theories (what we say we do) (Schon 1991). We may argue that because we are engaged in individualized care, an ethnomethodological examination could seek to examine such a claim by researching our speech, behaviour and conceptual frameworks in use.

Bowers (1992) suggests that through using an ethnomethodological approach it would be possible to examine how nurses and patients interact, and discover the commonsense categorizations used by nurses to organize their working lives. Theory here could be generated from practice and returned to practice as the everyday carrying out of practice would be uncovered and made explicit. Diers (1979) argued that research always begins with a problem, and research in nursing practice begins with problems in nursing practice.

Ethnomethodology assists in recognizing a problem because it asks us to consider the everyday 'swampy lowlands' (Schon 1991) of clinical practice, i.e. those 'indeterminate zones' where the use of strict scientific rule is useless in facilitating the right course of action, and where problems abound and need solutions not found in textbooks.

The next time you engage in practice, think of the commonsense understandings and assumptions you are using to carry out your job. You are not engaged in ethnomethodology but you are using its philosophical approach. Reflect and examine the forms of knowledge you use. If Polanyi (1964) is correct that we know more than we can say, then it may be that we will never fully grasp the thought processes that are in use by ourselves as nurses. However, by focusing on the micro-processes of nursing work we hold up a mirror to those thought processes and forms of knowledge in use.

As previously mentioned, the intention of this chapter was to describe and explore ethnomethodology, with the aim of presenting it not as the correct way of studying social situations, but as an alternative perspective which could be of value to research-minded health professionals. The critical and alternative approach adopted by ethnomethodology leaves those who adopt it with more questions but fewer assumptions. Such a state should not be a problem for the research-minded practitioner.

REFERENCES

Atkinson J 1971 Societal reactions to suicide. Cited in Haralambos M 1985 Sociology themes and perspectives. Bell and Hyman, London

Atkinson J 1978 Discovering suicide. Macmillan, London

Becker M, Rosenstock I 1984 Compliance with medical advice. In: Steptoe A, Mathews A (eds) Health care and human behaviour. Academic Press, London

Benner P 1984 From novice to expert: excellence and power in clinical nursing practice. Addison-Wesley, Menlo Park, California

Benson D, Hughes J 1983 The perspective of ethnomethodology. Longman, London

Bircumshaw D 1990 The utilization of research findings in clinical nursing practice. Journal of Advanced Nursing 15: 1272–1280

Bowers L 1992 Ethnomethodology 1: an approach to nursing research. International Journal of Nursing Studies 29(1): 59–67

Capra F 1984 The turning point. Pelican, London

Carper B 1978 Fundamental patterns of knowing in nursing. Advances in Nursing Science 1(1): 13–23

Cash K 1990 Nursing models and the idea of nursing. International Journal of Nursing Studies 27(3): 249–256

Chamberlain D, Vincent R 1984 Coronary care. In: Gerson G (ed) Intensive care. Heinemann, London

Cuff E, Sharrock W, Francis D 1992 Perspectives in sociology. Routledge, London

Diers D 1979 Research in nursing practice. Lippincott, Philadelphia

Durkheim E 1952 (first published 1897) Suicide: a study in sociology. Routledge, London

Fairclough N 1989 Language and power. Longman, London

Ford M, Walsh P 1992 Nursing rituals, research and rational action. Heinemann, Oxford

Friere P 1987 A pedagogy for liberation: dialogues on transforming education. Macmillan, Basingstoke

Garfinkel H 1967 Studies in ethnomethodology. Prentice-Hall, New Jersey

Giddens A 1976 New rules of sociological method. Hutchinson, London

Griffin A 1983 A philosophical analysis of caring nursing. Journal of Advanced Nursing 11: 661–670

Habermas J 1984 Knowledge and human interests, 2nd edn. Heinemann, London

Helman C 1990 Culture, health and illness, 2nd edn. Wright, London

Heritage J 1984 Garfinkel and ethnomethodology. Prentice Hall, Englewood Cliffs, NJ

Hilgard E, Atkinson R L, Atkinson R C (eds) 1979 Introduction to psychology, 7th edn. Harcourt Brace Jovanovitch, New York, p 248

Kelly G 1955 A theory of personality—the psychology of personal constructs. Norton, New York

Kelly P, May D 1984 Good and bad patients: a review of the literature and a theoretical critique. Journal of Advanced Nursing 7: 147–166

Kessen W 1991 The American child and other cultural inventions. In: Woodhead M, Light P, Carr R (eds) Growing up in a changing society. Routledge, London

Kuhn T 1962 The structure of scientific revolutions. University of Chicago Press, Chicago

Lambert C 1993 Plato, sociology and nursing. Nurse Education Today 13: 445–450

Lawler J 1991 Behind the screens: nursing somology and the problem of the body. Churchill Livingstone, Melbourne

Mitchell J 1984 What is to be done about illness and health? Penguin, Harmondsworth

Morris M B 1977 An excursion into creative sociology. Columbia University Press, New York

Parsons T 1950 Illness and the role of the physician. American Journal of Orthopsychiatry 21: 452–460

Polanyi M 1964 Personal knowledge. Harper & Row, New York

Rogers B 1989 Concepts, analysis and the development of nursing knowledge: the evolutionary cycle. Journal of Advanced Nursing 14: 330–335

Roper N, Logan W W, Tierney A J 1980 The elements of nursing. Churchill Livingstone, Edinburgh

Royal College of Nursing 1982 Promoting research mindedness. RCN Publications, London

Rutter M 1979 Maternal deprivation re-assessed. Penguin, Harmondsworth

Schon D A 1991 Educating the reflective practitioner. Jossey-Bass, Oxford

Schutz A 1972 The phenomenology of the social world. Heinemann, London

Selye H 1956 The stress of life. McGraw Hill, New York

Shilts R 1987 And the band played on: politics, people and the AIDS epidemic. St Martin's Press, London

Sudnow D 1967 Passing on: the social organisation of dying. Prentice Hall, Englewood Cliffs, NJ

Tilley N 1982 Popper, positivism and ethnomethodology. British Journal of Sociology 31(1): 28–45

Tizard B 1991 Working mothers and the care of young children. In: Woodhead M, Light P, Carr R (eds) Growing up in a changing society. Routledge, London

Walsh M, Ford P 1989 We always do it this way. Nursing Times 85(41): 26–35

Webb C, Mackenzie J 1993 Where are we now? Research mindedness in the 1990s. Journal of Clinical Nursing 2: 129–133

The media and research

Wladyslawa Czuber-Dochan
Linda McBride   Julie Wilson

7

■ KEY ISSUES

- **The close relationship between investigative journalism and research**
- **The media's potential to provide a powerful mechanism for the teaching of research and the dissemination of research findings**
- **The opportunities provided by the media to promote new ways of thinking to challenge and change practice**

INTRODUCTION

This chapter concerns the promotion of research mindedness within the context of a learning experience. It acknowledges that throughout their lives individuals learn in diverse ways, other than through formal classroom teaching. Learning can be dynamic, creative and magical. It can also have a darker more mysterious side when solutions to problems are sought. This chapter describes our own learning experiences which built upon our personal knowledge and experience of research. We achieved this by moving away from the confines of textbooks and the written word and turning towards media presentation. More specifically, we wanted to adopt a case study approach using the principles of reflection to demonstrate how a peer-led seminar based on a television documentary was used to develop the **concept** of 'research mindedness'.

This approach enabled us to learn in two ways. Firstly, we learnt by organizing and presenting the seminar. Secondly, we learnt through the written analysis of that experience. The influence that the media can have on individuals is evident in the statement made by Romiszowski (1974) in Box 7.1.

■ BOX 7.1

Television is a more powerful medium than the cinema ever was—not because more people watch television, but because people accept its message more readily, get more involved emotionally and are participants rather than observers.

During the seminar we explored how far the media, in this instance television, could be used to promote the concept of research mindedness. The documentary chosen to explore this issue was a Channel 4 programme called *Preying on Hope*. The programme was shown in January 1994 and looked at the perceived exploitation of individuals with acquired immune deficiency syndrome (AIDS). It was part of a series entitled *Undercover Britain*, which comprised several 30-minute programmes that had been recorded by a hidden camera. The programme we chose was a genuine attempt to discover what was happening in the real world of AIDS and its treatment. It was presented by a young man who had tested positive to the human immunodeficiency virus (HIV) in the previous year. He and his partner visited several doctors and alternative therapists who had advertised a cure for the HIV virus. One of the doctors prescribed shark's cartilage as a cure. The doctor, who had a reputation as a nutrition expert, practised in the prestigious Harley Street. When his 'prescription' was investigated microscopically, no evidence of shark was found. Further enquiries revealed that the doctor was not medically qualified. The programme illustrated how other false claims were being made about miracle cures. As a result of these discoveries, further investigations were undertaken by the Department of the Environment and the British Medical Association.

During the seminar we used the documentary to raise the following issues:

- concepts of research and research mindedness
- the role of the media in portraying research and research mindedness
- the need to critically evaluate the media using recognized approaches
- the extent to which the undercover investigation of the documentary could be described as research.

Our concept of research

In order to clarify our concept of research in preparing for the seminar we undertook a literature review. According to Macleod Clark & Hockey (1989, p 4), research is 'an attempt to increase the body of knowledge, i.e. what is currently known about nursing by discovery of new facts and relationships through a process of systematic scientific enquiry'. They also see that the essential characteristic of research is its scientific nature. For the Department of Health (DoH 1993) research is also broadly defined as the acquisition of knowledge, which includes gaining information, clarification and illumination as well as translating it (research) directly into policy or practice.

Drawing on these and other texts we concluded that research could be conceptualized as:

- a process
- scientific
- **objective**
- systematic
- problem solving
- advancement of knowledge
- exploration of facts and relationships
- an enquiring attitude.

As the list indicates, we adopted a broad concept of research because we saw it as being representative of the 'real world' of nursing. We believed that conceptualizing research in this way would provide opportunities to embrace both the art and the science of nursing knowledge. It would also support the notion that nursing, like research, was a diverse activity that takes place in a variety of settings. We also perceived that this broad approach to research would enable our colleagues within the seminar to engage in more lateral thought processes, promote a deeper understanding of research and support a different way of thinking.

Furthermore, we believed that Macleod Clark & Hockey's (1989) definition of research was particularly significant to the seminar because it reflected a desire to increase the body of knowledge and also emphasized the scientific nature of research. Within the seminar, the advancement of knowledge was expressed in the form of the media as a means of discovering new facts, the promotion of AIDS awareness and the exploration of a **qualitative** documentary using a predominantly scientific analysis.

Our concept of research mindedness

We believe that the concept of research and the concept of research mindedness are linked because both activities imply a problem-solving process. This process demands a number of skills which are part of becoming research minded. For us research mindedness means having the following attributes and skills:

- an enquiring attitude
- ability to apply research in practice
- critical evaluation skills
- a research awareness
- a logical approach.

Through our seminar we aimed to promote all of the above attributes and skills. One of the key questions we asked was: 'How far can investigative journalism be described as research?' This was a broad question but it demanded that we do a number of things within the seminar. Initially, we asked our colleagues to consider what they believed was meant by the term 'research'. We wanted them to see how far the journalistic enquiry advocated by the documentary actually supported or refuted their original thoughts and ideas. Finally, in order to find an answer to our key question, the group needed to engage in research-minded behaviour. This could be described as part of a logical approach to problem solving. They needed to ask questions about the research process, the **validity** and **reliability** of the research findings and the **ethics** of what they saw. This could be described as part of the skill of critical evaluation. Here the group needed to identify whether generalizations could be made as a result of the documentary in order to apply them to practice. In this context, research mindedness could be seen as a prerequisite for the implementation of research findings (O'Brien & Heyman 1989).

RESEARCH APPROACHES AND METHODS

In preparing for our seminar we had read a number of texts about research because we saw reading about research as an important part of the relationship between research, practice, management and education. Whilst we were not asking our colleagues to read a piece of research, they were being asked to engage in research activity using the media as a learning resource. We anticipated that the seminar presentation could provide an alternative means of enabling students to understand the issues that the documentary raised about research and AIDS. The research **approaches** and **methods** under review in this chapter include investigative journalism, research critique and **ethical issues**, each of which we shall discuss separately.

Investigative journalism

Gantz & Greenberg (1990) make the point that the use of television as an instructional tool is an exciting, realistic approach to providing continuing education for professional nurses. Gantz goes on to suggest that carefully crafted television programmes can stimulate changes in knowledge, attitudes and behaviours. We believed whilst planning our session that a television documentary would provide an exciting, thought-provoking way of exploring a very real area of concern for people with AIDS. We believed that the journalistic style of the documentary would encourage the group to consider their own attitudes and behaviours to the issues presented, as well as towards the researchers (in this case the television presenter and his partner). We saw that the development of these attitudes and behaviours corresponded to the development of research mindedness, suggesting that the media have a part to play in the promotion of research mindedness. Palmer (1988) states that 'television has a unique contribution to make in the world-wide effort to stem and manage the spread of AIDS. It can inform and motivate decision makers who control community actions'.

Gunter et al (1993) make the point that television has played a prominent role in many AIDS campaigns. In a survey of public interest on the coverage of AIDS, it was found that a majority of people believed that television had a responsibility to inform people about AIDS. This could suggest that the documentary is an appropriate mechanism for the advancement of knowledge. It can also be viewed as a learning resource readily available to patients and their carers.

An important point to be made here is that if television is to be used as a means of disseminating knowledge, it must take full responsibility for this. Television producers and print journalists very often use investigative journalism as if it were research. Indeed, investigative journalism has much in common with some aspects of research, and there are substantial areas of overlap, particularly in some of the methods used to collect data (Campbell 1989). An example is participant observation in qualitative research, a favourite of journalists. The main differences are that research often has a policy and practice relevance—being there not only to attract general interest but also to provide information on which decisions are made.

Shilts (1987), writing about AIDS, demonstrated how it is possible to combine investigative journalism with scientific rigour. He made the point that within journalistic enquiry it is important to adhere to scientific principles. Shilts, as the first openly gay reporter on a major US daily newspaper, was able to trace the historic developments both of the gay community in San Francisco and the spread of the AIDS epidemic. Out of his journalistic endeavours came the celebrated book *And the Band Played On*, which recognized the powerful status of science in tracking the origins of the deadly disease.

During the seminar we pointed out how journalistic knowledge should be recorded accurately and without **bias**. Journalists, like scientists, should also consider the moral implications of their actions because of their potential to influence or change the provision of the health care of tomorrow. Presenting knowledge in a neutral way may pose difficulties for journalistic enquiry, given the need to be hard hitting in order to attract both readers and viewers. Periodically, stories arise about epidemics, like the 1994 stories of killer bugs in Britain (Day 1994) or the 1995 Ebola fever scare in Zaire.

Perhaps you have had to cope with patients or clients who were worried about their health as a result of information disseminated by the media. Such an incident arose for one of us whilst visiting a patient. This incident is described in Box 7.2.

■ **BOX 7.2**

This is an account of a personal experience whilst working as a district nurse. It took place during the 1994 scare over necrotizing fasciitis, which had been given high coverage by the press as 'the killer bug'. I was visiting Sally, who required daily visits, when I noticed that she had a reddened patch on her ear. There was also a plug of cotton wool in her auditory canal. I asked her if her ear was sore. Sally replied that it was and had been for several days. She had waited until that morning to call out her GP who on examining the ear had diagnosed eczema, prescribing a steroid cream. Because Sally and the staff often teased each other I commented light-heartedly, 'At least you are not being eaten alive'. At that point the conversation took a serious turn and Sally confided in me that for the past few days she had thought that she was indeed being eaten by the killer bug.

Such an incident really shows just how careful we have to be when talking to patients and the need to be aware of the current news stories on health that may be affecting them.

Research critique

When reviewing any piece of research it is vital to expose it to critical analysis. It follows therefore that for any practitioner or teacher to be research minded it is essential to be equipped with the skills of critiquing. Treece & Treece (1986, p. 56) define critique as 'a critical evaluation of the strengths and weaknesses of any work'—in this case research. In their view, the term refers to a process rather than an attitude. The skills of critique, which promotes a questioning approach, supported our previous notions of what research and research mindedness mean for us.

For the purpose of the seminar we based our approach to critique on the guidelines set out by Treece & Treece (1986) and presented in Box 7.3. We deliberately identified a critique that was designed to evaluate **quantitative** research. We did this because we felt it would be interesting to see whether a piece of investigative journalism would survive the rigours of conventional scientific critique. We also thought this approach to be appropriate, given the experimental aspects of the documentary. We have already mentioned the microscopic examination of the drug claiming to contain shark's cartilage. By choosing a quantitative critique we were making a conscious stand to counterbalance the highly emotive subject matter of the programme.

■ BOX 7.3

Elements of critique (adapted from Treece & Treece 1986)

1. Research question(s):
   a. Were the question and the purpose clearly stated?
   b. Does the author differentiate between the general question and the specific one?
   c. Was the nature of the question practical or theoretical?
   d. What was the background to the question?
   e. Does the background logically lead to the question by identifying gaps in the knowledge?
   f. Was the relationship between the question and the previous research clear?
   g. What is the significance of the question for future research (value of the research)?
   h. Were independent, dependent and other variables clearly defined?

2. The literature review:
   a. Was the literature review specific to the purpose of the study?
   b. Were the investigators qualified to conduct the particular type of research?
   c. Did the authors provide adequate information for the reader to gain understanding of the topic?
   d. What is the date of publication and the date of research?
   e. Did the material include professional journals, books and literature and background material?
   f. Was the review logically and clearly organized?

3. Research design:
   a. Population and sample:
      (i)   Was the population identified and described?
      (ii)   Was the sample size appropriate?
      (iii) Was the sample random or non-random?
      (iv)   What measures were taken to protect the rights of the subjects?
      (v)   How was the sample selected (selection bias)?

    b. Methodology:
      (i)   Were the methods for collecting data appropriate for the study?
      (ii)   Were all the steps of the methodology included so that another researcher could replicate the study (reliability)?
      (iii) Did the researcher(s) obtain the data they sought (validity)?
      (iv) Was the procedure standardized?
      (v)   Was an effort made to control the variables?
      (vi) How many researchers were involved in obtaining the data?
      (vii) Was the researchers' bias reported?
      (viii) If the study was conducted by observation, was the researcher a participant or observer?

    c. Storing of information:
      (i)   Were the results of the statistical tests or the descriptive measure reported correctly?
      (ii)   Would the method of storing data allow the researcher to analyse the data objectively?

4. Analysis of data
    a. Were the findings and data interpreted correctly?
    b. Was the level of significance reported?
    c. Was the hypothesis accepted or rejected?
    d. Were the limitations of the research methods acknowledged?
    e. Were the tables, diagrams set up correctly?
    f. Were sufficient visual aids used to make the findings easily understood?
    g. Were there suggestions for further research?
    h. Were the implications of the findings for practice described?

5. Structure of the report, conclusions:
    a. Was the title appropriate to the study?
    b. Were the important variables mentioned in the title?
    c. Were the conclusions supported by the data?
    d. Did the conclusions follow from the stated purpose of the study and the hypothesis?
    e. Were the conclusions stated clearly and concisely?
    f. Were strengths and weaknesses discussed by the writer?
    g. Were the grammar and writing style conducive to making the report interesting and understandable?
    h. Was the abstract included? (The abstract should state the purpose, hypothesis and results. It should provide answers to the questions: who, what, where, when, how and why?)
    i. Does the report attract readers?

You will have another opportunity to consider approaches to research critiques in Chapter 9.

Ethical issues

Ethical issues are at the core of research and investigative journalism, irrespective of the approaches taken. There is, however, no clear agreement among researchers as to what is considered to be good ethical practice (Holm & Llewellyn 1986). Investigative journalists often face serious journalistic and ethical decisions (Patterson & Russell 1986) and the documentary *Preying on Hope* was a very good example of this. The sensitivity of conducting research associated with AIDS is acknowledged by the introduction of special guidelines on how to do ethical AIDS research (Bulletin of Medical Ethics 1991).

Furthermore, more general ethical issues such as deceit on the part of the researcher and the absence of informed consent on the part of the participants were at the core of the documentary. If you recall, the presenter posed as a patient seeking a cure for HIV and had a hidden camera to record what went on during the consultations between himself and the various 'experts'.

The question of ethics in relation to both selection of topic and the way in which research is conducted are extremely important areas for the research-minded practitioner and teacher. The use of deception in research violates the subject's **autonomy** to make informed decisions and is unethical (Rogers 1990). There are many examples of research which has dubious ethical status. However, some researchers believe that, at times, covert methods are required, as the following statement illustrates: 'The use of covert methods reflects the nature of social reality. Sneaky and deceptive methods are necessary to do good social science because social order rests on deceitfulness, evasiveness, secrecy, frontwork and basic social conflicts' (Warwick & Douglas; cited in Punch 1986, p. 29).

Covert methods are often used to justify research on 'deviants'. In cases of criminal behaviour, you might ask whether the researcher protects his/her subjects or uses the information collected to expose deviant activities to the authorities. To a certain extent, the position of the researcher is determined by his/her initial moral stance (Punch 1986). In the case of *Preying on Hope*, the presenter clearly spelt out his moral position at the outset. He was out to expose those people who were 'preying' on AIDS sufferers by taking their money for what were useless and often dangerous 'cures'. Therefore the investigator felt he had the right to invade the confidentiality and privacy of unscrupulous practitioners.

It is with regards to the ethics of covert methods that research and investigative journalism overlap. Some researchers, such as Jack Douglas and the San Diego 'school' of sociologists, believe that it is the job of research to expose the powerful, who prey on the weaker members of society (Punch 1986). In their view, secretive techniques are justified, to penetrate the 'fronts' erected to protect the powerful. Generally, however, researchers have been severely criticized for undertaking research in a covert and secretive manner, usually as undeclared participant observers. Sometimes the research has actually harmed vulnerable members of society as illustrated by Laud Humphreys' deceit in infiltrating the gay community whilst studying male homosexual behaviour (cited in Punch 1986). Humphreys undertook research with a hidden camera in men's public toilets to record the sexual practices of gay men. He also noted their car registration numbers so that he could follow them to their homes. This example illustrates the double dilemma of morals and ethics since the men were completely unaware of Humphreys' presence and intentions.

The documentary allowed us to explore similar key ethical issues and conflicts. The issue of participant observation, with the presenter an 'AIDS-sufferer' desperately seeking a cure, touches upon one of the key problems of participant observation. Because of its very nature, researchers in participant observation have to be deceitful to achieve acceptance in order to observe and monitor what is going on without changing the environment (Cormack 1991). The programme, therefore, exposed us to some very problematic and sensitive issues which can be met in many research situations, and as such was a good teaching tool about ethics.

Preying on Hope highlights the debate and the real uncertainty about whether the ends of the research justify the means. Did the ends of uncovering unprofessional and dangerous behaviour justify the covert methods that the presenter employed? Should the principle of informed consent, that the subject of the research should be aware that he/she is being studied, be applied throughout research? Clearly, if this were the case, much valuable work might not have been done (Holm & Llewellyn 1986) and the benefit derived from the research would have been lost (Rogers 1990). You will be able to pursue these issues further in Chapter 10, which is devoted to ethical considerations in research.

CASE STUDY

The following discussion puts our seminar in context as a teaching session. In order to explore an alternative approach to research mindedness, we used the example of investigative journalism to examine the skills required to understand the research process. We chose to explore a documentary concerning AIDS because we believed it had relevance for practitioners. We also felt that because it was emotive it would provoke discussion about certain aspects of the research process. We were personally aware of the potential power of the media over individuals' behaviour.

An individualized and student-centred approach to teaching is not a new idea but is not always easy to achieve, especially when teaching a notoriously difficult topic such as 'research'. This is why we need to employ fresh and innovative approaches. As professional health workers we have many opportunities for teaching and educating a whole variety of people on different communication levels, from doctors to patients. By using examples from the media we may find it easier to put across our learning messages. In teaching about research mindedness, the use of the media can be an ideal way of identifying problems and issues that are topical and difficult, and which require further investigation.

For the purposes of the seminar we asked our colleagues to watch the video and make any notes that they felt were relevant. We asked them to consider the following questions:

- How far can the documentary be described as research?
- What are the ethical issues involved?
- What is the most effective means of conveying: (1) the issues that the programme raises; (2) the implications of the findings?

At the end of the viewing we used Treece & Treece's critiquing guidelines.

Prior to the session we were aware that one of the major weaknesses of the documentary was its poor coverage of the formal procedures involved in the investigation. For example, there was little information about **sampling**, collection of background information and analysis of the substances purchased. However, despite the weaknesses, the programme offered us an opportunity to examine the issues surrounding sampling a small and fairly diverse population. The main sampling problem related to the difficulty of determining the scale of malpractice and the number of criminal acts associated with the alternative treatment of AIDS from which to draw a representative sample.

The sampling was done in a variety of ways, such as through the personal knowledge of the presenter, through seeing advertisements in the press, and through the 'gay grapevine'. These types of samples, known as **'convenience'**, **'opportunistic'**, **'purposive'** and **'snowballing'**, are all examples of **non-random sampling**. They are often used in situations where the total population is difficult to establish (Mann 1985). Furthermore, the use of the researcher's personal knowledge of what is 'out there' is not unusual when approaching potential research subjects (Hockey 1985).

Preying on Hope shows the viewer that small samples should not be discounted, as they can provide insight and understanding at a local level as well as generating ideas for more systematic large-scale research.

The next element of the documentary that we considered was whether the analysis and presentation of data answered the research question. In the programme, experts were invited to analyse and comment on the various medications being prescribed as cures for AIDS. However, the procedures were not standardized, which helped us to become aware of the required rigour in data analysis.

There was no way as viewers that we could verify the accuracy of the statements that were being made. We could only take the word of 'experts' that the substances being sold were harmful.

Furthermore, we were not presented with data, only a summary of the findings. An analysis and presentation of data is very important to make the research findings believable for other people and to confirm their validity and reliability. This highlights the need for the precise presentation of research findings in order to make implementation of research in practice possible. For findings to be utilized, it is important that the research can withstand rigorous critique.

As a group, we had a variety of research experience, which added to the richness of the debate concerning the quantitative/qualitative nature of the investigation. Some people questioned the guidelines we had selected to critique the documentary, suggesting that a qualitative approach would have been more appropriate. But we found that debating the research process in this way enhanced our research mindedness.

For example, the documentary helped us to understand that the qualitative experiences of making the programme were a very real representation of the presenter's situation as a young gay man seeking a cure for HIV and AIDS. We also wanted to rigorously explore how he had gone about his investigation to assess whether a documentary could follow a systematic line of inquiry and be exposed to scientific rigour. Indeed, as we have already noted, a number of attempts were made within the documentary to follow scientific principles, particularly in relation to the testing of treatments.

The critiquing framework adopted demanded that the group try to quantify essentially qualitative experiences. As a result of this it could be argued that using this framework meant that participants could not (rather than would not) see the documentary as research because they had become emotionally involved, making it difficult to adopt an attitude of science and objectivity.

If you look back to Box 7.1, you can see how our reaction to the documentary mirrors Romiszowski's statement about the power of television to involve viewers emotionally so that they become participants rather than passive observers.

In answering the question of how far investigative journalism can be described as research, it could be argued that a solution to this problem is dependent upon individual perceptions of what is meant by research and research mindedness. As a group we believed it would be particularly difficult to establish any form of consensus. This was because we were aware that the question had created personal conflict within many of the seminar participants. It had challenged their theoretical and sometimes taken-for-granted notions that research equals science. But the question had also promoted research mindedness as a problem-solving approach to apply to new situations.

Finally, the documentary demonstrated for us that qualitative and quantitative research approaches share a common goal—an understanding of the world in which we live. Rather than seeing them as being in opposition, we began to see quantitative and qualitative research as compatible and complementary.

REFLECTIONS FOR PRACTICE

How do investigative journalism and research relate to nursing practice and research mindedness? Investigative journalism is about communication. The knowledge that journalists generate is published in the media in order to raise public awareness of what is happening in the world. As Patterson & Russell (1986) suggest, investigative journalists may not always be telling the public something new. However, they play an important role in raising the public's awareness of many important issues. Investigative journalists communicate facts and ideas to the public at large.

Because nurses care for the public they are also required to communicate on a wide range of levels. Peplau's model of nursing reflects this view. She identifies nursing as a 'significant, therapeutic, interpersonal process' (p 51), with communication being one of the nurse's fundamental tools (George 1990). Thus, communication can be identified as a tool common to both the media and nursing. Communication also plays a crucial role in research, as part of the process and also in disseminating the findings. One of the reasons nursing research is difficult to disseminate is because many nurses do not read those journals (such as the *Journal of Advanced Nursing*, *International Journal of Nursing Studies*) that contain research reports (Polit & Hungler 1989, Couchman & Dawson 1990). Research reports are also discussed at conferences, which many practising nurses do not attend for a variety of reasons. In the current climate within the National Health Service (NHS), the availability of conference attendance for nurses may well be reduced because of the increasing pressure on resources, time and funding and the reluctance of many managers to see research as part of the nurse's function.

Taking into account the problems of making research findings available to practising nurses, it can be seen that the media do have a part to play in raising the research awareness of nurses as well as the general public. An example of how the media can raise awareness is given in Box 7.4.

■ BOX 7.4

In October 1981, the *Horizon* television programme entitled *Hunt for the Legion Killer* reconstructed the United States Centers for Disease Control search to identify the source of the hitherto unidentified legionnaires' disease. In 1976, the pneumonia-like disease struck down hundreds and killed dozens of military veterans shortly after attending a convention to commemorate the American Declaration of Independence. The cause of the disease was eventually traced to a bacterium that flourished in air conditioning systems (in this case in the hotel where the veterans had stayed). Karpf (1988) points out that, thanks to television, a far greater number of people were given access to how the search for legionnaires' disease took place and the results that were found.

The link between research awareness and the media has been made specific in nursing literature. Bond & Bond (1982) undertook a Delphi survey aimed at establishing the priorities for clinical nursing research, as viewed by nurses working in the North of England. In the concluding discussion to the article they acknowledge that the media played a part in shaping the results. Tierney (1994) acknowledges that most people are aware of research and that this in part is due to media coverage.

According to Clifford & Gough (1990), the ability to understand research is one of the main factors influencing research mindedness amongst nurses. Understanding may be inhibited by style and presentation of research papers and the jargon used. Polit & Hungler (1989) urge all practising nurses, not just students and research nurses, to read research articles and utilize the results.

There are different kinds of knowledge that are valuable to nursing and it is important to remember not to concentrate only on research that is based in the technical world. Carper (1978) identified four patterns of knowing in nursing:

- empirical—the science of nursing
- aesthetics—the art of nursing
- personal knowledge
- ethics—the knowledge of morality and ethical issues.

This broad base of knowledge provides ample justification for regarding the media in general, and investigative journalism in particular, as a valuable tool for the facilitation of research mindedness.

The use of the media and investigative journalism may facilitate a better understanding of the research process without the added stress of technical language and research terminology. In this sense, the media can reduce the barrier which is present for many practising nurses between the theory of research and a practical knowledge of research, enabling them to identify the process and the application of research in the clinical setting. The role of the media in removing technical language and making research more accessible, thus leading to action, is illustrated in Box 7.5.

■ BOX 7.5

In 1982, Yorkshire Television showed a film called *Alice—a Fight for Life*. The programme focused on Alice, who was suffering from asbestosis. As a consequence of the film being shown, the legal limits for use of asbestos in buildings and industry were changed. According to Karpf (1988), until the film was shown, there had been limited action despite research in 1966 suggesting that asbestos fibre had carcinogenic properties. Further evidence of the cytotoxic capacity of asbestos fibre was reported in 1973 and 1974 (Stretton 1976), but over 8 years were to pass before Alice's story was told and higher legal limits on the use of asbestos imposed.

Another case which demonstrates the role of the media in getting information to the public is that of thalidomide. In the early 1960s, thalidomide was promoted as a wonder drug to prevent the miseries of 'morning sickness' in pregnant women. The babies whose mothers had taken thalidomide were subsequently born with congenital defects because the drug had crossed the placenta during pregnancy, damaging the fetus. *Welt am Sonntag*, a German newspaper, ran a story received from doctors, about the possible connection between the drug and the deformities. The manufacturers of thalidomide refused to accept responsibility for the children's plight, claiming that when thalidomide was being developed, tests were not required to investigate whether drugs could cross the placental barrier. *The Sunday Times* of London took up the battle on behalf of the affected children and their families. A postgraduate student was hired for 4 months to undertake a literature review of tests conducted to investigate drugs crossing the placenta. He found that such tests had been undertaken as early as 1917 (Sunday Times Insight Team 1979). As well as demonstrating the commitment of journalists to be thorough during their investigations, this example demonstrates the moral responsibility of drug companies to review and conduct **clinical trials** before marketing their products. In this case, it may have been that the company ignored the early evidence of thalidomide's side-effects for financial reasons.

Nurses have a responsibility for maintaining and updating professional knowledge and competence as part of their Code of Conduct (UKCC 1992). Nurses must not only be up to date with nursing research that has the potential to facilitate better patient care but also the results of the latest clinical trials. In many ways research mindedness can be paralleled with the nursing process in that it needs to be assessed for its value to patient care and should be planned. The implementation of research findings must not be confined to those who conduct the research, but is the responsibility of all practising nurses. Like patient care, when research results are implemented they should be constantly reassessed to ensure that they remain appropriate and up to date or if further research is needed.

The media, as we have identified, are one important source for promoting research mindedness. The media also have an impact on the belief systems of nurses, who, as members of the general public, are potentially vulnerable to misinformation. A recent report by the Royal College of Nursing states that nurses may be influenced by media exposure to the extent that their understanding of AIDS and HIV may be distorted (Scott 1994).

The media comprise a number of diverse institutions. Each institution, whether it is a newspaper or a television network, has its own agenda of important issues. This means that they will each publish or transmit different topics in a variety of ways. Figure 7.1 illustrates the coverage given to HIV and AIDS in the national press in 1988–90. The categories covered within that topic in three newspapers are shown in Figure 7.2, which demonstrates considerable variation in coverage among papers. *The Sun* gives a high profile to stories about celebrities with AIDS as opposed to

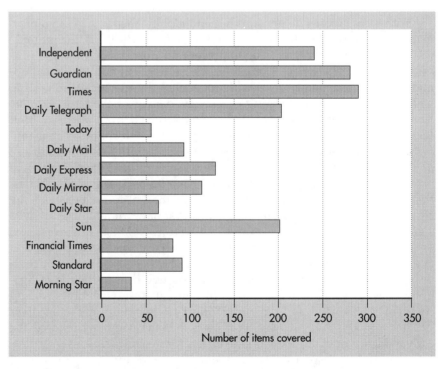

Figure 7.1 HIV/AIDS coverage in the UK national daily press 1988–90: number of items. (Reproduced from Eldridge J (ed) 1993 Getting the message across. News truth and power, by permission of Routledge.)

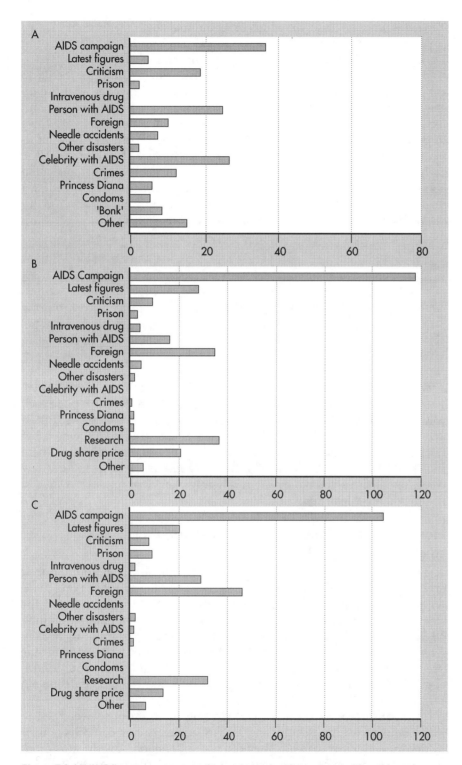

Figure 7.2 HIV/AIDS coverage: category of items during the 18-month period from November 1988 to April 1990; 'Person with AIDS' items are human interest stories about individuals with AIDS. (**A**) *The Sun*; (**B**) *The Times*; (**C**) *The Guardian*. (Reproduced from Eldridge J (ed) 1993 *Getting the message across. News truth and power*, by permission of Routledge.)

The Times and *The Guardian* which give minimal coverage. In contrast, the coverage of research related to AIDS ran at between 30 and 40 articles in *The Times* and *The Guardian* but did not feature in *The Sun*.

This divergence is important to remember when using the media to enhance research mindedness. We do not suggest, however, that broadsheet newspapers (as opposed to the tabloids) and BBC television and radio (compared with the independent channels) are the only sources able to promote research mindedness. Popular magazines often include information about research related to health. *Woman and Home* has a section each week of 'health news' which includes research as well as information about new products. Other magazines, including magazines aimed at a male readership, and other forms of media include information about research concerning health (for examples, see Box 7.6).

■ BOX 7.6

The February 1995 issue of *Woman and Home* included information about research suggesting that even polyunsaturated fats can cause 'furring of the arteries'. In contrast, monounsaturated fats may offer more protection. Monounsaturated fats are found in oily fish and olive oil.

The radio and television also cover health issues including research. This is highlighted by the *Radio Times* which includes a health page each week. Mark Potter, a GP who has a regular spot on *Good Morning* (BBC1) and *Classic Reports* (Classic FM radio), states that the media have a big impact on the public and should be used as a means of educating them (Potter 1994). If you think of programmes you have seen in the last few weeks and articles you have read, it is highly likely that research related to health will have featured.

How does this discussion about the media relate to clinical practice?

The media, by raising awareness of research, encourage both the public and nurses to consider and sometimes challenge the actions taking place within professional care. For example, after each discussion about the safety of the contraceptive pill, women ask questions at family planning clinics or of their GP about whether they should continue to take it. Even as we write, another scare about the contraceptive pill has hit the press. This time it concerns seven types of third generation contraceptive pill, which early research suggests increase the risk of deep vein thrombosis.

Newspaper reports about a new dressing made from seaweed led to many patients asking doctors and district nurses if they could have their ulcers dressed with seaweed. They did not understand how the new product worked and expected to have raw seaweed placed on their ulcers rather than a dressing derived from seaweed. Because of the positive media publicity about the dressings, patients were keen to try them.

When reading articles in the press or watching the television, we all become aware of the information being put across. On occasions it may cause us to question the topic being covered. This process is a form of reflection because it involves critical analysis of a situation (Atkins & Murphy 1993). In clinical practice, nurses are encouraged to be active in reflection. Schon (1983) suggested that reflection leads to better action and, in the case of nursing, improves patient care. In our view, reflection is akin to research mindedness, which also enriches patient care. There does not appear to be agreement within the nursing literature, however, that the effects of reflective practice can be measured. Yet the questioning approach encouraged by reflection appears to be valued by the profession, as does the need for nurses to adopt a logical, questioning approach as part of research mindedness. The overlap between reflection and research mindedness suggests the need to bring the two approaches closer together to investigate their impact on practice.

To what extent can nurses use the media in learning about research and research mindedness?

Can we as practitioners use the media to change nursing practice and improve patient care? The underlying view is that every nurse should be able to understand, interpret and evaluate research and thereby apply research findings for the benefit of nursing and the improvement of patient care. Although the documentary *Preying on Hope*, reviewed earlier in this chapter, was not strictly a piece of research, it highlighted issues that promoted discussion and developed research mindedness within our seminar group. Some of these issues can be found in Box 7.7. *Preying on Hope* acted as a springboard for discussion which demonstrated how the media can be used to develop the ability to critically assess research. In particular, this programme raised ethical issues that are often present but often overlooked in research.

■ BOX 7.7

Preying on Hope raised the following issues:

- how a research problem is identified and developed
- what research is and what it is not
- the process of collecting and analysing data
- qualitative and quantitative approaches to research
- problems and sensitivities surrounding ethics
- ways of advancing nursing knowledge
- communicating results and keeping up to date.

We found that the seminar was a valuable learning experience which demonstrated that as a group we had a good grasp of the research process in action. The use of the media to promote research mindedness illustrates that research relevant to nursing is not confined to the nursing press and need not always involve technical language and jargon. The language used in research reports is often off-putting to nurses new to research. Nurses need to be able to understand the issues involved in research early in their careers if their practice is to be research based, which in turn will enhance patient care. The media can provide an effective method for bridging the theory–practice gap, thereby removing the mystery and fear surrounding research.

We found that our seminar challenged some beliefs that had been held by members of the group for a long time. This demonstrates that the media can make a contribution to the learning of all nurses irrespective of their knowledge of and familiarity with research.

Alongside using the documentary *Preying on Hope* to promote research mindedness in a group of nurses and teachers, we also used it to further our knowledge base about HIV and AIDS. If the media are to be used to enhance research mindedness, the topic under review needs to be carefully considered. A topic seen as relevant to those involved in learning facilitates a better understanding of the process taking place. We only tend, for example, to watch those television programmes or read certain newspaper articles that we see as relevant to us. It is important to remember that in nursing and research, as in life, there will always be dilemmas that cannot be resolved immediately. Learning takes place constantly and not just within the formal classroom setting. In summary, this chapter has been used to illustrate how the media, in particular investigative journalism, can be used as part of life-long learning to develop research mindedness and broaden the knowledge base of nursing and health care.

REFERENCES

Atkins S, Murphy K 1993 Reflection: a review of the literature. Journal of Advanced Nursing 18: 1188–1192

Bond S, Bond J 1982 A Delphi study of clinical nursing research priorities. Journal of Advanced Nursing 7: 565–575

Bulletin of Medical Ethics 1991 How to do ethical research on AIDS. Bulletin of Medical Ethics 71(Sept): 8–11

Campbell D 1989 An investigative journalist looks at medical ethics. British Medical Journal 293: 1171–1172

Carper B 1978 Fundamental patterns of knowing in nursing. Advances in Nursing Science 1(1): 13–23

Clifford C, Gough S 1990 Nursing research, a skills based introduction. Prentice Hall, London

Cormack D 1991 The research process in nursing. Blackwell, Oxford

Couchman W, Dawson J 1990 Nursing and health care research: a practical guide. Routledge, London

Day M 1994 Galloping hysteria. Nursing Times 90(23): 18

Department of Health 1993 Report of the Taskforce on the Strategy for Research in Nursing, Midwifery and Health Visiting. DoH, London

Editorial 1995 Health news. Woman and Home, February, p 71

Eldridge J (ed) 1993 Getting the message across. News truth and power. Routledge, London

Gantz W, Greenberg B 1990 The role of informative television programmes in the battle against AIDS. Health Communication 2(4): 199–215

George J 1990 Nursing theories: the base for professional practice, 3rd edn. Prentice Hall International, New Jersey

Gunter B et al 1993 Public perceptions of the role of television in raising AIDS awareness. Health Education Journal 52/1: 19–27

Hockey L 1985 Nursing research: mistakes and misconceptions. Churchill Livingstone, Edinburgh

Holm K, Llewellyn J 1986 Nursing research for nursing practice. W B Saunders, London

Karpf A 1988 Doctoring the media. The reporting of health and medicine. Routledge, London

Macleod Clark J, Hockey L 1989 Further research for nursing. Scutari Press, London

Mann P H 1985 Social science research; research methods; survey methods, 2nd edn. Basil Blackwell, Oxford

O'Brien D, Heyman B 1989 Changes in nurse education and the facilitation of nursing research: an exploratory study. Nurse Education Today 9: 392–396

Palmer E 1988 Television role in communication on AIDS. Health Education Research 3(1): 117–119

Patterson M J, Russell R H 1986 Behind the lines: case studies in investigative journalism. Columbia University Press, New York

Polit D, Hungler B 1989 Essentials of nursing research methods, appraisal and utilization, 2nd edn. J B Lippincott, Philadelphia

Potter M 1994 Doctor at large. Radio Times, 15 October, p 57

Punch M 1986 The politics and ethics of fieldwork. Sage, London

Rogers B 1990 Ethics and research. American Association of Occupational Health Nurses Journal 38(12): 581–587

Romiszowski A 1974 The selection and use of instructional media—a systems approach. Kogan Page, London

Schon A 1983 The reflective practitioner. Temple Smith, London

Scott C 1994 The care and treatment of people with HIV disease and AIDS: a nursing perspective. RCN, London

Shilts R 1988 And the band played on: politics, people and the AIDS epidemic. Penguin, New York

Stretton T B (ed) 1976 Recent advances in respiratory medicine 1. Churchill Livingstone, Edinburgh

Sunday Times Insight Team 1979 Suffer the children. The story of thalidomide. Andre Deutsch, London

Tierney A 1994 An analysis of nursing's performance in the 1992 assessment of research in British universities. Journal of Advanced Nursing 19: 593–602

Treece E W, Treece J W 1986 Elements of research in nursing, 4th edn. Mosby, St Louis

United Kingdom Central Council for Nursing, Midwifery and Health Visiting 1992 Code of Professional Conduct. UKCC, London

Literature reviews

8

Janet Moir

☐ KEY ISSUES

- **Research mindedness**
- **Demonstrating problem-solving strategies through everyday examples and applying them to literature searching and reviewing**
- **Generating the appropriate references through topic identification and concept clarification**
- **Searching the literature and writing the review**
- **Exploring the relationship between the literature, knowledge and the research process**

PREAMBLE

As an educationalist, I was constantly amazed at the attitude of both staff and students towards conducting a review of the literature. The very notion appeared to generate high levels of anxiety or be regarded as something that had to be endured rather than enjoyed. Moreover, students were frequently discouraged from investigating a topic if it was thought that there was a dearth of literature or that the literature was difficult to obtain. This attitude appears all-pervasive, for as a practising health visitor I have heard my colleagues advise students to select a project that is perceived to be easy, rather than encouraging them to pursue a line of investigation that might be more challenging. It is my contention that reviewing the literature should become an integral part of nursing practice and that time and resources should be made available to enable nurses to do this. Indeed, such a practice is advocated by the UKCC in its fact sheets about post-registration education and practice (UKCC 1995a).

INTRODUCTION

I am sure that the following questions and comments about literature reviews will be familiar to many readers: 'How many articles do I have to read?'; 'What do I do with all the papers?'; 'Do I have to critique each article as I did for my research critique assignment?'; 'I cannot find any references, nothing comes up on computer'.

The purpose of this chapter is to attempt to address some of these issues.

I begin with a case study to illustrate the impetus for this chapter. I then demonstrate that we frequently use the skills necessary to review the literature in everyday life. This is a 'user friendly' guide which differs from other standard nursing texts on research in that it is intended to develop your expertise in critical thinking and problem solving as well as give some practical advice on the process of reviewing the literature. The book is about promoting research mindedness, therefore some of the exercises I give are intended to develop your powers of observation and curiosity. Cumpper and Say, in Chapter 3, argue that research mindedness should be perceived as an attitude rather than a process. I suggest that inquisitiveness and not assignments should direct nurses towards the library. Literature searching should be an adventure rather than a chore.

CASE STUDY

When I volunteered to lead the seminar on reviewing the literature for our research module, I did so out of a sense of frustration. In the two very different environments where I was working I was experiencing the same problems. Students and teachers perceived reviewing the literature as a mammoth task. They appeared particularly confused over the selection of suitable review material. Some students were advised that only 'research' papers were acceptable. This created further problems for the students who then spent time attempting to establish whether what they were reading was research. Personally, I cannot remembering facing similar dilemmas because I was lucky enough to have access to excellent library facilities and expert researchers.

For the purposes of the seminar, I decided to put myself in the position of many pre-registration students and review texts on nursing research, with particular reference to reviewing the literature, that were likely to be easily available to students. I limited my selection to texts by British authors since I found some students are alienated by American publications because of the unfamiliarity of the language and layout. I looked to see whether any of these authors addressed the questions students asked me. Almost all texts gave information about bibliographies, indexes, the use of computer technologies, etc. More recent texts took an interactive approach, giving students exercises in information gathering, using high technology as well as manually searching indexes and abstracts. None addressed the areas students appear to have problems with, such as what literature to review, and when and how to review it. What if there is a dearth of literature or nothing comes up on the computer search? My feeling was that the authors appeared to assume a level of knowledge that students who are unfamiliar with the research process may not have, hence the lack of information on these 'niggly' problems.

The issue of what to review has subsequently been addressed at length in the latest edition of Polit & Hungler's well-known textbook, *Nursing Research: Principles and Methods* (1994). All of the texts I reviewed followed a predominantly **biomedical paradigm** and the underlying philosophical **approaches** to research were not discussed in any depth. The methods of choice were assumed to be **quantitative**. The overwhelming impression given to the reader was that a review of the literature was the first step in the research process and a necessary component of any research proposal. The 'how' of reviewing the literature was not addressed. Although the texts might contain chapters on the mechanics of information gathering and critiquing the literature, there appeared to be very little advice on how to manage the information once it had been gathered or different avenues that might be followed in the event of a paucity of material. During the ensuing seminar, my peers raised the following issues for discussion:

1. Biomedical approaches and quantitative **methods** dominate nursing texts despite the interest shown in **qualitative** research by an increasing number of nurses over the last decade.

2. Literature reviews have low status as a stand-alone activity. My fellow classmates and I felt that reviews were usually associated with the research process and therefore only conducted if required for an assignment, a research proposal or as part of a research study. We felt that 'independent' reviews of the literature should be seen as a valuable resource for all practitioners and used to inform practice.

3. Funding bodies frequently require literature reviews as part of a research proposal. This may present a dilemma for those hoping to undertake a phenomenological study. This requirement serves to reinforce the notion that literature reviews are the first step in the research process, but, as noted by Corben and Stephenson in Chapter 5, phenomenologists often undertake the literature review once data are collected.

4. As more students have access to computer technology the perception is that literature searching will be easy. However, one problem seems to be that students and teachers are not proficient users of different databases so that, unless there is an expert librarian who is both accessible and approachable, students waste time trying to find their way around the system. The problem is often compounded by the fact that the technology is from North America, using North American terminology, referring to North American literature which may not be easily obtainable.

5. Some students experience difficulty in thinking creatively, hence the notion that if literature does not show on computer it does not exist.

It was this last issue that gave additional impetus to this chapter, i.e. the need for nurses to develop critical thinking skills and lateral thinking. It is my intention to address some of these issues in the rest of this chapter, illustrating them with examples from practice and indicating further reading.

PROMOTING RESEARCH MINDEDNESS

One of the problems discussed with my fellow classmates was the perception that research and literature reviews were the province of researchers and educationalists. We felt that the texts I reviewed perpetuated this myth and, therefore, it would be useful to demonstrate how research skills are used in everyday life. This section asks readers to reflect on everyday events in order to raise their awareness of how we are constantly utilizing research skills and reviewing the literature.

Example

How many of us have bought an expensive product without first considering whether we were getting value for money? One example I use to illustrate how both the skills and the process of research could be applied to buying any product is that of selecting a holiday.

When deciding on a holiday it would seem sensible to gather as much information as possible in order to make an informed choice. You are likely to begin with travel brochures. These may only give you information about flights and accommodation so that you may need to look further afield to get information about the place and the local facilities. If, like me, you are a cynic, you may be asking yourself if the skies are really so blue as shown in the picture? Is the place as idyllic as it looks, or is the company that is trying to sell its product omitting negative information? In conducting this investigation you have demonstrated the same data collection and critiquing skills as those necessary to review the literature.

Exercises to promote searching and critiquing skills

1. Advertisers through the media are constantly informing us that now is a good time to buy a car because competition dictates that companies are having to offer 'special deals' to attract buyers. You may wish to investigate these deals. Consider where you are going to get information about a car. What is that information worth to you? Is there a snag with these 'exceptional 'offers?

You could divide this exercise into two parts:
   a. gathering and evaluating information about the car
   b. gathering and evaluating information about financial arrangements.

List the skills used in this exercise to demonstrate your understanding of those required by a researcher. Re-read the introduction to Chapter 3 to remind yourself of what they are and their close association with being research minded. They can be summarized as being systematic, thoughtful, critical and enquiring when approaching new information.

2. A patient or client requests information about his or her condition, or about a product that has been recommended. Look around your work area and observe the type of information available to patients and clients. Consider who produced the information. Discuss with your colleagues the value and usefulness of the information.

By undertaking this exercise you are demonstrating your information-gathering and critiquing skills. With the increasing market economy and the change in the NHS, it is crucial that nurses become aware of what is being promoted and how. There has been a rise in 'health promotion/ health education material' sponsored by the pharmaceutical industries. Large companies frequently have a larger budget than the health authority or the Health Education Authority, and are able to produce very attractive materials. However, it is unlikely that companies produce these materials purely for altruistic reasons. Their aim is promote their products so that nurses are unaware of the hidden messages that are being relayed.

3. Collect several newspapers on one day. Consider how the same event is reported. Discuss with a friend which version you believe to be an accurate reflection of events and why?

E. H. Carr suggests that historians have a corpus of ascertained 'facts' available to them which they are able to collect, take home, cook and serve up in whatever style appeals to them (Carr 1961). Imagine how an historian might interpret the event in 50 years time. Consider what is a fact.

4. Try telling a friend about a film you have seen recently. Why was it worth trudging through the snow to see it? Conversely, why was it a waste of money?

These exercises are intended to demystify critiquing skills. However, my colleagues Barnes and Lewis will give you more in-depth knowledge on how to critique the literature in the next chapter. For those who are interested in sharpening their critical thinking skills, I would recommend Brookfield's *Developing Critical Thinkers* (Brookfield 1987).

I found it an incredible experience to read my thoughts in print. It was also a relief to be given 'permission' to 'legitimately' express my own thoughts in print and in assignments. I am sure many readers have struggled to write an assignment in what is perceived as academic language. Brookfield demonstrates how it is possible to be human in academic circles. His book invites and allows debate.

TOPIC IDENTIFICATION AND
CONCEPT CLARIFICATION

Topic identification and **concept** clarification relate to the problems of how to manage too much or too little information, i.e. what to do if nothing comes up on computer. It is also about clarifying your own thoughts and world-view. I feel that it is absolutely soul-destroying to research something that you are not interested in. Where there is a wealth of information you may have to be specific about the area you wish to review (see the exercise associated with Box 8.1). Where there is little information you may have to diversify your thinking (see the example below). Concept clarification can help clarify your thoughts and assist you in your decision about the area you wish to pursue.

This exercise is called hunt the concept. Identify and list the concepts discussed in Box 8.1.

■ **BOX 8.1**

Pain is a favourite topic of students because there is extensive literature but also because students have witnessed patients in pain. The volume of material means that students have to decide what aspect of pain they are interested in prior to beginning a search. A manager might be interested in the cost of analgesia or the effectiveness of pain control measures. A charge nurse might be interested in developing standards in pain control and will therefore be interested in the literature on quality assurance. Another nurse may decide to review the literature on complementary therapies. For students, their starting point might be to decide whether they are going to focus their review on a particular patient or client group or are going to address health professionals' attitudes and practice.

Example

A student wanted to write a research proposal about the possible relationship between restrictive clothing, manual handling of patients and back pain. She felt her uniform dress inhibited her movement and put her at risk of back injury. At the time, there was very little literature on the subject and other students had been discouraged from researching it. If we look at the concepts mentioned, she might have searched three topic areas:

* uniforms
* health and safety at work in relation to lifting patients
* back pain and injury.

In fact, references on the CINAHL CD-ROM (see p. 195) came up with American literature about fashions in uniforms. There did not appear to be any literature relating to the area under investigation. She may have given up there and then but for a small Royal College of Nursing leaflet on manual handling of patients. The leaflet mentions the need for unrestrictive clothing. This single line was the gateway to other literature. The leaflet referred to a study by the Confederation of Health Service Employees (COHSE). This study in turn generated more appropriate references demonstrating that inappropriate uniforms had caused concern in the past and that it was an area which required further research.

If the student had not been able to find any literature, she could have put forward a research proposal advocating a phenomenological approach to establish if others felt that a problem existed. Lack of literature is not a reason for not writing a research proposal, though clearly it does present problems for students who have been asked to write a review.

Concept clarification

Think of a topic that interests you and break it down into concepts that will assist you in your search. It is sometimes useful to do this exercise as a group. If you are thinking of actually conducting a search, it is also relevant to consider American terminologies at this stage, particularly if you have access to American indexes and computer databases. It is sometimes useful to display your ideas on a white board, chalk board, or poster so that others can add to them; Box 8.2 provides an example.

■ BOX 8.2

Topic: Breast-feeding
Concepts

* The physiology of breast-feeding
* The incidence of breast-feeding in the whole population or sectors of the population
* Societies' attitudes to breast-feeding
* Professionals' attitudes to breast-feeding
* The role of the pharmaceutical industry and advertising 'formula milks'
* The role of the professionals in promoting breast-feeding
* The experience of lactating women
* Health promotion and breast-feeding

The area that I decide to explore will be influenced by my reason for the study and, to a lesser extent, my own interest and personality. As a practising health visitor in a multicultural area I would be interested to undertake a phenomenological study of why Asian women bottle-feed by day and breast-feed at night. I have a dislike of 'number crunching' so I would be uncomfortable with more quantitative approaches. Health Service purchasers, on the other hand, are more likely to be concerned with statistical data that give information about the incidence of breast-feeding at birth, on discharge from hospital, at 6 weeks and at 4 months. They are also concerned to monitor the influence of health professionals on breast-feeding rates and are therefore collecting data about which hospital the infants were discharged from and into which health visitor's care. Both studies would be studies about breast-feeding but conducted from totally different perspectives. If each of us were to review the literature, I would look at the literature on culture and health whereas the purchasers may be more interested in studies that relate to the cost-effectiveness of health visitors or breast-feeding practices within maternity units.

You may have generated numerous concepts but be still unclear about how to manage them. I have found Beattie's (1986) fourfold curriculum model (Box 8.3) a useful framework for exploring ideas particularly as a prelude to writing a research proposal.

■ **BOX 8.3**

Key subject or words
Clarify the topic or key words.

Portfolio of meaningful experiences
This might be interpreted as exploring your philosophy of life. My own life experiences cause me to focus my thoughts on women and favour qualitative approaches in preference to quantitative methods.

Schedule of basic skills
Identify where, when and how, skills and resources.

Cultural issues
This is about identifying your own cultural biases and the influence these might have on your research.

Why Beattie's fourfold framework is a useful model

Key words or subject headings. Selecting key words or subject headings enables you to brainstorm your ideas.

Schedule of basic skills. Compiling a schedule of basic skills gives you an opportunity to consider your resources and how you are going to conduct your review. Do you have access to a good library? Can you use computer technology or do you have access to a good librarian who can? Are you likely to be able to obtain most of the literature referenced within the time and budget you have available? Might you be better to search the literature that is easily available to you in the first instance? Do you know how to search manually through abstracts and indexes or do you need to book a time with the librarian?

Portfolio of meaningful experiences. A portfolio of meaningful experiences promotes reflection and is an opportunity to consider your preferred way of knowing. It enables you to think about your own world-views and perspectives and to consider the research approach you are most comfortable with. The keeping of portfolios is becoming increasingly common amongst nurses, midwives and health visitors as an educational requirement for such initiatives as PREP (UKCC 1995b) and the Higher Award (ENB 1991).

Cultural issues. An agenda of important cultural issues could be interpreted as exploring your own culture and the effect of your emic perspective (way of understanding and interpreting a situation) on your study or it could be that you wish to explore cultural issues relating to your study population.

Example: Beattie's framework in action

I am interested in the subject of osteoporosis but I am uncertain of which aspect I wish to explore. Below I have compiled a map of key words, a

---

■ **BOX 8.4**

Map of key words	*Schedule of basic skills*
Menopause	A review of journals immediately available
Hormone replacement	Menopause clinic
Calcium	Line searches: CINAHL
Bone density scanning	Social science abstracts
Complementary therapies	Health promotion units
Women's attitudes	Books
Family traits	Self-help groups
Amenorrhoea	
Anorexia	
Ballerinas	
Teenagers	
Education	
Health beliefs	
Resources	
Nursing care	

Portfolio of meaningful experiences	*Agenda of important cultural issues*
My experiences of broken bones	That women have a right to information regardless of educational achievements or language
A family history of osteoporosis	
The medicalization of society	The choice of health professionals particularly women doctors
Osteoporosis as a women's issue	
Amenorrhoea and slimming	Epidemiology
Hormone replacement therapy (HRT) versus self-help	

schedule of basic skills required to carry out the review, a portfolio of meaningful experiences and an agenda of important cultural issues.

Looking at the list of key words, I may decide to focus my attention on the nursing care of patients with osteoporosis or, as a health visitor, I may decide to concentrate on health promotion issues. A schedule of basic skills enables me to identify the resources available to me. Am I confident to make my own search or will I need to make an appointment with the librarian? A portfolio of meaningful experiences directs my research interests towards women with amenorrhoea as a result of rigorous exercise and diet. As I work in a multicultural area, I am concerned that women receive care which meets their needs. I might therefore focus my research on the needs of Asian women in the hospital or community.

SEARCHING THE LITERATURE AND WRITING THE REVIEW

Getting started

A review of the literature is considered to be 'an extensive, exhaustive, systematic and critical examination of publications relevant to the research project.' (Grey 1990). The literature reviewed does not necessarily have to be published. It is acceptable to include unpublished dissertations and theses or reports. In fact a PhD thesis is often a very valuable resource in that the literature review may be more up to date than anything that is published.

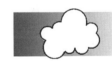

Consider why this might be so. Hint: look at a copy of the Journal of Advanced Nursing *and note the time-lag between when the article was written and the time it was accepted for publication.*

The process

The first step in reviewing the literature is to decide on the purpose of the review and the subject to be reviewed. Individuals conducting a review for their own interest or for the purposes of an assignment may not be concerned with clarifying the purpose of the review and therefore need only decide on the topic to be reviewed. However, researchers use the literature in different ways and for slightly different purposes, depending on the approach taken. Broadly speaking, a review of the literature enables the researcher to determine:

- what previous work has been done on the topic
- the level of knowledge and **theory** development relating to the subject
- the research **methodologies** employed and the strategies that might be employed during the proposed study.

There is some debate about the timing and purpose of the review, depending on the philosophical approach adopted by the researcher. For example:

• A phenomenologist is concerned with exploring the lived experience of people's lives: it is important that the researcher does not contaminate the study with preconceived ideas gleaned from the literature. However, if the phenomenologist has to present a research proposal he or she may use the literature to support the strategies that are to be adopted during the study.

• An ethnographer is interested in understanding culture and patterns of behaviour within groups. She or he may review the literature to give background to the study and to assist in interpreting the findings.

• In **grounded theory**, the literature may be reviewed in the beginning in order to raise the awareness of the researcher. As the study progresses, the researcher uses the literature to explain, support, or extend the theory generated by the research findings.

• An historian uses the literature as a source of data as well as for generating research questions. She or he may spend years finding and examining the literature.

• In philosophical enquiry, the literature serves to generate philosophical questions. The answers may be analysed from a variety of sources including the literature.

Deciding the topic

Successful searching and reviewing of the literature demands enthusiasm, curiosity and interest. It is deadly to pursue a subject that is of no interest because you think it is going to be an easy option. Most researchers start with a hunch which they then formulate into a research question. Those wishing to proceed with an experimental/quantitative design may formulate concise research questions, whereas those intending to use a naturalistic design may start with a broader focus. It is beyond the scope of this chapter to go into detail about formulating the research question (you will find that in Ch. 11) but the design of a study may influence the literature reviewed. The two positions were reflected in the textbooks I reviewed for my seminar. Some authors advocate that students begin their search with a narrow focus whereas others favour a broader perspective. I feel that it is more important for students to be clear in their own minds of what it is they hope to achieve. This can be done through concept clarification or by using Beattie's model. Another possibility is to ask yourself the following questions (Deploy & Gitlin 1993):

• What is it about this topic that is of interest to me?
• What about this topic is relevant to my practice?
• What about this topic is unresolved in the literature?
• What about this topic is of societal or professional concern?

Whatever subject you choose it must be of interest to you. If you are faced with the necessity of producing a literature review quickly because you have an assignment deadline and you have not thought about it or you do not know what to do, if you keep a reflective diary as suggested in Chapter 1, it may provide a source of inspiration. If not, you can set yourself an 'awareness' day and make a conscious effort to observe practice during the course of your daily activities. Life generates researchable questions so that an incident may happen, a question may be asked or something may be said that fires your imagination and gives you a topic.

Information gathering

Having selected a topic and identified the concepts that you wish to explore, your next step is to consider your resources in terms of local library facilities, time and finance. Most recent texts on nursing research tell us how easy it is now that computers can generate appropriate references. However, purchasers of systems may well find that their investments do not bring the benefits they had been led to expect if staff and users are not familiar with the information retrieval process. It takes a skilled librarian or investment in time to teach students and staff how to maximize the use of technology.

Beware: many databases are North American, reviewing predominantly American literature and using American terminology. Not only do you have to be familiar with retrieval mechanisms and terminology but you also need to consider whether you will be able to obtain the publications reviewed.

Example

When a college of nursing purchased a CINAHL compact disc, everybody suddenly became interested in literature searching. The excitement was short-lived when it transpired that no-one, including the librarians, had any idea how to maximize its use. A brave student decided to take on the challenge. She wanted to look at 'something to do with menopause'. She could not be more precise in her thinking since she was hoping the computer would generate sufficient references with abstracts to give her some ideas. She struggled for several hours and finally retrieved 10 references from North American journals. The most recent reference was published in 1990 (by now it was 1995). This student informed me that there was very little information on menopause. Out of curiosity I did a search on the RCN's database and retrieved 56 references from British journals that would have been easily available.

Activity

Explore what your local library has to offer before beginning your search. Most libraries will have facilities for manual searching of card indexes or microfiches, abstracts and bibliographies. It is sometimes useful to browse through the printed indexes and familiarize yourself with the language prior to using the CD-ROM. CINAHL, for example, is the CD version of Cumulative Index to Nursing and Allied Health Literature. If you are hoping to do an on-line search, it is crucial that you know exactly what to look for. On-line databases are frequently accessed via a PC with a modem (telephone connection) to the main computer, which may be thousands of miles away. It is very expensive to work on a system on a trial and error basis, so it is advisable to discuss your needs with a librarian who may help you to refine your search with the aid of published texts such as the MEDLINE.

An interesting exercise is to take a subject and see how it is written up in the abstracts, indexes and bibliographies. Abstracts usually give the most information, with bibliographies giving a few lines and indexes giving little more than a reference (see example below).

■ BOX 8.5

Pressure sores: references

Listed under tissue viability or pressure area care: NURSING BIBLIOGRAPHY September 1991
92/392 BOND M. Pressure sore point prevalence survey NURSING RESEARCH ABSTRACTS Vol14 No3 1992.
Decubitus Ulcer. INTERNATIONAL NURSING INDEX Vol27 No1 1992.

The Royal College of Nursing (RCN) bibliographies may be more useful than the computerized databases to nursing students since they concentrate on reviewing journals that are likely to be easily available as well as being more informative than the North American publications. The English National Board in Sheffield also offers a search service which some colleges may be able to access directly.

Like the RCN bibliographies, the journals are predominantly British publications and therefore more likely to be easily available. Some libraries have their own database and review all the journals that are stocked. This is particularly useful because it may mean you can actually get hold of them easily. In summary then, before beginning a literature search go to the library and find out what computer facilities are available to you. Consider when you might use them. Some examples are:

- CINAHL—reviews nursing and paramedical journals
- 'sociofile'—the North American sociology database
  (Sources: Sociological Abstracts and Social Planning Policy and Development Abstracts (SOPODA))
- 'PsycLit'—the compact disc version of Psychological Abstracts
- 'ERIC'—a database on education (Sources: Education Resources, Resources in Education, Current Index to Journals in Education).

Enquire about any British databases, including the library's own. Always start with the information that is immediately available. It is sometimes more useful in a small college of nursing library to go through the journals manually so that if you find an article you know it is there and has not been ripped out. Ask the librarian if there are any recent dissertations covering your topic. They are always a good source of references as are anthologies of current research. Students often make use of South Bank University distance learning packs as a source of references (Clark & Hinchliff 1992).

Do not be intimidated and always ask the librarian particularly for help with on-line searches and use of CD-ROMs. CD-ROMs often give abstracts with the reference, making it easier to determine the nature and usefulness of the paper. Whatever method of reference collection is used, it is crucial to note the full reference and gather as much information as possible about the literature before sending off for it.

Organizing information

Having acquired a list of references and numerous papers and books, you then have to consider a way of organizing the information. Findley (1989; cited in Deploy & Gitlin 1993) advocates reading all the abstracts of the journal articles and placing them in piles of 'highly relevant and absolutely must read', 'relevant', 'maybe relevant and will probably read', 'not relevant but will keep just in case'. He then carries out the same procedure for books, using the preface and contents page to judge the relevance. Having done that, the next stage is to classify the articles and books according to subject or concepts and begin to think of a framework for writing the review.

Individuals have different methods of taking notes from the written word; some write on index cards, others on a word processor. Whatever method you choose, be certain to keep a full reference list.

A very visual way of charting your information is to display it on the wall. Concepts or subjects are displayed on the horizontal axis and the source of the information on the vertical axis (see Box 8.6).

Example

A friend of mine had to write a review of the literature on the role of the practice nurse in caring for older people. There was very little literature about the role of the practice nurse with this client group. There was, however, a considerable volume of literature addressing the debate surrounding screening older people for unmet needs. It is this area that interested my friend since it was likely that she would be involved in offering a health assessment to all patients over the age of 75 years within the general practice where she worked. Several themes or concepts were identifiable throughout the literature: issues such as the costs and benefits of screening older people; who should do the screening; what should be screened (e.g. hearing, blood pressure) and what instrument should be used to do it; where the screening should take place; whether patients should be invited to be screened or screening sessions could be conducted opportunistically. Some of these issues are represented in chart form below.

■ BOX 8.6			
Sources:	Concept 1: the benefits	Concept 2: who will screen?	Concept 3: instrument used
Author/year of publication			

As you write you can check ideas, concepts and references against your wall chart. It offers you an instant holistic picture of what is going on in the subject area.

Writing up

My experience of facilitating students who are writing research proposals suggests that they have problems critiquing and synthesizing the literature simultaneously. It seems that students are often asked to critique a research paper as an assignment. The usual way to do this appears to be to answer questions posed in most research textbooks, such as 'How large was the **sample**?', 'Was the research question clearly stated?', and so on. You have had an example of this in Chapter 7 when a set of criteria in the form of questions about research studies were used to critique a video. This approach may yield a satisfactory critique of one research paper but students find it difficult to relate that process to reviewing several pieces of literature. Moreover, the questions posed often 'fit' more neatly for the purpose of critiquing a quantitative study rather than a qualitative study. Neither do they address the issues involved in critiquing sources that are not research based.

Example: reflections for practice

As a student teacher I taught two sessions on critiquing the literature. The first was with a mixed group of post-registration nurses doing a diploma in health studies. The second group were health visitors. I asked both groups to critique two papers using Cormack's guidelines (Cormack 1991). One paper reported a quantitative study and the other a phenomenological study.

Both groups of students were able to apply Cormack's criteria to the quantitative study but had more difficulty with the phenomenological study. The latter, carried out by Baillie (1993), was about health visitors' experience of mentoring project 2000 students. Using Cormack's guidelines, students might be forgiven for rejecting Baillie's study on the grounds of her sample size. The first group read the study quickly, went through the criteria and struggled to make bits of the study match the guidelines. The health visitors, by contrast, were engrossed in the study and were delighted to see their thoughts in print. They put aside Cormack's guidelines and allowed their spontaneous 'gut' reaction to critique the literature. I was completely taken aback by the health visitors' response. I had grown so used to the accepted practice of giving students a paper to dissect using a very structured framework like Cormack's (or the other sets of guidelines referred to elsewhere in this book) that I had never questioned the appropriateness of my actions.

The review

There is no set way to write a review. The style and presentation are likely to be influenced by the purpose of the review and the research methodology. However, most authors will include an introduction, some discussion of the concepts and/or theories addressed in the literature, and a critical evaluation of the current level of knowledge as well as identifying gaps in the literature. If you are writing the review as part of a research project, then you need to give an overview and justification for the study and design as well as indicating where your study will fit along the spectrum of knowledge of the topic. Whatever your reason for writing a review, identifying concepts and displaying information on a concept/**construct** wall chart will give a visual prompt about the issues involved and go some way to help you organize material.

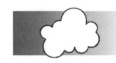

Take any short publication and try to identify the concepts. It does not have to be a nursing journal. You could do the same exercise with a magazine or newspaper article. As you read, be thinking about what the article is saying. Do you believe what you are being told? If so, why is the information credible? Are there gaps in the information given? Is there a hidden agenda? If you do not believe what is being reported, then why not?

Students are usually able to write a descriptive review of the literature but 'the icing on the cake' is the ability to demonstrate critical thinking throughout the review. Readers need to have some indication of the value of a particular study before spending time and money obtaining it.

CONCLUSION

Reviewing the literature should be an integral part of nursing practice if nursing is to become a researched-based profession. However, I would suggest that reviewing the literature is perceived as a feature of academia, only necessary for the purpose of an assignment or as a discrete activity for managers wishing to support policy prescriptions.

Reviewing the literature needs to be given a higher profile within the profession with more reviews being published to inform practice rather than as a necessary part of research. In my view, reading should become a legitimate activity, with nurses having easy access to libraries. Unfortunately, the market economy within the health service and within higher education appears to have resulted in more centralized library facilities with access limited to those who have paid for them.

As a nurse teacher, I observed that writing a review of the literature generated high levels of anxiety and conflicting advice. I hope that this chapter has gone some way to alleviating some of those problems. Many of the latest texts on nursing research address the problems I have identified. Decker & Blecke (1995) give a very comprehensive guide to North American CD-ROMs. Polit & Hungler (1994) go into some depth discussing the different types of data that might be reviewed. Hardy & Mulhall (1994) have an excellent chapter on the dilemmas of writing a research proposal for qualitative research. What is more difficult, is to ensure creative thinking in what we write. Nurses need to read a little, think a little and write a little every day—and question more.

REFERENCES

Baillie L 1993 Factors affecting student nurses learning in community placements: a phenomenological study. Journal of Advanced Nursing 18: 1043–1053

Beattie A 1986 Beattie's fourfold curriculum. In: Allen P, Jolley M (eds) The curriculum in nurse education. Croom Helm, London

Brookfield S 1987 Developing critical thinkers. Open University Press, Milton Keynes

Carr E H 1961 What is history. Penguin Books, Harmondsworth

Clark E, Hinchliff S 1992 Sociology, physiology and psychology in practice. South Bank Polytechnic Distance Learning Unit, London

Cormack D F S 1991 The research process in nursing, 2nd edn. Blackwell, Oxford

Decker S, Blecke J 1995 The literature review: search in research. In: Talbot L (ed) Principles and practice of nursing research. Mosby, St Louis

Deploy E, Gitlin L 1993 Introduction to research. Mosby, St Louis

English National Board for Nursing, Midwifery and Health Visiting 1991 Framework for continuing professional education and the higher award. ENB, London

Grey M 1990 The literature review. In: Lobindo-Woods G, Haber J (eds) Nursing research. Mosby, St Louis

Hardy M, Mulhall A 1994 Nursing research in theory and practice. Chapman & Hall, London

Polit D, Hungler P 1994 Nursing research: principles and methods. J B Lippincott, Philadelphia

United Kingdom Central Council for Nursing, Midwifery and Health Visiting 1995a Post-registration education and practice fact sheet. UKCC, London

United Kingdom Central Council for Nursing, Midwifery and Health Visiting 1995b Standards for education and practice following registration (PREP). UKCC, London

Critiquing the research literature

Donna Marie Lewis   Charmagne Barnes

9

◻ KEY ISSUES

- **Promoting research mindedness through research critique**
- **The nature of the critiquing process**
- **Acquiring effective reading skills**
- **An approach to critiquing quantitative and qualitative research**
- **Critiquing: an effective means of exploring the research process**
- **How research critique can be applied to practice**

RESEARCH MINDEDNESS

The challenge of appreciating and generating an enthusiasm for research concerns most of us involved in the delivery of health care. Promoting 'research mindedness' could be seen as a way of encouraging each other to meet such a challenge.

However, at this stage, it is important to share with you that we have not always been this enthusiastic about research mindedness because we associated it with doing research. We saw those involved in research as a remote elite. The following ditty captures our former feelings: 'Oh clever brilliant person how intelligent thou art! with all those questions and answers ... which we are delighted to have no part!!'.

Thus, for us, the process of research appeared extremely complex, understood only by the very few. Furthermore, we saw promoting research mindedness as the responsibility of those undertaking research, rather than anything to do with us.

We now see research mindedness as an exciting invitation to look at existing practices, giving the freedom to challenge knowledge constructively. When transferred to the context of health, research and its findings can improve the practice and knowledge base, which in turn should ultimately benefit patient and client care.

◼ BOX 9.1

For example, if you are a practitioner, identify existing practices in your area that you have decided to implement following critical evaluation of their effectiveness. Such an example may be the management of heel pressure sores in patients/clients with mobility difficulties using methods of prevention and enhanced heel care backed up by research (Zernike 1994).

Promoting research mindedness, be it in practice or in the educational setting, helps to demystify research by making it accessible and meaningful to all health care professionals. One way to achieve this goal is to learn how to critique research as we demonstrate in the next section. It can also encourage you to develop and maintain a long-lasting interest in the subject.

If research mindedness is incorporated into teaching, learning, knowledge and practice, it assists in the development of a knowledgeable consumer with the ability and agility of mind to evaluate research findings objectively. Thus a balance can be struck between those findings that are useful and those that require further development to implement in current and future practice.

For us, developing the ability and skills to question research articles 'critically' and ascertain the value of findings for our practice was a turning point. We realized that we did not necessarily have to undertake research to become research minded.

How then do you learn to critically evaluate research? In principle, most health care professionals would support the need to develop sound critiquing skills to ensure that research carried out in a particular field is instrumental in the development and maintenance of sound clinical practice. However, many of us feel we lack the skill to evaluate research reports effectively. How confident are you regarding critiquing a published piece of research?

We put this question to 20 lecturers, in a department of nursing studies. 15% of the respondents answered 'fairly confident'; but an overwhelming 85% admitted that they were not at all confident. Some of the lecturers even stated that they would be mortified if they had to teach students how to critique a research article.

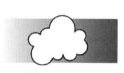

Why do you think they felt like that?

Well, for many the word 'research' was synonymous with statistics and mathematics; while others, even though they had a good knowledge of the research process, still had reservations about actually teaching it.

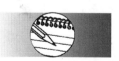

Can you list four reasons why you may avoid reading published research articles?

You might find your reasons are similar to those of the lecturers. When they were pressed to pinpoint the reasons for their fears and apprehensions about reading and critiquing research, the most frequently cited reasons were:

- fear of the statistical content of many published research articles
- inadequate knowledge of the research process
- a lack of understanding of the language used—some stated that 'too much jargon' was used
- some concepts were difficult to master and not always applicable to practice.

Although these results are random and somewhat crude, they are very much in agreement with published research about the attitudes of nurses towards the research process (Rees 1992).

In this chapter we hope to allay many of your fears by taking you on a journey through the critiquing process. It is hoped that at the end of this experience you will be much more enlightened and confident in evaluating and using published research.

APPROACH

The following section will show readers the importance of acquiring sound critiquing skills by linking the research process to clinical practice and everyday life situations. It will also demonstrate how to evaluate **quantitative** and **qualitative** research articles, outline approaches to help readers to become 'critical users of research' and finally illustrate how to use the critiquing process as an effective means of exploring many issues relevant to the research process.

The nature of critiquing

In one sentence summarize your understanding of the word 'critiquing' and compare it with the definition below.

'Critiquing' is an American term, which has gradually crept into the language of British nursing journals. 'Evaluation', although broader, is another term that conveys the same meaning. However, for the purposes of consistency, 'critiquing' will be the word of choice throughout this chapter.

Unfortunately, many people equate critiquing with the words 'criticize' and 'critical'. The Oxford dictionary defines 'critical' as: 'Looking for faults; pointing out faults'. This definition left us with the distinct impression that the main objective when reading a piece of published research was to search judiciously for errors and minute slip-ups inadvertently made by the researcher. The next stage was to write a highly destructive account of the research.

This is not what critiquing a published piece of research is about, however. It entails having an objective and balanced approach when evaluating any piece of research by highlighting both its merits and limitations, in much the same way that a broadcasting company such as the BBC endeavours to do.

■ BOX 9.2

For example, listen to the *Today* programme on Radio 4 between 6.30 and 8.45 a.m. on weekdays and note how the interviewer maintains objectivity and balance. One example is when representatives from each of the major political parties are invited to the studio to discuss a current political issue, say a by-election result. The interviewer should give politicians equal time to give their comments and views on the results.

To include

The following definitions embody what the critiquing process entails:

A critique is an objective evaluation of the quality of the written report or article, the strength of the research design and the adequacy of the author's interpretation of the findings.

(Ryan-Wenger 1992)

A critique is a judgement about the merits and/or value of a piece of research.

(Morrison 1991)

Indeed Morrison (1991) goes on to state that a good critique should be:

- objective
- constructive
- unbiased.

The critique must also demonstrate:

- penetrating analysis
- decisive analysis of the quality of the research.

Dwelling on the negative aspects of a research report does nothing to inspire the confidence of the reader in the findings.

It is of course necessary to acknowledge limitations within the study but the positive findings should be highlighted first. You should also adopt a similar approach to writing your own reports about research or clinical practice. As Oberst (1992) points out, neophyte researchers often emphasize and are over-critical of the limitations of their work at the expense of positive findings.

You can of course learn from limitations and errors, which should be stated, and make appropriate suggestions of how to overcome them.

For examples of when research goes wrong and how you can learn from mistakes, read Professor Emeritus Lisbeth Hockey's (1985) *Nursing Research: Mistakes and Misconceptions*. One example of particular interest described by the author on pages 71–72 was when she stated in a report on her research on the relationships between general practitioners (GPs) and district nurses that: 'In spite of the obvious advantages of working alongside nursing staff, half the GPs did not want such an arrangement. This statement was pounced on by the newspapers who reported that GPs don't want to work with nurses'.

The newspaper was enabled to quote out of context because the author had omitted to present all the results in her report. In addition, she had incorporated her own views on the findings. This example graphically illustrates how authors can inadvertently (or by design) introduce their own **biases** into the reporting of their study.

The literature review is another example of where critiquing skills should be in evidence. David Benton & Desmond Cormack in their chapter on 'Reviewing and evaluating the literature' in *The Research Process in Nursing* (Benton & Cormack 1991) refer to a review undertaken by Pam Smith entitled *Learning to Care* to demonstrate the components of a good literature review. *Learning to Care* clearly demonstrates many of the features that constitute a well-written literature review. It is logically presented, the impetus and rationale for the study are clearly outlined; but most importantly the author presents a well-balanced and critical analysis of the method, content and theoretical perspective of previous findings. The one criticism Benton & Cormack have is that the author introduces a completely new **concept** (Donabedian's 'structure process outcome' quality framework) in the concluding paragraph of the review. In academic work including essay writing, you should never introduce completely new concepts into the conclusion.

By way of comparison, Peter Mackereth's (1989) literature review, contained in his article entitled *An Investigation of the Developmental Influences on Nurses' Motivation for their Continuing Education*, lacked flow, mainly because he jumped from one topic to another and used several very long direct quotations which should have been paraphrased. In addition, the review was mainly a descriptive narrative with little or no evidence of critical analysis. Watch out for this. An author should never leave readers to do all the work of interpreting quotations or descriptions without providing commentary to assist them make sense of text or data.

The importance of having sound critiquing skills

This section will explore further the reasons why health care workers need to acquire sound critiquing skills, leaving the reader in no doubt as to why this is fundamental to the nursing profession.

Make a list of the times during your professional career in which you have had to evaluate and utilize research findings.

You could have mentioned any one of a number of incidents including: implementation or reviewing new procedures within the clinical setting, for example the introduction of electronic thermometers to replace mercury glass ones; being a member of a journal club or an ethics committee; having to complete an assignment for a course.

The purpose of this exercise was to illustrate that in almost every aspect of our professional lives we are constantly, or we should be, evaluating research findings in order to improve our practice. In short, information is being obtained in order to make an appropriate decision. Indeed, if research is to be instrumental in the development and maintenance of sound clinical practice, then critiquing the findings of published research has to be an essential skill to be mastered by nurses from all specialities.

Can you think of an example where changes in clinical practice were made, based on poorly evaluated research findings?

■ BOX 9.3

A useful example is the introduction of 12-hour nursing shifts. Initial studies demonstrated many positive advantages including continuity and improvements in patient care and the overall enthusiasm of staff for the shifts because it afforded them more days off duty and time for further education. However, many of these studies were small and often carried out in North American countries; hence limited generalizations could be made without carrying out larger comparative studies in the UK. In spite of these factors, many hospitals, driven by potential economic rewards, have enthusiastically implemented these shifts. Over the last few years, more and larger studies carried out in the UK have shown that in general the quality of patient care was adversely affected during 12-hour shifts and, overall, nurses disliked them.

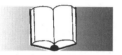

You might like to refer to research on the impact of 12-hour nursing shifts by Todd et al (1989). This is an excellent example of a large-scale comparative study of the effect of a 12-hour shift system on the provision of nursing services. It also contains a very good literature review on 12-hour shifts.

The key to a well-written literature review is the development of sound critiquing skills. Indeed, Cormack (1991) goes even further by stating: 'If you are to become a nurse researcher, or you are to practice from a research base, it is essential … to proficiently conduct a critical review of the literature'.

Furthermore, critical analysis and synthesis of related research will help you to avoid many pitfalls if you intend to carry out your own research. Evaluating related research can also give new insights and generate new ideas for future projects.

Good critiquing skills prevent nurses from blindly accepting inept research findings. This is particularly pertinent, for not all of the plethora of publications produced each year are of high quality. Furthermore, researchers are after all just human beings conducting research in an imperfect world, therefore there is every likelihood that mistakes will be made, bias introduced, important findings not identified or fairly attributed. It is only by allowing research to be evaluated, debated and **replicated** that its true worth can be appreciated and fraudulent practices exposed. This is an issue we return to in our case study.

With the integration of research into the curriculum of pre- and post-registration courses (ENB 1989), nursing is at last moving towards what the Briggs' Committee (DHSS 1972) recommended 25 years ago 'A research based profession'. Thus, there is a particular onus on nurse educators to incorporate research into their teaching of an ever-expanding student body that includes experienced practitioners as well as students new to nursing. Indeed, we contend that learning by critiquing is an extremely effective strategy to facilitate an understanding of the research process. Clinicians, educators and managers need to be adept at evaluating research publications in order to be involved in their field. Whichever approach is chosen to promote research mindedness, either reviewing the literature, writing proposals or learning by doing research, critiquing skills are essential to all these activities.

Over the last few years, nurse lecturers in particular have found that research has become an integral component of their job description. However, not everyone is able to carry out this aspect of their work effectively.

As discussed earlier, many lecturers feel inadequate and insecure about their knowledge of the research process and thus shy away from incorporating it into practice. Perhaps confidence could be enhanced by adopting a positive and determined attitude towards teaching research. Indeed, this was precisely what we did in our seminar. First, we identified the gaps in our knowledge, and second, we took on learning about the research process as a head-on challenge. We did this by planning and presenting a seminar on how to evaluate a published piece of research. We also improved our critiquing skills in the process. Because we found the seminar such a positive experience, we decided to write about it.

Finally, critiquing sessions can be an effective means of exploring or clarifying many other issues of relevance to the research process, as illustrated later in the chapter.

QUANTITATIVE AND QUALITATIVE RESEARCH

Before reading the next section, which guides you through the critiquing process, you might like to consider how it relates to the world-views and concepts underlying quantitative and qualitative research as discussed in Chapter 2. As an aide-mémoire, their key features are summarized in Table 9.1.

Table 9.1 Comparison of quantitative and qualitative research designs

	Quantitative	Qualitative
Philosophical origins	Logical positivism	Interpretivism Critical social theory
Main concerns	To test hypotheses and theories	Discovers, describes and verifies; in short, identifies patterns that can lead to development of theories and hypotheses
Research objectives	Quantifying/comparing individuals or groups (Objective sense data) 'the whole is equal to the sum of the parts'	Holistic approach. Interested in views, feelings and perception of individual. Focus on whole process (Subjective data) 'the whole is greater than the sum of the parts'
Research design	Logical predictive framework Experimental or descriptive	Framework not always predictive, i.e. phenomenology, historical, grounded theory, ethnography
Research instruments	Structured, i.e. questionnaire, structured interviews, non-participant observer, critical incidence	Unstructured and open, i.e. interviews, participant observer, personal/historical documents
Presentation of findings	Statistical data (descriptive or inferential)	Narrative, i.e. extracts from interviews/diaries
Sampling	Random	Non-random
How knowledge obtained	Deductive	Inductive

To recap, quantitative research is derived from the **logical positivist** view of scientific knowledge (Moody 1990) whereby knowledge can only be obtained by objective analysis of the world. The individual is perceived objectively, acontextually, quantifiably and reductively. In short, people are seen as only the sum of their parts.

The 1960s saw the emergence of a new world-view with philosophers of science such as Kuhn & Laudan (cited in Silva & Rothbart 1984) challenging the logical positivist approach to obtaining scientific knowledge. Indeed, some nurse theorists (Leininger 1969, Watson 1981) were derisive about the dominating influence of the logical positivists on the profession. They argued that such an approach was too narrow and cold, and in effect dehumanized the individual. Kuhn & Laudan contended that scientific knowledge is not derived solely from objective data but comes from a variety of contexts influenced by intuition, values, psychological and social forces, history and traditions.

As you will have gathered from Chapters 2, 5 and 6, qualitative research has no interest in quantifying or reducing the individual to separate parts. On the contrary, the qualitative researcher is interested in in-depth studies of human concerns. The opinions, perceptions and feelings of the individual are sought in order to understand them fully: in other words, an **inductive** approach is adopted. It is only through understanding the feelings of clients and patients that nurses will be able to intervene effectively. As shown by the examples of phenomenology and ethnomethodology, the qualitative researcher views individuals holistically, seeing them as much more than the sum of their parts. Teachers may be particularly interested in consulting Bull's (1992) account of using qualitative methods in teaching undergraduate students research.

We should add at this point that both quantitative and qualitative research have the same ultimate goal, which is to compile an account of the nature of knowledge and understanding to improve and advance nursing and, ultimately, patient care. Furthermore, you will be becoming increasingly aware from other chapters in this book that many researchers actually incorporate both approaches and see them as a continuum.

For the purposes of this chapter, 'quantitative' research, as the word implies, attempts to test **hypotheses** and theories by designing studies and using data collection methods to measure and quantify **variables** of physical **phenomena** and target populations. If you refer to Chapter 3, you will be able to identify the enzyme 'rennin' as an example of a physical phenomenon and 'patients with leg ulcers' as an example of a target population. Examples of variables include different temperatures and their effects on rennin; and, for the target population of patients, the type of dressing and its effect on leg ulcers.

As we saw in Chapter 4, the findings derived from quantitative studies are presented numerically using **descriptive statistics** (e.g. averages and frequencies) which summarize data, and **inferential statistics** (such as correlations) through which inferences (informed guesses) are drawn from the data. Findings are often presented as tables, **histograms** or graphs, followed by discussion, interpretation and explanation. Statistical tests are used to justify findings and conclusions and to make generalizations to populations outside the study.

In Chapter 3 we saw examples of two types of **study design**. One was an experimental design by which an intervention (variation in temperature) was tested in an experimental group and compared with a **control** group (normal body temperature); the second type of design compared two types of intervention (wound dressing) between two groups. In each case, the groups were matched to be as similar to each other as possible. Devices can be used, such as 'cross-over' and 'double-blind' studies, to ensure that the intervention, rather than other factors such as the researcher, is influencing the results.

The article you are about to critique, *Helping People to Stop Smoking: a Study of the Nurse's Role* (Macleod Clark et al 1990), is an example of a descriptive case study design.

GUIDELINES FOR CRITIQUING
RESEARCH STUDIES

Most of us have access to research through published articles rather than the original research report. We have chosen one such article written from a quantitative perspective for you to critique. Having revised some of the issues associated with conducting quantitative research, we now build on that knowledge by taking you step by step through the article, which is reproduced in Appendix 2, and asking you questions. These questions will be used to guide you through the critiquing process.

Before embarking on the critiquing journey it is appropriate at this juncture to review some essential and effective reading tips.

Reading tips

It can be an extremely daunting task trying to decide which of the 200 references obtained from your successful literature search will be of most benefit. Do you spend several weeks in the library reading each one word by word, use up half of your grant cheque/wages photocopying all the articles so that you can read them at home in comfort, or do you devise a systematic approach to help you select the ones which will be most relevant to your topic? Most people, given the choice, would select the last option. However, we suspect that many readers, because they lack the necessary skills, tend to opt for the first two.

A strategy which will help you to be selective about reading material as well as improving your ability to study and remember material is the 'SQ3R' system (Taylor 1992). SQ3R stands for 'survey, question, read, recall, review'. It is a fairly well-known method, which is based on three basic principles for improving memory, i.e. organization of material, elaborating the material and practising retrieval (see Atkinson et al 1990). We shall now review each component of the SQ3R system in turn.

Survey

Surveying will give you an idea of the topic, content and structure of the study. The most useful approach is to read the title and the abstract, then scan the text. Focus on the headings of the main sections, diagrams, tables and summarized sections, especially the main findings of the study. This technique will assist you in organizing the study in your mind. At this stage do not attempt to make any notes or highlight sections.

Question

Next sit back and reflect on the information you have gleaned from the study; then ask yourself how it might enhance or add to your knowledge of the area you are studying. Ask yourself which part of the article you may need to re-read to assist you in making your decision. It might be helpful at this stage to write down any important points that spring out at you.

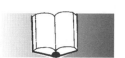

Imagine you were considering 'strategies to prevent people smoking', as part of thinking about the nurse's role in meeting the 'Health of the Nation' targets to reduce cardiovascular disease and strokes. In this function, review the article in the appendix entitled Helping People to Stop Smoking: a Study of the Nurse's Role. *Use the techniques of surveying and questioning discussed above to decide on the usefulness of the study for your purposes.*

The exercise should have taken about 10–15 minutes and it will have been well spent. In this short period you will have obtained an overview of the topic and decided whether it is worth in-depth reading. If you had read the whole article, including re-reading sections which were unclear, it might have taken well over 1 hour or more. You would have wasted valuable time and at the end of that period the study might not have added anything to your investigations.

Read

If you have concluded that the article will add to your topic of interest, then you should now read the study thoroughly. Most people find that they have to read the report several times to gain full understanding.

It is useful to highlight main points as you read. For example, you could use a fluorescent pen to highlight short (rather than whole) sections of relevant text. Asterisks (*), vertical lines and short notes in the margin are other useful techniques. Taylor (1992) *Study Skills for Nurses* and Wilson (1987) *Introducing Research in Nursing* are two very useful texts for practical hints in reading for understanding.

Another way to enhance comprehension is to get into the habit of writing down any words you do not understand and ascertaining their meaning. The advice we usually give to people when they are new to a topic, such as life sciences, is to compile a glossary of words and terminologies that they can refer to quickly. Like anatomy and physiology, research has its own language. People coming to any new subject or situation have to learn a new language by gradually building up a vocabulary in order to become fluent.

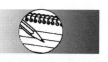

Finally, write a short note in your own words about the piece you have been reading; this is perhaps the ultimate test of comprehension. If all else fails, clarifying issues with colleagues and teachers can be very beneficial.

Critiquing quantitative research

The study that will be used to try out the critiquing process is the one by Macleod Clark et al (1990), mentioned above.

The approach used to critique the article is based on guidelines devised by Ryan-Wenger (1992) and outlined in Table 9.2. These guidelines for critiquing quantitative research show areas of overlap with Treece & Treece's (1986) framework adapted by the authors of Chapter 7 to review a television documentary. Ryan-Wenger asserts that there are three main types of variable or characteristic that nurses should ascertain when critiquing research articles: the credibility, integrity and replicability of the report findings. A summary of the credibility and integrity variables and their associated criteria can be found in Table 9.2. In her article, Ryan-Wenger divides the variables into those that are important, credibility variables, and those that are essential, integrity variables. However, such a division may be seen to be artificial because the important variables overlap and also influence the essential ones.

Important reminders for successful critique

- Maintain a balanced and objective approach when critiquing an article.
- Approach each section of the report with a number of pertinent questions. We suggest you use the criteria for meeting the integrity and credibility variables of the report as a basis for these questions.
- Knowledge of the research process and the structuring/writing of a research report is necessary.
- Have a good research textbook at hand, such as Cormack (1991), *The Research Process in Nursing*, to refer to any unfamiliar terms.

Having completed the first three steps of the SQ3R method—survey; question; read—you should now be able to answer the following question about the article.

What is the research approach used in the above report?

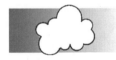

This article reports a quantitative descriptive study. It will be evaluated therefore against quantitative research standards derived from principles of hypothesis testing, statistical methods and ethical procedures.

We reached this conclusion because the article follows the standard format used for many quantitative research reports outlined under Ryan-Wenger's integrity variables (Table 9.2) such as: 'Theoretical framework'; 'Review of literature'; 'Research questions or hypotheses'; 'Sample'; 'Subject concerns' (ethical standards); 'Procedure' (data collection methods, validity issues); 'Analysis'; 'Results' (or Findings); and 'Interpretation' (Discussion). As will be discussed later, not all reports adhere to this format, especially qualitative research.

Credibility variables

We shall now use Ryan-Wenger's credibility variables presented in Table 9.2 to ask questions about the article.

Table 9.2 Variables essential for the credibility and integrity of a research report (adapted from Ryan-Wenger 1992)

	Variable	Criteria
Credibility variables	Writing style	Well-written, organized, subheadings
	Author	Appropriate clinical and research expertise
	Title of report	Describes study design, variables measured and/or manipulated, and target population
	Abstract	Accurate reflection of the research study, not only the significant findings
	Problem	Scope and significance of problem are documented
Integrity variables	Logical consistency	Congruence among the theoretical framework, review of literature, purpose, research questions or hypotheses, design, operational definitions, analysis, and interpretation of findings
	Theoretical framework	Introduced promptly; clearly and adequately explained; documented by primary sources
	Review of literature	Logical organization; critical analysis and synthesis of related literature, including strengths and limitations
	Research questions or hypotheses	Clearly stated; congruent with current level of knowledge
	Sample	Target population described; method of selection and inclusion and exclusion criteria reported; nonparticipation and attrition rates provided; adequate sample size; random assignment to groups when appropriate
	Subject concerns	
	Human	Evidence of informed consent, freedom from harm and coercion, protection of privacy and confidentiality or anonymity
	Animal	Evidence of humane care and treatment of animal subjects
	Procedure	Method of data collection clearly described; threats to internal and external validity are identified or controlled
	Operational definitions	Provided for all variables measured or manipulated; congruent with conceptual definitions; evidence of adequate reliability and validity of measures, particularly for the study sample
	Analysis	Statistics are congruent with type of research questions or hypotheses and level of data
	Results	Summary scores and extent to which assumptions of statistical procedures were met are provided; statistical significance reported; no post hoc analyses unrelated to the original research question or hypotheses
	Interpretation	Discussion of findings in relation to the theoretical framework and previous review of literature; incorporation of strengths and limitations of the study; examination of practical versus statistical significance; caution in research and practice implications without evidence of replication of findings

Writing style. What about writing style? Is the report well structured and systematic? Whatever the research approach the author is coming from, as a critical reader you will be seeking to establish whether the report is well structured and systematic throughout. This standard has been achieved by the authors of the article. It is clear and systematic, with appropriate headings and subheadings, leaving the reader with the impression that the authors have clarity of thought and are well organized.

Author. After scanning a report we note the author(s)' qualifications and experience. You can ascertain this by scanning the bibliography for previous publications in the area being investigated. If the criteria for this variable (Author) are satisfied, one's confidence in the authorship of the report is increased. It may, however, mean that studies undertaken by new researchers are at risk of being overlooked.

The authors of this report are indeed well qualified. All are graduate nurses, including the principal author Jill Macleod Clark, who has a doctorate. These factors indicate that the authors should be knowledgeable about the research process. A quick scan of the reference list will also establish that Macleod Clark has published a number of papers relating to smoking and its effects, indicating a certain level of expertise on the topic. In addition, she also works in a well-respected institution—the Nursing Department of King's College, London University, which has an excellent reputation for the quality of nursing research produced there and which achieved a high grading in the 1992 university research assessment exercise described in Chapter 11.

However, a word of caution. Although good academic qualifications may encourage you to trust the researchers' judgement and enhance the credibility of the research, it does not guarantee it. The scientific literature is littered with fraudulent practices, some of them committed by very respected researchers (Lock & Wells 1993). Many are forced to falsify information because of the pressure to achieve quick results. In fact this was one of the issues which was discussed at length during our critiquing teaching session and will be developed further in the case study section of this chapter.

Title of report. Look at the title of the report: *Helping People to Stop Smoking: a Study of the Nurse's Role*. What information does it convey about the study?

The title is very specific in that it conveys that the article will describe the nurse's role amongst a clearly defined target population—people who smoke. Ryan-Wenger asserts that the title of the report is the door to opening the report, since without a clear and informative title the study is liable never to be read. Furthermore, Ryan-Wenger contends that esoteric and ambiguous titles only 'detract from the credibility of the work'. We would argue, however, that a slightly odd or obscure title may well attract the enquiring reader.

Abstract. Does the article's abstract convey a clear but succinct account of the study, state the results obtained and the implications of the findings? The researchers were not explicit about how the data were collected. On the positive side, the study design was clearly stated (i.e. a case study) as were the major variables—patients, clients' characteristics, smoking history, health beliefs, and motivation to stop smoking. The main results were highlighted and the implication for nursing practice stated.

Problem. In the abstract of the article, the researchers only implied the nature of the problem under investigation, i.e. 'Sixteen trained nurses from various clinical backgrounds participated in a project designed to describe the process and assess the outcome of their attempts to help a range of patients and clients to stop smoking'. This statement raises the question of why they were doing this. The abstract did not clearly convey that there is a dearth of research regarding nursing interventions in relation to education about smoking. Overall, however, the abstract gave a reasonable insight into what the report was about.

The specific problem which provided the impetus for the research was not alluded to until the final paragraph in the introduction to the article. We felt the research problem which identified the need to develop effective smoking cessation strategies given the limited knowledge of nurses' role in relation to this process should have been introduced earlier in the article. Instead, the authors discussed at length the general problem of the effects of smoking within different groups of the population, which in our view detracted from the focus of the report. However, the necessity for the study was conveyed and the problem substantiated with adequate background information.

Integrity variables

Consult Table 9.2 in which the variables that are required to support the scientific integrity of a research report, and the criteria by which to judge them, are outlined. Use them together with our commentary to evaluate the main body of the article.

Logical consistency. Logical consistency refers to the overall presentation of the report and whether each integrity variable follows through from one section to the next.

Theoretical framework. The theoretical framework used by the authors in this article is a modified version of the health belief model (Becker 1974) and the nursing process. However, the authors made only a fleeting reference to the framework. In particular the relationship between the health belief model and the nursing process could have been explained in more detail in order to give readers more insight into how the researchers planned to use them.

Why does a theoretical framework enhance the integrity of a research report? Parse (1987) states that theories are 'specific tools which guide research and practice'. Thus by using a theoretical framework the researchers are in effect testing out the **theory** and its relevance to practice. They can clarify issues relating to the theory, add to the existing body of knowledge or use the findings as the basis for further research.

Literature review

Read the introduction to the article and literature review. Put it aside and take a few minutes to reflect on what you have read in response to the following questions.

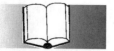

- *Has the impetus and rationale for the study been clearly stated?*
- *Has the problem to be investigated been clearly introduced and defined?*
- *Have the authors carried out a balanced critique of the literature with reference to the following:*
  - *—discussion of the problem from the general to the specific*
  - *—related research problems*
  - *—identification of the need for further research in the area or replication of previous research?*
- *Will the study extend existing knowledge?*
- *Has a theoretical framework been identified and clearly explained?*

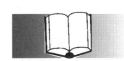

Overall, the introduction and literature review fulfilled all the necessary criteria. The authors initially discussed the effects of smoking in the population of the UK. They then narrowed the focus by reviewing the statistics relating to the smoking pattern amongst nurses. However, at this stage we felt that if we had not read the abstract this section would have misled us into thinking that the report would be investigating the effects of smoking amongst nurses. In short, we felt this section did not add anything to the problem under investigation. The authors made readers aware of the many smoking cessation strategies which have been devised, directing them to an appropriate review article (Schwartz 1987) rather than restating its content and risking their own literature review becoming very lengthy. They then focused on the particular strategy that the study would be using. Finally, the authors discussed the dearth of research available concerning the role of nurses in smoking cessation strategies, highlighting the positive and negative aspects and where the gaps in knowledge existed. Thus, they quite clearly demonstrated the need for further research into the topic. The following extract states explicitly the aims of the study and how it will add to existing knowledge: 'The study ... was therefore designed to explore in detail the process and outcome of nurses' interventions in relation to smoking cessation, and thus broaden the approach taken in the studies described above'.

Before discussing the next integrity variable it would be useful at this stage in your reading to summarize succinctly your findings and impression of the study so far. This exercise will help you to develop your ability to analyse and integrate your findings. In short, it tests your ability to put your own interpretations on what you have gleaned from the report.

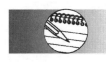

Sample. The sample of nurses, midwives and health visitors recruited to the study seems to have been selected non-randomly. They were not representative, therefore, of the nursing population as a whole. Thus this would limit the degree to which the findings could be generalized. However, the purpose of case study designs is to focus on a small number of subjects to look at many different variables in order to obtain an in-depth picture of the topic under investigation.

Procedure. The research procedure was clearly outlined by the authors. They were quite explicit from the beginning of the report that they would be using a case study design. Consequently, they immediately gave the reader some insight into the structure and format of the article. From previous experience, the reader would consider that a case study does not make any attempt to determine cause and effect by designing a study with an experimental and control group. Rather, it involves an in-depth exploration of a specific topic, in this case the role of a group of nurses, midwives and health visitors in helping their clients/patients to stop smoking. The framework for the study and how it would be adapted to obtain the desired information, including the use of **structured interviews** and the training programme which the nurses had to undergo before the patient interventions began, was described in detail.

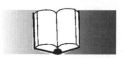

Read the next section of the article—'Data collection'. A brief outline of each method is given and the rationale for choosing it.

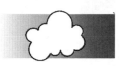

Why do you think the methods of data collection were so varied?

We do not think it surprising that a wide range of data collection tools were required, given the the need to investigate thoroughly the diverse variables associated with the nurses' educational interaction with their clients. The information collected ranged from demographic (age, gender, social class and race) and biochemical (carbon monoxide and cotinine levels), involving the use of biomedical equipment, to more subjective data such as the client/patient perception of nurses' interventions.

Despite identifying ineffective communication skills amongst the nurses, the researchers did not carry out a pilot study to improve them. Neither did they allow sufficient time for these nurses to improve their communication skills. Given that good communication between nurse and client/patient was the key to the success of the study, we felt the researchers should have made every effort to ensure that those fundamental skills were present at the outset. Perhaps they should have specifically recruited nurses with these skills.

In general, however, the description of the procedure for data collection was clear and succinct.

Operational definitions. Ryan-Wenger describes **operational definitions** in her paper in the following way: 'As a rule of thumb, all nouns in the research questions or hypotheses should be operationally defined' (p. 398). Put another way, an operational definition means that for the purposes of research, a concept is translated into something which can be observed and measured. In this study a check list was devised to assess and thereby '**operationalize**' the patients' motivation, worries and feelings about stopping smoking. Physiological measures of carbon monoxide levels in their expired air and urinary cotinine were also used to confirm physiologically that the patients had stopped smoking.

No mention was made regarding the **reliability** and **validity** of these or any of the tools used in the study. We suspect that because some of the measuring tools (e.g. the 'Bedfont' carbon monoxide monitor) had been used in previous studies, the researchers did not re-evaluate them. The fact is that they probably should have done, since, as Cormack (1991) points out, 'neither reliability nor validity is constant—both change over time'. Perhaps the information was included in the original report and omitted from this scaled-down version; but an article should contain enough information for the reader to adequately assess and evaluate the authors' interpretation of results obtained. Assessing the reliability and validity ensures that the instrument actually measures what it says it does and that a degree of accuracy is maintained over time and between subjects and settings.

Can you think of ways in which a researcher could ensure some degree of validity and reliability in the tools used to measure variables?

An example from one of the authors' own experience involved ensuring **content validity** for a questionnaire she had designed to assess the documentation of nursing care plans. In order to do this she consulted a lecturer with expertise in the research and development of nursing care plans.

In relation to reliability, consider the problems of obtaining inter-rater reliability in health education interventions between nurses and clients.

What is meant by **inter-rater reliability**? An example from clinical practice will aid your understanding of the term. If several nurses in succession measure the blood pressure (BP) of the same patient, providing the results are adjusted for physiological/psychological effects on BP under these circumstances, the results obtained should be within very similar limits. In other words, accuracy of the instrument should reduce to a minimum the influence or bias from the nurses taking the measurement (Cormack 1991). In the Macleod Clark study, the same patient received health education from the same nurse throughout. It is much more difficult, however, to standardize and measure the effects of an educational intervention, although the training programme the nurses went through was designed to do this.

Subject concerns (ethics). Ryan-Wenger describes subject concerns as protecting the rights of humans and animals against harmful research effects. Macleod Clark and colleagues obtained ethics committee approval for their study and the patients involved in the health education programme signed a consent form.

Ryan-Wenger does not, however, consider the effects sponsorship may have on subjects taking part in a study.

How relevant do you think it is to establish who sponsors a research study? For instance, the sponsors of the study we are critiquing was the Health Education Council (now the Health Education Authority).

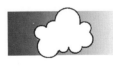

It is extremely important to ascertain who the sponsors are because the findings may be biased towards their interests. Well-known examples in nursing are studies sponsored by the manufacturers of transparent dressings used to cover intravenous infusion sites and pressure-relieving devices. If nurses are not astute and discerning when reading research reports or advice from company representatives, then inadequate or inappropriate equipment may be purchased. In the long run this may be very costly for patients and the NHS in financial, physical and emotional terms. Objective evaluation of a product should always be sought.

Analysis. Data from the study were analysed using SPSS (Statistical Package for the Social Sciences) which was a wise decision in view of the quantity of material that needed to be analysed, thus reducing the possibility of error in the calculations. On the whole, the statistical tests/analysis were appropriate for the type of data obtained. Most of the data in this report lend themselves to univariate statistical analysis, which basically entails the analysis of individual variables (Marsland 1992). **Univariate statistics** describes the frequency and distribution of a variable; thus it measures proportions (i.e. percentages), central tendency (i.e. **mean, mode, median**) and **variability** (**standard deviation**). In this study, variables such as the percentage of the sample in respect of social class, and beliefs and worries about effects of smoking and smoking behaviour, were presented and explained.

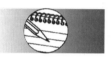

List three other approaches, besides tables, which the researchers could have used to display and describe their data.

You might have considered any one of the methods described in Chapter 4, such as **pie charts**, **histograms** and **bar charts**.

The **Spearman's correlation coefficient** was applied by the authors to test the relationship between the level of motivation and health consequences such as breathlessness. The Spearman's correlation coefficient is a statistical test which is used to assess the relationship between two different variables. It was applied in the article to demonstrate that there was a significant relationship between these two variables with a P value of $< = 0.01$. (Do you remember from Chapter 4 what the 'P' value signifies?)

In other words, participants became more motivated to stop smoking if they thought smoking would cause increasing breathlessness or conditions such as bronchitis. Although the information gleaned from this test is less sensitive than other types of statistical analysis, it was suitably applied to the data which used an **ordinal** level of measurement. Ordinal data provide only fairly general information in the first instance. Again, you can revise your understanding of what we mean by **levels of measurement** by referring to Chapter 4. The ordinal level of measurement is often used by nurses to assess patients. For example, the Norton pressure sore risk assessment tool is based on an ordinal scale. The level of measurement one decides to use when collecting data is crucial to the type of statistical tests that can be applied and consequently will limit the amount of information obtained and level of precision which is obtained from these tests.

Results. The results were described succinctly in a logical order and clearly laid out. For example, because of the nature of the report—a case study—many variables were examined, and it was therefore helpful that the researchers summarized all these variables in table form. A quick scan of the tables reminded the reader of all the areas being measured. The alternative would have been to plough though the whole report. The use of subheadings when discussing each finding also assisted in a logical flow and clarity.

Discussion

Read the discussion once. Then reflect upon what you have read. Read it a second time, asking yourself the following questions:

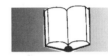

- *Does it adequately discuss and analyse the important findings of the results? If not, which aspects do you think should have been explored further and why?*
- *Are the results discussed in relation to the aims of the report (i.e. exploration of the process of information giving and the outcome of nurses' interventions on whether their clients stopped smoking or not)?*
- *Are the limitations of the research discussed and suggestions made regarding how to overcome them?*

Although the discussion dealt in part with the above questions, there were also a number of issues which we would have liked to have been explored in more detail. For example, we would have liked more background information on the nurses taking part in the study in relation to their own smoking habits and their motivation to participate.

The rising incidence of smoking amongst women and the higher prevalence among lower socioeconomic groups was highlighted in the introduction. The majority of subjects in the study represented these two groups. Because of this, it would have been interesting if the researchers had given further information on the impact of socioeconomic conditions and gender on their subjects' smoking behaviour. This question arose during classroom discussion and we discuss it further in our case study below.

The other aspect that could have been explored further is why health visitors and midwives appeared to have a higher success rate in encouraging their clients to change their smoking behaviour than the nurses in acute wards. The researchers surmised that the success rates of the health visitors and midwives were probably due to the continued contact and support their clients received. The nurses in acute settings had much briefer encounters with their patients. The authors made no suggestions or recommendations, however, for how nurses working within acute settings could ensure that their patients continued to have support after discharge.

You might find as we did that as you read you want to make your own recommendations for practice and future research. We, for example, would suggest that a shared care approach between hospital and community staff might be an effective way of ensuring that, after discharge, patients receive positive reinforcement and support to follow up any health education advice. Alternatively, referring patients to smoking cessation support clinics might also be beneficial. An idea for future research might be to set up a comparative study to ascertain the relative effectiveness of these two approaches to patient support.

You have now completed your journey through the critiquing process and acquired a set of skills with which to build up your proficiency and expertise.

See the summary below for points to consider when critiquing research or any written material for that matter. Tip: keep a copy of these points in a place (say your diary or an index card) where you can refer to them readily whenever you embark on a critique.

SUMMARY

- What have I learnt from reading this paper?
- What descriptive information is to be learned from it?
- To whom does the information apply?
- What explanatory conclusions can be drawn and how general are they?
- Does this research replicate a previous study?
- Can the results be applied to other settings including my own practice?
- What major gaps remain in my knowledge and how do I fill them?
- Does the research contain cautionary tales or make recommendations for future research or practice?

Critiquing qualitative research

The literature abounds with information about critiquing quantitative research. However, there is a dearth of material pertaining to qualitative research. Why does this situation exist, especially when research based on qualitative methodologies is increasingly used by nurses? There are a myriad of reasons for this, but the ones which are often cited in the literature are the confusion which exists about what exactly constitutes qualitative research (Cobb & Hagemaster 1987) and the influence of the logical positivists' view of science on nursing. Consequently, qualitative research is often evaluated inappropriately, using quantitative criteria derived from principles relating to the scientific method (Morse 1991). Morse contends that this situation has in part arisen because qualitative researchers have failed to formulate and develop evaluation criteria based on the principles and assumptions underlying the approach.

The aim of this section, therefore, is to highlight the need for qualitative research to be evaluated against its own criteria. To this end we give a brief overview of qualitative approaches on which to base them. Additional references on this topic are given in the list of further reading at the end of the chapter.

What are the concepts underlying qualitative research?

Qualitative researchers derive knowledge contextually from subjective data about values, intuition, psychological and social forces, history and traditions. The qualitative researcher is interested in the views, opinions, perceptions and feelings of participants as a means to understanding the topic under investigation. The outcome of qualitative research is the identification of patterns which may lead to the development of theories and/or hypotheses to expand nursing's knowledge base.

Qualitative research is usually criticized for lack of rigour when evaluated using quantitative criteria. In order to address this situation qualitative researchers need to develop their own set of guidelines. Beck's (1993) article *Qualitative Research: the Evaluation of its Credibility, Fittingness and Auditability* clearly and succinctly discusses the importance of these concepts as a basis for establishing rigour in qualitative research. The terms 'credibility, fittingness and auditability' are the qualitative equivalent of validity and reliability in quantitative research. Indeed, in a study of the lived experience of post-partum depression, Beck (1992) demonstrates the auditability of her study by giving a clear account of the research process. First, she describes how she chose appropriate research participants (women who had recently given birth); second, she asked them to review the findings, which included direct quotations; and third, she sought an expert in phenomenological research to assist in the data analysis. Auditability is required in order for the reader to evaluate whether the study is dependable or not. **Dependability** is the qualitative equivalent of reliability.

Credibility with its connotations of 'truth' confirms the validity of a study when readers recognize the situation being described in a research report as closely related to their own experience. Another interpretation of credibility is when readers recognize an experience in their practice setting which they have previously only read about in a research report.

Transferability of a qualitative study, also referred to as 'applicability', is the quantitative equivalent of **generalizability**. It is also associated with 'fittingness' since a study is judged to be transferable if the findings are able to 'fit' into other contexts. In order to be able to judge the fittingness or applicability of the study to other contexts, the readers need to have enough information about the research setting to do this.

In a well-known and frequently quoted paper, Sandelowski (1986) eloquently explores the factors which contribute to the misconceptions about rigour in qualitative research. These factors include: the many types of qualitative research approaches and **methods** available; the evaluation of qualitative research using inappropriate quantitative criteria; the artistry involved in qualitative inquiry; and the indistinct boundaries which exist between qualitative and quantitative research.

Sandelowski also gives guidelines on how to achieve rigour in qualitative research by which she devised the notion of the 'decision trail' as a means of assisting researchers to indicate clearly from where and how their findings have emerged. Subsequently, the reader is able to 'audit' the research process detailed in the report and understand its underlying logic.

In conclusion, it is hoped that the above discussion has dispelled one of the common misconceptions about qualitative research—its lack of rigour. As the reader may have discovered, although qualitative research is based on different philosophical assumptions from quantitative research, achieving a high degree of rigour in the research process is equally important.

Indeed, if one understands the differences in philosophical assumptions underlying different research approaches, it follows that the criteria for critiquing them must also differ.

We think that Knafl & Howard (1984) made an interesting point when they stated the following: 'We ask readers of qualitative research to evaluate that work in the context of the overall study purpose. We ask writers to state their purpose explicitly so that the reader can formulate realistic expectations'.

CASE STUDY

This section of the chapter is based on the seminar we presented to our colleagues on 'Research critique' as part of our 'Promoting research mindedness' module.

We chose the article *Helping People to Stop Smoking: a Study of the Nurse's Role* by Macleod Clark et al (1990) which we discussed earlier in this chapter. The article was chosen for the seminar because we felt that the subject area was of interest to today's nursing students, educationalists and practitioners.

The Project 2000 document (UKCC 1986) that examines nurse training in the light of changing patterns of health needs, sees health promotion and disease prevention as one of the main issues for ensuring effective health care in the next few decades. The nursing role in health promotion, based on clear frameworks and up-to-date research and evaluation studies, is highlighted. Current nurse training focuses on health and prevention of illness to reflect a broader vision of health care needs. Consequently, health promotion and disease prevention are its main themes.

Smoking is also a significant issue at both a political and public level, with smoking still being the largest cause of preventable disease in the UK (Macleod Clark et al 1990). The Government tries to discourage smoking through its policies on cigarette taxation, public education and information, but it has a hard job since the tobacco industry spends at least £100 million each year on advertising to promote smoking (DoH 1991).

The critique of the article was carried out using a discussion group approach to learning (Quinn 1988), rather than a formal lecture. We posed questions in order to encourage the group to focus on a particular point or analyse a section of the article more thoroughly. Although some authors (such as Quinn 1988) dismiss lectures as being too mechanistic for teaching research, others such as Cormack (1991) suggest: 'A lecture can be instructive … and fun to hear, whilst learning by doing … can be a perplexing muddle'. We tend to agree with Cormack when teaching groups new to research, but our colleagues were not.

We both felt that given the rich knowledge base and diverse experience that our colleagues had of practice, education and research, this approach to critiquing would promote self-direction, critical thinking, confidence and the sharing of ideas. This was indeed the case, resulting in a lively session that was essentially learner rather than teacher centred. Our role was that of facilitator to enable our colleagues to learn through discovery.

Our colleagues' participation throughout the session was dynamic, with questions asked and listened to, opinions offered that were accepted and disagreed with and issues raised that were thought to be vital and relevant to nursing practice. This contributed to a lively and enjoyable session for all of us.

Our colleagues appeared stimulated by the issues raised from the critique, at times so much so that we had to use our skills and knowledge of facilitation to draw their attention to a particular point that had been missed, or invite them to analyse a step of the research process more thoroughly, such as validity and reliability issues.

Our group discussion raised a number of other important issues which we thought were relevant to you, the reader. We share a number of them with you, to give a flavour of how research critique can stimulate many issues relevant to clinical practice and also dispel the common misconception that research is irrelevant in the 'real' world.

One significant point that was raised was the importance of being constructively rather than destructively critical. There is a danger of communicating research and its application whilst critiquing in a manner that might leave one with the impression that a critique is an attempt to find fault with the work presented. Rather, we wanted to convey an appreciation of the complexity of the research enterprise and an **objective** assessment of the work. The negative aspects associated with research critique have implications for the reader who is involved in transmitting such knowledge. If we are to appreciate, analyse and apply research, the information and knowledge that a piece of research generates should be conveyed positively whilst acknowledging its limitations.

Regarding our seminar, we gave out the article 2 weeks in advance. We all agreed that this gave us the necessary time to go through the article in sufficient detail to digest the information being presented and formulate our thoughts on the merits and limitations of the study. This in turn enhances understanding, participation and confidence during group discussion so that critiquing research can be an enjoyable experience. We cannot emphasize enough the importance of giving yourself enough time to read and reflect when preparing a research critique or any piece of written material for that matter.

We felt that the value of 'learning through discussion' encouraged expression of thought, ideas and free speech from each group member, and promoted personal growth and confidence in all of us. We achieved this by creating an environment where we all felt safe and relaxed so that learning could take place.

Reflect on your favoured style of learning for a minute. For example, do you prefer lectures, discussion or being taught by your peers? Do you enjoy learning in a group or individually?

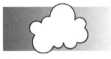

These reflections are important, given the importance of clinical supervision and mentorship in nursing, and might be worth exploring whenever you find yourself in the role of teacher or learner with patients or colleagues.

An issue raised from the study itself was that of health promotion as the remit of the nurse. We unanimously supported the role of the nurse as health promoter in that we saw it as part of caring. However, we felt that current NHS financial cutbacks and restraints on resources limited the time staff had to engage in health promotion interventions. The result was that lip service was paid to promoting health rather than engaging in it. This observation is significant in the light of the recent White Paper

'Health of the Nation' (DoH 1991), which describes and sets targets for improved health performance. The focus of the document is on health promotion by individuals being encouraged to be responsible for their own health and supported by the active participation of health professionals.

We also highlighted that it appeared that health intervention strategies adopted by the nurses in the study helped patients to stop smoking. We suggested that they might have been even more effective if they had been better prepared for their role as health promoters. For example, communication skills together with a sound understanding of the anxieties regarding cigarette smoking cessation and how to help the patients control these anxieties would have enhanced their role.

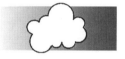

Do you agree with our observations? From your understanding or experience of health promotion how might the nurses in the study have been more effective?

To us, it appeared that the hospital nurses did not have adequate time to establish the necessary relationship for health promotion at an individual level. This led us to question further whether nurses are adequately equipped in terms of training and resources for their role as health promoters. However, the results of the study did show that the health visitors and midwives enjoyed a higher success rate than their hospital colleagues. We surmised that this finding was due to the continued contact and support the midwives and health visitors were able to give their clients.

From the hospital nurses, midwives and health visitors within our group came the suggestion that a shared approach between hospital and primary care teams would be one way of ensuring patients/clients receive the reinforcement and support they require to stop smoking.

Another suggestion made by one member of the group was based on an article she had read by McBride & Moorwood (1994) who recommend the need for a hospital-based health promotion facilitator to motivate, coordinate and support staff in their health promotion strategies and activities. The article describes a study to evaluate the role of a health promotion facilitator within the hospital setting, using the model of a primary care facilitator developed by Fullard and colleagues (1984). The study was carried out on three wards and the use of the primary care facilitator model was thought to be also appropriate to the hospital setting. The evaluation revealed that there were significant changes in ward staff's attitude to and increased activity in health promotion.

We asked our colleagues for their opinions regarding the theoretical framework on which the study was based. It was highlighted by two colleagues, with an interest in sociology and psychology respectively, that the health belief model used in the study is a prescriptive approach to health promotion which research suggests is of limited value (Davison 1994). The model is not fully effective because health educators do not take into account the social and cultural context of their clients/patients. We noted above that the rising incidence of smokers amongst women and lower socioeconomic groups was highlighted in the introduction to the study of Macleod Clark et al (1990). We also noted that the patients and clients who participated in the study came from these same groups. Studies have shown that many women use smoking as an essential coping mechanism against the stresses of rearing children in poverty (Graham 1994). We felt from our nursing and life experiences that it is far more effective to empower people to change their own lifestyle by raising self-esteem, listening and taking on board their needs, and working to their agenda, a point supported by Tones et al (1990). In short, the health educator works in partnership with the clients and their families. If the nurses in the study had focused their health strategies on understanding why these individuals find it difficult to stop smoking, more than 17% might have been still not smoking at the 1-year follow-up.

Fraud and misconduct defined by Morrison (1990) as 'disreputable science' was another key issue that emerged from our lively discussion. In spite of the **ideology** of seeking scientific truth, we argued that dishonourable science does exist. It includes fraudulent acts such as falsifying and manipulating data, plagiarism and even reporting research that has not been carried out.

Morrison's article provides more insight into the issue of fraud and misconduct. These issues of fraud and misconduct ranged from personal to organizational and professional causes which are discussed briefly in the article.

Let us not forget the example of scientific misconduct in relation to female scientist Rosalind Franklin, who played a significant role, with male colleagues Watson and Crick, in discovering the double helix structure of DNA. Her findings made a major contribution to this scientific discovery but the fact that she was one of the few women in a male-dominated world marginalized her from mainstream discussions and publications. An article written in *Women's Studies International Forum* (McDaniel et al 1988) examines the social–structural and cultural barriers that women in the modern world experience. The authors endorse the view that women entering traditionally male preserves such as science, regardless of their academic credibility, 'are seen as inadequate in comparison to men'.

You might like to consider how this view can be translated into the nursing arena where the majority of nurses are women and traditionally dominated by the male medical hierarchy. Nursing research has been heavily influenced by medical science and yet now nurses need to play their part in developing multidisciplinary research.

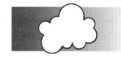

Morrison advocates methods to detect scientific misconduct which should be carried out by peers, co-authors, journal editors and reviewers alike. This approach she emphasizes is essential for the advancement of nursing as a science.

As health care workers about to enter the culture of higher education, we felt that personal and organizational factors might play a part in fraud and misconduct. Whilst personal factors relate to being trustworthy, professional or organizational factors could relate to elitism and the pressure to publish. The ethical implications of these pressures are discussed further in Chapter 10.

We felt that there is a personal responsibility to be aware and make fellow professionals, including doctors, aware and alert to the possibilities of disreputable science if we are to be respected and recognized as carers and researchers within a profession which places a great emphasis on trust.

This class experience, which we have endeavoured to share with you through this case study, hopefully gives you an insight into our chosen method for teaching the process of critiquing research and encouraging critical analysis. It was for us a very enjoyable session that reflected learning, both for our colleagues and ourselves as facilitators.

We hope that the issues that our discussion raised will have helped you recognize the relevance of research critique in drawing out questions and thoughts for current and future practice, which in turn paves the path for the questioning, confident research-minded practitioner.

REFLECTIONS FOR PRACTICE

Application of knowledge and skills about the research process gained through the journey of research critique is perhaps the biggest challenge facing us. It is evidence of being research minded and research aware. Whilst the importance of research-minded educators is acknowledged so that the link between theory and practice in nursing can be made and accepted, practitioners are at the forefront of that challenge, applying research useful to their personal and professional development that ultimately leads to improved patient and client care.

There are many opportunities for lecturers and practitioners to improve both their knowledge base and practice. Below is a list of tips (adapted from Davis 1990 and Rees 1992) for how to go about this.

Tips for improving nursing's research base
- Teachers and practitioners can increase their research skills by giving priority to reading and evaluating research articles, and attending appropriate conferences, courses and study days.
- Teachers and practitioners can use students' research critiques as a resource.
- Research interest groups, journal clubs and self-help groups can be set up among colleagues to improve research skills.
- A resource folder with relevant research articles can be kept in coffee rooms to share with colleagues.

We would now like to suggest how learning to critique research and use critical thinking skills in particular, can be applied in practice by teachers, practitioners and students.

Learning through discussion groups
Learning through discussion groups (LTD; see Quinn 1988, pp. 167–168) is the approach we used to learn about critiquing with our colleagues. This approach is particularly appropriate for groups with lots of experience of the research process.

You can use the critiquing process for other subject areas besides research. For example, one of us conducted a session on the complications of intravenous (i.v.) cannulation. Project 2000 students were asked in advance to critique research articles on the subject in small groups and feed back to the main group. The students not only learned about the problems associated with i.v. cannulation, updated research into the area and recommendations for safe practice, but also utilized effectively their critiquing skills. In addition, the positive comments and enthusiasm this approach generated from the students was evidence that the topic could be taught successfully using the LTD approach. It will also reinforce the fact that research is essential in all areas of nursing.

Seminars/peer group teaching

This approach creates 'safe' space and is effective in consolidating knowledge of the critiquing process amongst groups with a shared interest.

We would further suggest that in order to ensure effective use of the critiquing process, creating the right learning environment, which was highlighted previously, is vital to both mentor and mentee. Another tip that might prove both useful and enjoyable is if learners are allowed to begin their journey through the critiquing process by choosing articles of interest to them.

Journal clubs

Within the ward setting these are an exciting and powerful way of enhancing critiquing skills and keeping up to date with research within both your practice area and the nursing profession. Indeed, research has demonstrated that becoming involved in journal clubs does improve critical appraisal skills significantly (Linzer et al 1988; cited in Tibbles & Sanford 1994). You can refer to Tibbles & Sanford for guidelines on how to develop and manage a research journal club.

Applying research findings to your area of practice

Clarifying/making decisions about controversial areas of practice. Concerns about the standard of documentation of care plans within a ward area provides an example of the approach. On our particular ward we had vague thoughts about why our documentation was not adequate, so a few of us decided to form a working group and critique the literature about care plans and documentation and present the data to the rest of the team. This initial step actually led to a change and improvement in the type of documentation that was used on the ward.

Writing standards for everyday nursing procedures. Knowledge of the critiquing process will enable you to review the available literature, decide on its merits, judge its transferability to your area of practice and help you in writing standards of care for your patient/client.

Undertaking small projects within the ward area. Before the project outlined above which set out to change the nursing documentation was carried out, a questionnaire was designed to find out if the problems identified from our critique of the literature also applied to our ward area and what type of documentation the staff would favour. Thus we redesigned our care plans based on the result of the questionnaires.

On a final note, we recognize that whilst we have reiterated the value and need to apply appropriate research findings to your area of practice, it may not always be easy and trouble-free. Encouraging team members to become research minded, especially if senior to yourself, may take some working out. In addition, your recommendations may require changes in other departments which are outside nursing's control. For example, following a critical review of the literature you may want to change oral hygiene procedures on your ward. This course of action may involve the central sterile supply department (CSSD) changing some of the items in the oral hygiene pack. One objection to the change might be that the new contents of the oral hygiene pack will cost more than the existing ones. Finances may not be available or the budget holders will need convincing that the money spent would not be better utilized elsewhere. Our suggestion is to enlist the help of others with sound clinical judgement and financial and organizational abilities so that together you can work out the best way of tackling the change process.

Poster presentations

This is an effective, interesting and fun strategy for developing critiquing skills. You are asked to critically appraise a published piece of research and present it succinctly and graphically in the form of a poster (see Sweeney 1984, Kleinbeck 1988, Scorensen & Boland 1991 for further details).

Poster presentations can be particularly beneficial if used within the clinical setting, not only to the individuals involved in preparing them but to all members of the multidisciplinary team. For example, one of the authors and a colleague whilst working on a coronary care unit produced a number of posters that summarized the findings of several studies of great interest to all members of the ward team. The studies we presented were the International Studies of Infarction Size (ISIS) trials. For each trial we had a succinct introduction, a number of colourful graphs, pie charts, histograms or bar charts and captions, which illustrated the relevant results.

Finally, the main findings and recommendations were summarized using bullet points. On average, the posters took about 6–8 weeks to prepare. You might say that this seems like a fairly long time but we were meticulous in preparing them and sought help and guidance from the graphics department of our hospital who laminated each display for us. We consulted our colleagues for their opinions about what they gleaned from the posters and whether they found them easy to read, eye-catching, informative, practical and relevant to their practice. It was a very rewarding experience to find that the posters were a great success, and we were congratulated by both our nursing and medical colleagues. Another advantage of poster presentations is that they can be moved for short periods to other related areas such as, in our case, medical and surgical cardiology wards and the cardiac investigations and outpatient department.

SUMMARY

This chapter has looked at critiquing as an effective means of exploring the research process, whilst emphasizing the value and importance of acquiring effective reading skills. We have also attempted to demonstrate ways in which this can be achieved in various clinical settings. Transferring these skills to areas and aspects of practice further emphasizes the value of critiquing for the consumer of research as part of research mindedness and research-based practice in health care.

REFERENCES

Atkinson R L, Atkinson R C, Smith R R and Bem D J 1990 Introduction to psychology, 10th edn. Harcourt Brace Jovanovich, London

Beck C T 1992 The lived experience of post-partum depression: a phenomenological study. Nursing Research 41(3): 166–170

Beck C T 1993 Qualitative research: the evaluation of its credibility, fittingness and auditability. Western Journal of Nursing Research 15(2): 263–266

Becker M H 1974 The health belief model and sick role behaviour. Health Education Monographs 2: 409–419

Benton D, Cormack D F S 1991 Reviewing and evaluating the literature. In: Cormack D F S (ed) The research process in nursing, 2nd edn. Blackwell Scientific Publications, Oxford, pp 96–97

Bull J M 1992 Using qualitative methods in teaching undergraduate students research. Nursing and Health Care 113(7): 378–381

Cobb A K, Hagemaster J N 1987 Ten criteria for evaluating qualitative research proposals. Journal of Nursing Education 26(4): 138–142

Cormack D F S (ed) 1991 The research process in nursing, 2nd edn. Blackwell Scientific Publications, Oxford

Davis B 1990 Research-based teaching. Nursing Standards 4(48): 38–40

Davison C 1994 Conflicts of interest. Nursing Times 90(13): 40–42

Department of Health 1991 Health of the nation. HMSO, London

Department of Health and Social Security 1972 Report of the Committee on Nursing (Chair: Professor Asa Briggs). HMSO, London

English National Board for Nursing, Midwifery and Health Visiting 1989 Project 2000: a new preparation for practice. Guidelines and criteria for course development and the foundation of collaborative links between approved training institutions with the NHS and centres of higher education. ENB, London

Fullard E, Fowler G, Gray M 1984 Facilitating prevention in primary care. British Medical Journal 289: 1585–1587

Graham H 1994 When life's a drag: women, smoking and disadvantage. HMSO, London

Hockey L 1985 Nursing research: mistakes and misconceptions. Churchill Livingstone, Edinburgh

Hunt M 1987 The process of translating research findings into nursing practice. Journal of Advanced Nursing 12: 101–110

International Council of Nurses 1990 How the ICN is promoting nursing research. International Nursing Review 37(4): 295–298

Kleinbeck S M V 1988 Poster sessions bring research to the OR. Association of Operating Room Nurses Journal 47(5): 1299, 1301–1304

Knafl A K, Howard J M 1984 Interpreting and reporting qualitative research. Research in Nursing and in Health 7: 17–24

Leininger M M 1969 Ethnoscience: a promising approach to improve nursing practice. Image: Journal of Nursing Scholarship 3: 2–4

Lock S, Wells F 1993 Fraud and misconduct in medical research. British Medical Journal, London

McBride A, Moorwood Z 1994 The hospital health promotion facilitator: an evaluation. Journal of Clinical Nursing 3: 355–359

McDaniel A S, Cummins H, Beauchamp S R 1988 Mothers of invention, meeting the role of mother and worker. Women's Studies International Forum 11(1): 1–11

Mackereth P 1989 An investigation of the developmental influences on nurses' motivation for their continuing education. Journal of Advanced Nursing 14: 776–787

Macleod Clark J, Haverty S, Kendall S 1990 Helping people to stop smoking: a study of the nurse's role. Journal of Advanced Nursing 16: 357–363

Marsland D 1992 Methodological inadequacies in British social sciences. Cason Hall, London

Moody L 1990 Advancing nursing science through research. Sage, Newbury Park, London, vol 1

Morrison P 1991 Critiquing research. Surgical Nurse 4(3): 20–22

Morrison S R 1990 Disreputable science: definition and detection. Journal of Advanced Nursing 15: 911–913

Morse M J 1991 On the evaluation of qualitative proposals. Qualitative Health Research 1(2): 147–151

Oberst M T 1992 Warning: believing this report may be hazardous. Research Nursing and Health 15: 91–92

Parse R 1987 Nursing science, major paradigms, theories and critiques. Saunders, Philadelphia

Quinn F M 1988 The principles and practice of nurse education, 2nd edn. Chapman & Hall, London

Rees C 1992 Practising research-based teaching. Nursing Times 88(2): 55–57

Ryan-Wenger N M 1992 Guideline for critique of a research report. Heart and Lung 21(4): 394–401

Sandelowski M 1986 The problem of rigor in qualitative research. Advances in Nursing Science 8(3): 27–37

Schwartz J L 1987 Review and evaluation of smoking cessation measures. US Department of Health and Human Services, Washington DC

Scorensen S E, Boland D 1991 Use of the poster session in teaching research critique to undergraduate nursing students. Journal of Nursing Education 30(7): 333–334

Silva M C, Rothbart D 1984 An analysis of changing trends in philosophies of science on nursing theory development and testing. Advances in Nursing Science 6(2): 1–13

Sweeny S S 1984 Strategies for teaching nursing research: poster sessions for undergraduate students: a useful tool for learning and communicating nursing research. Western Journal of Nursing Research 6(1): 135–138

Taylor J 1992 Study skills for nurses. Chapman & Hall, London

Tibbles L, Sanford R 1994 The research journal club: a mechanism for research utilisation. Clinical Nurse Specialist 8(1): 23–26

Todd C, Reid N, Robinson G 1989 The quality of nursing care on wards working eight and twelve hour shifts: a repeated measures study using the monitor index of quality of care. International Journal of Nursing Studies vol 26(4): 359–368

Tones K, Tilford S, Robinson Y 1990 Health education, effectiveness and efficiency. Chapman & Hall, London

Treece E W, Treece J W 1986 Elements of research in nursing, 4th edn. Mosby, St Louis

United Kingdom Central Council for Nursing, Midwifery and Health Visiting 1986 Project 2000—a new preparation for practice. UKCC, London

United Kingdom Central Council for Nursing, Midwifery and Health Visiting 1992 Code of Professional Conduct, 3rd edn. UKCC, London

Watson J 1981 Nursing's scientific quest. Nursing Outlook 29(7): 413–416

Wilson H S 1987 Introducing research in nursing. Addison-Wesley, Menlo Park, California

Zernike W 1994 Preventing heel pressure sores: a comparison of heel pressure sore relieving devices. Journal of Clinical Nursing 3: 375–380

FURTHER READING

Study design

Campbell J 1989 Dietary treatment of infant colic: a double-blind study. Journal of the Royal College of Practitioners 39: 11–14

Crichton N 1990 The importance of statistics in research design. Complementary Medical Research 4(2): 42–50

Fulton M, Raab G, Thomson G, Laxen D, Hunter R, Hepburn W 1987 Influence of blood lead on the ability and attainment of children in Edinburgh. Lancet i(8544): 1221–1226

Levels of measurement

Tierney A, Atkinson I, Anderson J, Murphy-Black T, Macmillan M 1988 On measurement and nursing research. Nursing Times 84(12): 54–55

Qualitative research

Aamodt M A 1983 Problems in doing nursing research: developing a criteria for evaluating qualitative research. Western Journal of Nursing 5(4): 398–402

Holloway I M 1991 Qualitative research in nursing: an overview. Journal of Advances in Health and Nursing Care 1(2): 39–58

Health of the nation

Jacobsen B, Smith A, Whitehead M (eds) 1991 The nation's health – a strategy for the 1990's. A report from an independent multidisciplinary committee. King's Fund Centre, London

Ethical issues

10

Joy Lyon   Caroline Walker

█ **KEY ISSUES**

- **Ethical theories and principles in everyday practice**
- **The knowledge base of ethics as related to nursing research**
- **The role of ethics committees**
- **Promoting research mindedness through ethical awareness**

Nursing research is more likely to be designed, completed and used in an ethically sound way if nurses understand and have thought through the implications of ethical principles which are relevant to nursing research. The identification of the values which guide their actions and the relationship of these to ethical principles is a prerequisite.

(Royal College of Nursing 1993, p. 10)

PREAMBLE

Nursing as a discipline in its own right requires its own unique knowledge base. Research can help in the development of nursing knowledge, but it is important that in our enthusiasm for professional development, both as a professional body and individually, we are aware of, and responsive to, the ethical issues involved. Consideration of ethical issues is a hallmark of professionalism; furthermore, nurses have a professional responsibility to remain both academically and clinically up to date (UKCC 1992). As such, they need to base practice on the latest available research findings. Practice based on tradition or myth may at best provide unnecessary care, at worst may do actual harm, which is an ethical issue in itself. Practice based on unsound research may be harmful, and unnecessary care has financial implications in today's market-led health service. Current nurse education emphasizes the nurse as a 'knowledgeable doer', which implies a research-based practitioner, able to 'demonstrate an appreciation of research and use relevant literature and research as an aid to practice' (UKCC 1986, p. 41).

INTRODUCTION

In choosing **ethics** as our topic for the research mindedness seminars from which this book evolved, we were coming from a position of recently having undertaken small-scale research projects as part of academic studies.

Both projects involved the collection of primary data, one via a postal questionnaire to health visitor clients, the other via questionnaire and interviews with colleagues. One of us had the experience of submitting a research proposal to a nursing ethics committee, the other felt the medically dominated local ethics committee inappropriate for the chosen methodology (**ethnography**). The resultant discussion and planning for the seminar raised our awareness of the complexities of the **ethical issues** surrounding research, which we wanted to convey to our colleagues. The seminar was planned as an interactive session, focusing on the following key points which we identified from the Taskforce Report on nursing research (DoH 1993):

- 'The term research is at times used in a rather loose and general way to describe a variety of activities and processes. We use the term research to mean rigorous and systematic enquiry, conducted on a scale and using methods commensurate with the issue to be investigated, and designed to lead to generalizable contributions to knowledge.'
- '... research into the practice of nursing can only be of real value if it is located within a systematic process designed both to improve and utilize knowledge.'

Given our recent experience of undertaking small-scale research projects as part of an educational course, we were interested in the Taskforce's view that: 'Such work is to be commended when it is undertaken with due regard for practical and ethical considerations and within a good supervisory and research structure. However, it must not be seen as a substitute for the generalizable and cumulative research which we would place at the heart of a strategy for advancing research in nursing' (DoH 1993, p. 6).

Lively debate followed with two main areas of interest emerging:

- the knowledge base of ethics as related to nursing research
- the promotion of research mindedness in nursing through ethical awareness.

This chapter draws on the seminar discussion, personal exploration and further debate between ourselves and the book editor, Pam Smith. Our debates were particularly lively because of our very different clinical backgrounds (acute cardiac nursing and primary health care), which influenced our ethical perspectives. We feel that many of the ethical issues raised during the seminar and whilst writing this chapter, although primarily concerned with research, were also applicable to clinical practice. We decided therefore to use examples from clinical practice to stimulate readers to explore ethical theories and principles as part of being research minded.

Seedhouse (1988) says that issues requiring specific ethical decisions are just the 'tip of the iceberg', and that there are a variety of other issues that are not necessarily recognized as having ethical implications. Seedhouse also describes a general level of ethics that we use in our daily lives for making decisions. For us, therefore, because ethics pervades all aspects of our lives, ethical knowledge is fundamental to being research minded. More specifically, with the growth of nursing research, an increasing number of nurses, midwives and health visitors are becoming involved in research activities. Our participation in such activities may be as consumers and evaluators of research; as implementors of change informed by findings; involvement in studies as both researchers and subjects; or as advocates for patients who are research subjects. Whatever our participation, we need to be able to justify our decisions from a sound ethical knowledge base. This knowledge will not only enable us to be more articulate in debate but more effective practitioners. Ethical knowledge will also empower us as professionals and put us on an equal standing with other health care professionals. However, because the situations which provoke ethical questions and concerns are often very complex, there may be no definitive answers. The outcome for this chapter, therefore, is not to provide answers but to stimulate the reader to further ethical debate and exploration and question both practice and research.

WHAT IS ETHICS?

This section aims to provide the reader with a framework within which to consider some ethical aspects of health care research. We hope to enable readers to identify and articulate appropriate questions and develop further discussion. We have offered guidance with this process but not definitive answers.

The term ethics refers to the study of morals, although the two terms are often used interchangeably. Originating from Greek and Latin respectively, they relate to the issues of right and wrong in the theory and practice of human behaviour (Thompson et al 1988). Popkin & Stroll (1993, p 1) define ethics as 'a code or set of principles by which people live'. These principles provide a framework for inquiry about norms, values, beliefs, right/wrong, and good/bad, within which decision making and actions may be critically examined.

Moral philosophers have the luxury of uncertainty, but in the real world, uncertainty does not determine practice, which requires decisions. Different areas of knowledge may be used for practical decision making, compared with academic philosophical discussion (Eraut 1985). Practitioners, by the nature of their work, have to make decisions in order to take action. Ongoing changes in society and advancing technology have increased debate regarding the appropriateness of some decisions being made in health care. One example is the prolonging of life by artificial means, regardless of the quality of that life. Such a decision may go against the intuitive, commonsense decision that a patient should be allowed to die with dignity. You may recall the circumstances surrounding the case of Tony Bland, the young man who was severely brain damaged following the Hillsborough Football Stadium disaster. Tony was kept alive for 4 years by artificial means. He was little more than a human vegetable, being unable to communicate in any way with his family. Eventually a court decision was taken on behalf of his parents to withdraw the 'artificial means' which were keeping Tony physically alive and let him die peacefully and naturally.

Often opposition to such a decision may be expressed by people with values based on a different ethical theory, which may result in confusion. Developing an understanding of ethical theories, principles and rules can help to clarify such confusion, and enable decision makers to articulate the rationale for their actions and judgements.

Beauchamp & Childress (1989, p. 7) describe a hierarchy of moral rules, principles and theories. Particular judgements and actions are justified by moral rules which, in turn, are justified by principles, which can be defended by an ethical theory. We use a similar framework to the one used by Beauchamp & Childress. Readers are advised to refer to these authors if they wish to explore this framework in more depth.

ETHICAL THEORIES

There are two generally accepted ethical theories in western society: **utilitarianism** and **deontology**. The utilitarian viewpoint considers that the end justifies the means, suggesting that an action is justified if it produces the greatest good (and also happiness) for the greatest number. Proponents of utilitarianism include the philosophers David Hume (1711–1776), Jeremy Bentham (1748–1832), and John Stuart Mill (1806–1873).

Deontology (from the Greek *deon* duty) suggests that some actions are right or wrong in themselves, not merely as a result of their consequences but because of their actual characteristics; for example, telling lies is always wrong irrespective of the consequences. Immanuel Kant (1724–1804) was a well-known deontologist who advocated the 'categorical imperative', this is that a basic law will apply without exception; for example, always tell the truth. Other deontologists take a more flexible approach by accepting more than one basic law, with circumstances determining priority.

These philosophers were writing during a period of great change in society associated with the Industrial Revolution and need to be considered with this in mind. Similarly, the ethical considerations of today need to be viewed within the climate of current changes in health care towards a market-led service divided into purchasers and providers.

A flavour of the life and times of philosophers associated with utilitarianism and deontology

The views of individuals may be more or less acceptable to society according to prevailing social norms of the time. The social context within which individuals live may also influence their views. The philosophers associated with ethical theories (Hume, Kant, Bentham and Mill) lived during a period of rapid transition from an agricultural to an industrial economy— the Industrial Revolution began around 1750. The working and home environment of large numbers of people became an industrial town rather than a village or farm. Factories were built close to rivers (later coalfields) for access to the power required to operate the rapidly developing machinery. Industrial towns sprang up around these new factories. Conditions within the factories were often intolerable: working hours were long; children were employed; low wages were paid; and health and safety of employees were of low priority. Communication systems improved over the timespan of these philosophers (1711–1873). Canals and railway networks were developing, and the penny post was instituted in 1840.

Kant spent much of his life teaching in the university of his native town, while Hume spent all but 3 years of his life in London or Edinburgh. In contrast, Bentham travelled widely until his retirement to the country at 56 years of age where he was a prolific writer on politics and ethics. Bentham is, however, portrayed as an extremely shy and sensitive person and, while he wrote copiously, he published little of his own volition. Friends would force him to publish or surreptitiously publish work for him. Compare this picture with today's world of rapid travel and communication networks via computer, telephone and fax linking large areas of the world in seconds. How successfully could a shy, insecure person express his views in today's world of mass media publicity?

■ **BOX 10.1**

Here is a list of some world events that occurred during the life span of these philosophers. Readers may find it helpful when picturing the world in which these great thinkers were living.

The French Revolution 1789
Washington elected the first US President 1789
The Battle of Trafalgar 1805
Abolition of the slave trade:
  —in the British Empire 1807
  —in the US 1865 (following the Civil War 1861–1865)
First British Factory Act 1833
Queen Victoria ascended the throne 1837
Charles Darwin published *Origin of Species* 1859

Readers may also like to consider the impact economic aspects had on the thinking of these philosophers, and how they compare with economic aspects of health care in today's NHS. Why is it, for example, that the British Government no longer provides sufficient state funding to enable the health service to provide universal coverage and 'cradle-to-grave' access irrespective of ability to pay?

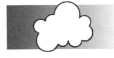

Economists attribute these changes to the 'New Right' thinking of conservative politicians who are committed to individualism, privatization and free market enterprise rather than collectivism and state ownership of industries and services (Hutton 1995).

How do the theories of utilitarianism and deontology apply to everyday clinical practice and research?

From a utilitarian perspective, because small-scale projects can benefit the researcher but contribute only minimally to the overall knowledge base, such projects may be considered unethical. Utilitarianism could be considered to support research into problems affecting large numbers of people as opposed to research into the less common, but perhaps more interesting or prestigious, topics. For example, research into preventing coronary heart disease through lifestyle change may from a utilitarian perspective be more acceptable than research into cardiac surgery, in that lifestyle change may benefit a greater number of people than costly surgical interventions carried out on a much smaller number. However, more resources may go into researching cardiac surgery because of its status as an elite medical speciality. It is difficult to predict the long-term outcomes of such surgery, and research on such a costly intervention may be seen to be justifiable from a utilitarian perspective if in the long term the results can be used to benefit the greatest number.

■ BOX 10.2

Clinical example 1

Jane, a health visitor, is approached by a client who says she has a problem she would like to discuss. Jane is aware that if she stops to talk to this person she will be late for her health assessment clinic. She also knows that this is someone who does not readily use the health visitor service and notices that she looks anxious.

In making a decision Jane has to weigh the needs of one person who has seen her opportunistically against the needs of several people who have booked appointments. Looking at the dilemma from a utilitarian perspective, Jane could decide not to accommodate one client's needs in order to accommodate the greater number who have appointments. Looking at the dilemma from a deontological perspective she may decide that she has a duty of care to this anxious person irrespective of the consequences to the larger number of people.

Thus two different decisions could be made, each of which could be justified by a theory that guides ethical thinking. In reality, the uniqueness of the situation at that particular point in time will influence practice. In health visiting, the current emphasis on needs-based care (as opposed to routine contacts) and empowering clients may influence Jane towards the latter decision. However, managers might take a utilitarian viewpoint because of the pressure on them to make financial savings. Jane could have found herself in a similar situation to a health visitor interviewed for a research project on organizational changes in the NHS. This health visitor told the researcher that she felt 'money has replaced the patient in our focus of care' (Traynor & Wade 1994).

■ BOX 10.3

Clinical example 2

Mary, a health visitor, has been told in confidence by Mrs X that her husband is drinking heavily and sometimes becomes violent. Mrs X's 4-year-old daughter is brought to the health centre with bruising that does not seem typical for a child of that age. Because the child may have sustained a non-accidental injury, Mary has the dilemma of whether she should discuss her concerns with her nurse manager and the social worker.

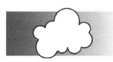

In this situation, is confidentiality a 'categorical imperative'? In other words, must Mary keep confidence at all costs?

Again, Mary's decision will be influenced by current thinking such as the rights of the child, the 1989 Children Act (DoH 1989), and her employer's policy on child protection. In this situation, she may well decide that she has a duty of care that involves breaking confidentiality. However, she may also decide to inform the client of her decision in order to maintain honesty and openness in line with current health visitor thinking. It is also important for us to be aware that our personal philosophies and experiences may influence our decisions.

Furthermore, personal and societal feelings tend to run high around child abuse and alcoholism and we must guard against them clouding our judgements in emotive situations. We may jump to conclusions that the child has sustained a non-accidental injury because her father is a heavy drinker, without checking the circumstances carefully to give him the benefit of the doubt. In practice, our decision making may not fit neatly into utilitarian or deontological perspectives. The use of ethical principles rather than theories may be more helpful in everyday ethical decision making.

ETHICAL PRINCIPLES

Following Beauchamp & Childress (1989) there are four main principles:

- respect for autonomy
- nonmaleficence
- beneficence
- justice.

Let us consider each of these principles in turn.

Autonomy

Autonomy, derived from the Greek for self and rule, refers to the ability of people to choose freely for themselves and direct their own lives (Seedhouse 1988). Respect for autonomy therefore involves respecting people's right to make decisions based on their personal values and beliefs, free from the controlling influence of others. For researchers, autonomy may be influenced by employers and funding agencies, whilst for research subjects, autonomy may be influenced by information (or lack of information) and unequal relationships.

If the principle of autonomy is to be safeguarded during research, unless agreed otherwise, confidentiality and anonymity of research subjects must also be respected. This principle applies to organizations as well as individuals and requires assurance that research subjects have sufficient information on which to base an autonomous decision on whether or not to participate in the research. In order to make that decision, they need to be fully aware of any risks or consequences of participating in the research (RCN 1993). Research subjects may also be acting autonomously in choosing not to have the information. If, however, researchers are party to information they consider either morally or legally wrong, they may feel obliged to tell the subjects. Only then are the subjects in a position to make informed choices. If, on the other hand, subjects disclose sensitive information, researchers may be faced with the dilemma of whether they should break confidentiality or not. Munhall (1988) suggests that in such circumstances it may be better to dissuade the subject from imparting information outside the parameters of the study.

Conflict may also arise if the researcher is a care provider. The RCN (1993) addresses this issue by suggesting that the nurse researcher should be aware of such conflicts and be prepared to resolve them if and when they arise. Munhall (1988) refers to the two extremes of this conflict as the therapeutic imperative (the duty to care) versus the research imperative (the advancement of knowledge). In reality it may be difficult to decide at what point the therapeutic imperative is being compromised by the research imperative. The researcher aims to generate knowledge that will benefit future patients (the utilitarian view), whereas the carer aims to benefit current patients (the deontological view). Munhall (1988) takes the deontological view by suggesting that the therapeutic imperative (the duty to care) takes precedence over the research imperative (the advancement of knowledge). In other words, advocacy on behalf of current patients to ensure they come to no harm takes precedence over advancing knowledge for the greatest good; for the nurse as carer, the end cannot justify the means. Lelean (1975) gives the following clear-cut example. In research on the effectiveness of communication systems within the hospital nursing team, nurses were employed as non-participant observers. This meant they were not allowed to take part in any nursing care of patients. Lelean describes two occasions when the nurse researchers could not keep to their research brief:

> The first was when a patient who was mentally confused was about to drink her hand cream. The observer removed it and shifted the bedside locker so that the hand cream could not be reached (no nurse was in the ward at the time). The second occurred five minutes before the end of a day's observation period. A patient, who was walking with the aid of crutches, fainted as she was passing the observer. The observer caught her and called for a nurse.

> (Lelean 1975, p. 38)

If the observers had been taking a utilitarian viewpoint they may have preferred to wait and see what the outcome of these two incidents might have been without their intervention. However, the therapeutic imperative suggested that the observers should intervene, since the two patients may have suffered harm if they had not. It is also interesting to speculate in the second incident whether the observer put herself at risk by catching the falling patient. It is well known that nurses can suffer serious back injury by putting patients' safety needs first in such situations.

Nonmaleficence

The notion of **nonmaleficence**, the duty of not inflicting harm, is another important consideration in research. We can see, for example, that if the observers had not intervened in either of the incidents recorded by Lelean, they would have indirectly been inflicting harm on the two patients by not preventing them harming themselves. Nonmaleficence therefore is not necessarily as straightforward as it at first appears. It is important to remember that harm takes many forms: it can be emotional as well as physical and varies considerably between individuals.

Research interviews or questionnaires, whilst initially appearing harmless, may cause distress by raising emotional issues or causing disclosure of previously private experiences. Aspects of research subjects' lifestyle or past life may be uncovered or relived, leaving them feeling uncomfortable or confused with no means of resolving the issues. If the researcher, having obtained the required data, ignores or is oblivious to what is left behind, the principle of nonmaleficence is not being met.

As discussed in Chapter 2, feminist researchers stress the importance of the research being for the benefit of the research subjects and the development of an equal relationship with the researcher. Sharing experiences, however, makes the researcher vulnerable in the same way that research subjects are vulnerable (Webb 1993). Whilst this could reduce exploitation of the research subject, to what extent it can actually be achieved is open to debate (Webb 1993).

In order to apply the concept of nonmaleficence (i.e. the duty of not inflicting harm) to ethical judgements about clinical and research situations, it is necessary to establish a standard of care due to individuals which practitioners and researchers are obliged to provide. The duty of care may require prevention or removal of harm as part of normal practice, and, therefore, by not preventing harm (as we saw in the examples above) the principle of nonmaleficence has been violated. Standards of due care are usually determined by role and general societal expectations. If the nurse has a duty to act as an advocate for patients, then not to intervene if research appears to contravene ethical principles would in itself contravene the principle of nonmaleficence. Patients who have not been given all the information regarding **clinical trials**, or are felt not to understand the issues, will not be fully autonomous. Yet many patients may consent in order to help the researcher, who they respect and trust and perhaps feel in awe of. They may also have an altruistic motive in that they see their participation in the research as helping society at large. In order to act as advocates, nurses may need to challenge colleagues, but they cannot do this effectively without the ethical knowledge base.

Beneficence

Beneficence builds on the principle of nonmaleficence in that it goes beyond preventing or removing harm to actually doing or promoting good. Looking at beneficence in this way also suggests that nurses have a responsibility to act as advocates for patients who are subjects of research conducted by others, as well as complying with the principle in their own research. The principle of beneficence could also lead to questioning the ethics of research that is purely for the benefit of the researcher (for example as part of an educational programme) but will not benefit the research subject. From a purely utilitarian perspective, this could be justified if the experience makes the researcher more research minded and as a result a better practitioner, so benefiting the greater number in the long term.

Fulfilling one ethical principle may conflict with fulfilling another, however, since 'good' and 'harm' are rarely inseparable. For example, achievement of a good outcome may inevitably be accompanied by one that inflicts harm. When this happens it is referred to as the 'double effect'. In clinical practice, the provision of physiotherapy to prevent chest complications such as atelectasis following open chest surgery may have a good effect or outcome. But, in the process, the physiotherapist may cause pain and discomfort to the patient (bad effect or outcome). One way to resolve this conflict is by seeing that the overall outcome of physiotherapy is to maximize good (i.e. by preventing atelectasis and other complications) but also to minimize harm by ensuring that the patient receives adequate analgesia prior to the treatment.

Justice

The principle of **justice** (being fair) is based on Aristotle's concept that how individuals are treated relates to their position and worth within a given society. Individuals will be treated therefore in proportion to their standing (Beauchamp & Childress 1989). This is a complex principle, since it suggests that not all individuals are equally valued within society. Arguments can be made for distribution of resources according to need, welfare or merit and for fairness and impartiality. Justice is particularly relevant when considering the distribution of scarce resources at all levels in health care and, as such, is part of the equation when justifying the cost involved in setting up and conducting research studies. Gillon (1986) suggests that medical need is often the criterion on which the principle of justice is judged. If this is the case, then it is possible that certain patients, depending on their race, age, gender, sexual orientation or social status, are being discriminated against when decisions are made about who is most worthy of receiving a high-tech medical treatment.

In research terms, judgements about who should be included in research studies and, indeed, who and what should be studied in the first place may be based on similar criteria. For example, the now infamous Tuskegee Syphilis Study, set up in 1932, satisfied none of the requirements for ethical research (Caplan et al 1992). The subjects of study were 400 black men in Tuskegee, Alabama. The unethical conduct of the study still has repercussions for the African American community today, who not surprisingly profoundly distrust the motives of both public health services and research.

The study was set up to 'determine the natural history of untreated syphilis' (Caplan et al 1992, p. 29). 400 black men with syphilis were recruited and matched against 200 black men who were not infected with the disease. Subjects were subject to spinal taps to investigate the neurological effects of syphilis under the guise of 'special free treatment'. Informed consent was not obtained from the recruits. They were given the standard heavy metal treatment for syphilis that was available when the study began, but were denied penicillin when it became available as an effective treatment in the 1940s because it would interfere with the 'natural' history of the disease. The study, which was funded by the US Federal Government, continued until 1972 when a public health official expressed his deep concern about its morality to a newspaper reporter. Following media exposure, the study was finally discontinued and a series of law suits followed on behalf of the subjects.

A number of ethical issues are raised by the Tuskegee study, including two key questions. First, should the results of an unethical study continue to inform the clinical knowledge base on syphilis? Second, how should groups already discriminated against be protected from such unethical invasions as well as being adequately represented in and benefiting from clinical trials?

The exposure of the study in the US led to the setting up of a National Commission for the Protection of Human Subjects of Biomedical and Behavioural Research in 1974. The Commission laid down rigorous ethical requirements which continue to serve as guidelines in the US for the conduct of present-day research on human subjects.

Ethical principles and emotions

When considering ethical principles, it is important to acknowledge that emotions may influence our decision making. For example, the reporter who exposed the unethical conduct of the Tuskegee study did so because of the deep concern he felt about the morality of the research.

The work of Gilligan (1982) can help the reader appreciate how the concepts of logic and justice, which form the implicit basis of commercial and legal ethics, may be at odds with emotion and conscience, which are the guide for most individuals. Gilligan suggests that depending on how situations are perceived, different solutions may be proposed, resulting in different outcomes. In particular, Gilligan proposes a different theory of moral development from the established theory proposed by Kohlberg based on the principle of justice. Gilligan subsequently identifies a 'different' or 'female voice' that determines individual values and decision making based on care and responsibility, which enables situations to be viewed as a 'narrative of relationships that extends over time'. By comparison, the male voice sees situations 'like a math problem with humans'. Gilligan continues: 'The different voice I describe is characterised not by gender but theme. Its association with women is an empirical observation, and it is primarily through women's voices that I trace its development' (Gilligan 1993, p. 2).

Harbison (1992) explores the relevance of Gilligan's female voice to the voice of nursing and shows how nurses may be unwilling to make decisions on clinical scenarios presented in classrooms because they recognize the need for contextual information in order to make clinical decisions. They also need to draw on the emotional aspects of the caring relationship that is fundamental to expert nursing practice. This example suggests that nurses make their decisions on the basis of an ethic of care and responsibility rather than logic and justice. The vignette below will help you to consider some of the factors that influence decision making.

■ **BOX 10.4**

Clinical example 3

A patient has died in a specialist high-care area. His relatives have been visiting frequently and have become familiar with the setting and the variety of carers. They have been prepared for his death but are distressed when told by telephone that he has actually died. They are on their way to the hospital to see the deceased and the staff on duty. It is anticipated that they will arrive on the unit in approximately 30 minutes. An emergency admission for a patient undergoing surgery is requested by the medical staff. Consequently, a bed is required urgently and it is suggested that the deceased patient be moved to the mortuary on the grounds that nothing more can be done for him. On the other hand, the survival of the patient undergoing surgery may be influenced by access to specialist facilities.

Consider:

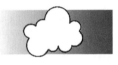

- *the effect that 'knowing' the deceased and his family, and the anonymity of the emergency patient and his family, has on your feelings about this situation*
- *the duty of care you have to the deceased patient and the emergency patient*
- *the relationships involved in this situation: deceased patient and his relatives; emergency patient and his relatives; nurse caring for deceased; nurse about to care for emergency patient (who may in fact be the same nurse); colleagues in theatre; medical colleagues; other staff and patients within the unit*
- *how these relationships impact on how you feel and on the decisions you make.*

From this example the reader may perceive how the emotional impact of caring may conflict with the logical aspects which suggest that priority should be given to ensuring the survival of the live patient. The reader can explore alternative solutions that may meet both emotional and logical needs.

Consider the range of options below:

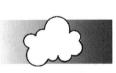

- *Can the emergency patient remain in the operating theatre to recover for a period of time?*
- *Can operating theatre or unit staff be released to accommodate the needs of relatives (and staff)?*
- *Can another bed space be generated for the emergency patient?*
- *Can another space be found for the deceased and the nurse who has been caring for him released to meet the relatives' needs?*

Alternative solutions may require imaginative use of available resources, recognition of the relationship between individuals and health care teams, and identification of the long-term effects of decisions. The latter may include the bereavement process of relatives; the perceived quality of service delivery (do we have a duty of care only to the patient or does this include the family as well?); and the professional and personal satisfaction of staff working within the unit.

Although in this section we have been looking at the application of ethical principles to clinical practice, many of the situations we have described apply equally to research. In neither case can the ethical principles be viewed in isolation from each other or from the context within which the clinical practice or research is taking place. When principles conflict, priority is likely to depend upon the context and the uniqueness of the situation, as well as being influenced by our emotions and relationships with the people involved.

THE ROLE OF ETHICS COMMITTEES

This section aims to discuss ethical issues and research through an exploration of ethics committees.

Background

Research ethics committees are generally accepted as a forum for assuring that all research involving human subjects is carried out in an ethically sound manner. Their development stems from concerns following the use of human subjects in research by the Nazis during the Second World War and the subsequent Nuremberg Trials. Following the trials between 1946 and 1947 of 20 physicians who had conducted extreme human experiments in the concentration camps of the Third Reich, the Nuremberg Ethical Code was formulated. The experiments were often fatal and usually involved non-consenting inmates (Shevrell & Evans 1994). They exposed people to extremes of altitude, temperature and a variety of poisons. Subjects were also deliberately injected with bacteria of a range of diseases in order to develop vaccines and treatments. One experiment was performed by an eminent German neurologist who attempted to establish a viral cause for multiple sclerosis. Shevrell & Evans (1994, p. 350) write:

> The focus, both at the trials and now, has been on human experimentation in the camps. As noted by Caplan, this had the unfortunate effect of (1) fostering the 'comforting myth' that only fanatic, marginal physicians and scientists carried out these unethical experiments and (2) minimizing the role played by more 'mainstream' elements of medicine in providing scientific legitimacy to Nazi policies. Within the context of a state and society that systematically devalued the intrinsic worth of certain classes of human beings, unethical experiments did occur within the ivory tower of academic medicine.

Since the Nuremberg Trials, the World Medical Association's Declaration of Helsinki governs biomedical research using human subjects with an emphasis on freely given informed consent and the premise that the interest of the subject must always prevail over the interest of science and society (Gillon 1986). There are parallels here with the setting up of the

National Commission for the Protection of Human Subjects of Biomedical and Behavioural Research in the US following the exposure of the Tuskegee Syphilis Study.

The setting up of such safeguards suggests that of the two types of ethical theory previously discussed, deontology rather than utilitarianism takes precedence. The precedence of deontology is reiterated in the research guidelines published by the Royal College of Nursing which state:

The research subjects entrust themselves to the researcher who has an obligation to safeguard them and their welfare in the research situation. Any nurse researcher must decide at what point ethical requirements necessitate an intervention in order to maintain the safety of the patients/clients, whatever the consequences for the research.

(RCN 1993, p. 8)

The following recommendation is also made: 'there must be safeguards for protection against physical, mental, emotional and social harm' (RCN 1993, p. 12).

In order to ensure the deontological ethic is maintained, all research activities involving human subjects should be submitted to a research ethics committee (RCN 1993, Neuberger 1992, RCP 1990). The role of the committee in protecting research subjects and offering informed and independent advice is clear as outlined below.

The committee has a role in relation to:

- the value of the research per se, which is perhaps more suggestive of a utilitarian ethic
- applying ethical principles to all stages of the research process, including interpretation and dissemination of results.

The legal power and liabilities of ethics committees once research proposals have been approved are less clear. Since nurses are relative newcomers to research, ethics committee members may be unused to considering topics and **methodologies** favoured by nurse researchers. Because of this, some health care institutions have set up separate ethics committees for nursing research.

A critical consideration of the membership, organization, power and responsibilities of ethics committees is therefore an essential component of research mindedness for nurses. It will enable them to act as the patient's advocate from an informed knowledge base when research is being carried out in clinical areas.

When evaluating research reports, it is helpful to check whether ethical approval has been granted. If it has, this will give ethical credibility. However, the critically aware practitioner will want to consider the ethical implications of the research and how they have been addressed, by applying the four ethical principles discussed above. It is not always easy to do this since research articles in journals often do not give sufficient detail for readers to evaluate the ethical implications fully. They have to be reassured, therefore, that the research is ethical because it has been approved by an ethics committee. Many professional journals will only accept research reports for publication if ethical approval has been granted.

Membership of ethics committees

Every district health authority is required by the Department of Health to set up local research ethics committees and there are clear guidelines for membership. A range of health care professionals including nurses is suggested, along with a minimum of two lay members. However, Neuberger (1992) in a survey of 222 ethics committees found that 12% had no nurse representation and that 52% of the total membership were hospital doctors. This finding could question the suitability of some committees for assessing the ethical component of nursing research.

The medical dominance of ethics committee membership could result in **quantitative** research methodology and experiments being considered more favourably than **qualitative** research methodologies such as phenomenology, which some nurse researchers consider are more appropriate to the study of nursing (Jasper 1994, Kiikkala & Munnukka 1994). Pollack & Tilley (1988), in a small study, found that nurses' negative encounters with ethics committees included the committees' lack of understanding of qualitative methodology and competence to evaluate such studies. The Royal College of Physicians (1990, p. 42) suggest in their guidelines that the committee should: 'be satisfied that the research activity is a worthwhile one, and should examine the overall design of the proposed research'. This could indicate a medically orientated approach to research methodology.

The issue of research being worthwhile is interesting since a proposal may be considered ethically sound from a deontological perspective but not from a utilitarian perspective, especially if it is not seen to be producing generalizable knowledge. If there are conflicts between the two perspectives, should the proposal be approved? It could be argued that all knowledge has value and, until the research is complete, its value in contributing to generalizable knowledge is unclear.

The current medical dominance of ethics committees could discourage nurses from submitting research proposals and result in studies being carried out that had not received ethical approval. Pollack & Tilley (1992), in a study of factors that influenced whether nurses submitted their proposals to ethics committees, found that a key factor concerned gaining access to subjects. The ethics committee was seen to have a gatekeeping function in this respect. The perceived 'hassle factor' associated with submitting proposals also influenced nurses' decisions to submit or not. These factors might imply that nurses did not make their decisions on ethical principles but rather responded to the need to get the research started as quickly as possible. It is possible, therefore, that nurses who do not see the need to submit their research to the scrutiny of an ethics committee lack ethical awareness but neither are they being supervised or guided by experienced researchers.

The need for ethical approval of research exists whether the subjects are patients, nurse colleagues or students. Assurance that consent is freely given could be compromised if the researcher is in a more powerful position than the subject. This is invariably the case for patients, who may feel dependent on doctors and nurses for their treatment as well as being research subjects. Often nurses do not see the need to seek ethical approval for research with colleagues and students. Researchers may, however, have power over their subjects, as is the case of lecturers over students and ward sisters over junior staff. This situation could impinge on the principle of autonomy in that students or junior staff members may feel unable to refuse to take part in research conducted by their seniors. The ethics committee, therefore, has a role in assuring that potentially vulnerable subjects are not exploited. Smith (1994) found that 'nurses as subjects' was a predominant theme in nursing research, although she does not indicate whether there was an issue of unequal relationships between researchers and researched or whether ethical approval had been sought. The Royal College of Nursing (1993, p. 8) gives clear guidelines about: 'researchers being aware of exploiting relationships that are unequal'.

If research has not been scrutinized by an ethics committee, the researcher may be unaware that the same or similar settings and subjects are being studied. Consequently, the value of the research may be open to question as well as there being ethical implications of overload on research subjects and possible violation of the principles of nonmaleficence and beneficence. We shall return to this issue in 'Reflections for practice' later in this chapter.

Separate nursing ethics committees

The difficulties described above lead to consideration of whether it would be appropriate to have separate nursing ethics committees (Hunt 1992). This is the situation in one authority known to the authors where the increasing volume of nursing research proposals has precipitated the setting up of a separate nursing research ethics committee. Proposal forms have been designed which are more appropriate to nursing research than to medically orientated clinical trials. The setting up of this committee coincided with the integration of nursing education into higher education in the authority. In the 5 years since its formation the number of proposals submitted to the committee has increased from one per month to five to 10 per month. The majority (80–90%) of the submissions were from nurses undertaking degree studies (M Ross, personal communication, 1994).

One of the drawbacks of setting up separate nursing research ethics committees is their potential to separate nursing research from other health service research. Such a separation may narrow nursing's perspectives and reduce the likelihood of multidisciplinary collaboration to develop an integrated health service research strategy. The value of integrated research is stressed by the nursing research Taskforce (DoH 1993). In fact, the nursing ethics committee described above has expanded into a social science committee, to become multidisciplinary rather than have a purely nursing membership. Unless there is good communication between committees and/or some joint membership, it is possible that research that uses the same clinical areas will be approved, risking subject overload. Perhaps a committee with true representation of a range of health care professionals would be more ethical, independent and appropriate than one that has either medical or nursing dominance; specialists could be co-opted as necessary. However, the increasing amount of nursing research has implications for ethics committees, whether joint or separate, in terms of increasing workload and training needs. Neuberger (1992) suggests that one nursing ethics committee member should be a nurse who has regular patient contact. This has implications for clinical nurses and emphasizes the importance of ethical and research mindedness for nurses. Neuberger (1992, p. 19) argues for the presence of 'hands on rather than senior nurses' on ethics committees, because these nurses are seen as being closer to patients than their medical colleagues. The recommendation indirectly emphasizes the clinical nurse's advocate role. However, if, as Bage (1992) indicates, rights and liabilities of ethics committees stem from the individual committee members, it is crucial for members to understand their obligations and responsibilities from a sound ethical knowledge base. Whilst a legal case involving an ethics committee has not been recorded, with increased consumerism in society this may well happen in the future.

Legal powers

The lack of legal power of ethics committees is a concern for Neuberger (1992), who recommends that health authorities should make it a disciplinary offence to conduct research without ethical approval. At present, research ethics committees do not have the power to insist that all research carried out within the health authority is presented to them, and they are not the final arbiters of whether research can go ahead. Nurses need to bear this in mind when critically analysing research reports and performing their patient advocate role. The Department of Health guidelines relate to the NHS but not to research carried out in the private sector, which could be of concern for the many nurses who work there. Neuberger (1992, p. 45), in her review of the role of ethics committees, made a clear recommendation for more legal powers. She said: 'the major recommendation of this report is that there should be legislation to strengthen research ethics committees' role, and to empower them to carry out their genuine tasks properly, with the support and training they require'.

Research or audit?

What constitutes research that requires ethics committee approval and what constitutes audit, which generally does not, may be confusing. Usually, audit involves data or subjects that the 'auditor' has access to through her/his normal working role. Audit involves review and evaluation of current care or services, often by routinely obtaining consumer feedback rather than setting up special studies. Results are not usually published outside the organization for which they have been obtained. The current health care reforms mean that more audit is taking place because of the emphasis on cost-effective services. Whilst more audit must be applauded if it leads to the consumer's voice being heard and improvement in services, it could lead to overload for the subjects if there is no coordination between research and audit activities. From the patients' or clients' perspective, a questionnaire or interview for either audit or research purposes may be very similar; both may be intrusive and leave them feeling uncomfortable about the process.

Because of the confusion surrounding the difference between audit and research you might like to consider the following situation.

■ BOX 10.5

Clinical example 4

A health visitor has been running a weaning group. She would like to evaluate the effectiveness of the group and is interested in finding out if group attendance influences dietary behaviour. She is also undertaking degree studies and feels that this has potential for her research dissertation.

A project is designed to compare the weaning practice of group attenders and that of parents from a neighbouring practice where no such group exists. It involves a random sample from both areas, which will involve gaining access to the names and addresses of clients who are not on her caseload. Data are to be collected via a postal questionnaire. She feels that the results could be of interest to other health visitors and hopes to publish them in a nursing journal.

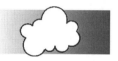

Do you think that this project is research or audit?

Do you think that the health visitor should present the project to an ethics committee for approval?

You could consider your answer using the following guidelines:

- the research sample—who they are and how they are to be accessed
- how the results are to be used.

You will probably decide after considering these two points that the project is research rather than audit and that the proposal should be submitted to an ethics committee. Suppose she had decided on one of the different approaches for her project outlined below.

■ BOX 10.6

Clinical example 5

- The sample used was drawn entirely from her own caseload, comparing the weaning behaviour of parents who had attended the group with those who had not attended.
- It was a collaborative project between health visitors in two different practices.

Either of these last two scenarios may begin to sound more like audit than research because they were set up to evaluate and review the effectiveness of current practice. For the clients included in either Clinical example 4 or Clinical example 5, their involvement would be identical, but in example 4 they would have the 'protection' afforded by an ethics committee scrutinizing the project, whilst in the other situation they would not. On the other hand, the results of the study would be published in example 4, whereas in example 5 the results would be used internally by the practitioners to improve the service. One basic difference between research and audit is that they are set up for different purposes which must be declared to the participants.

This example is intended to highlight the complexity of the issues and the potential confusion. The ethically aware, research-minded nurse will, it is hoped, seek guidance from experts both in research and audit before proceeding with any projects involving patients, volunteers or health authority staff (including students). However, in reality, those with deadlines for studies may be put off by the possible delays and the anxiety that the experts may not approve their proposal or may put restrictions or conditions on it.

Ethics committees and the research process

At the beginning of this chapter we said that the ethical component of being research minded applies to all aspects of the research process. If this is so, we would suggest that ethics committees have a role in assessing the ethical implications of all stages of that process in the proposals they receive. Committee members would need to be assured that the applicants are adequately qualified, experienced and supervised; the methodology and methods used are appropriate; results are accurately analysed and interpreted; and results are disseminated in a way that is likely to generate knowledge and improve practice. Researchers would need to report back to the committee on their progress and with their results. This would have enormous implications for the committee's workload and may seem unrealistic and unnecessary. The reader may like to consider whether the committee can fully fulfil its function of assuring that all research involving human subjects is carried out in an ethically sound manner without such feedback.

Suggested learning activity

In preparation for the seminar which inspired this chapter, one of the authors met the chairperson of an ethics committee and attended a session as an observer. This proved a valuable learning experience and is something the reader may like to consider doing.

Find out about your local research ethics committee by asking the following questions:

- *Is there a separate nursing ethics committee?*
- *Who are the committee members?*
- *What is the ratio between medical, nursing and lay membership?*
- *How often does it meet?*
- *How many nursing research studies are submitted to the committee?*
- *Have a look at the application form, is it suitable for nursing research?*
- *Where does the committee meet ?*

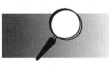

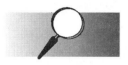

If you are able to attend one of the meetings you could choose one of the ethical principles and consider how the researchers are meeting it. For example autonomy: how are the researchers assuring informed consent is being obtained before the commencement of the research?

REFLECTIONS FOR PRACTICE

Since the Briggs' Committee (DHSS 1972) proposed that nursing should become a research-based profession, nurse teachers have been developing methods of teaching research effectively. Research is a complex subject, and it may be that the only way to learn about it is to do it. Traditionally, nurses undertaking degree studies have completed a small-scale project as part of their educational development. Greater numbers of nurses undertaking degrees has resulted in an increase in the amount of small-scale project work. As mentioned in the introduction to this chapter, a debate has now arisen around the assumption that this is the best way in which to learn about research.

We have already referred to the Department of Health Taskforce on the Strategy for Research in Nursing, Midwifery and Health Visiting in which the issue of small-scale projects was raised (DoH 1993). The report states: 'Research skills and experience need to be far more widespread than at present in the nursing professions' and continues: 'not … all practitioners should be carrying out research as part of their role or development; indeed, the proliferation of inadequately supervised, small scale projects should be curbed'. The Taskforce Report recommends in Section 3.3.1 that greater numbers of nurses should be able to use research appropriately, with a smaller number able to carry it out:

> *the proliferation of inadequately supervised small scale projects should be curbed. However, every practitioner does need to develop a capacity for critical thought and to acquire analytical skills; a small number—but far more than at present—require research training to enable them to engage in research while retaining their clinical base or to bridge the worlds of research decision making, practice development and policy.*

The Taskforce Report considers research literacy to be essential for all practitioners, but we also ask whether the skills for understanding, critiquing and using research are the same as those required for doing research. To some extent, Mander (1988) answers these questions in her review of the options available for making nursing research based. She discusses three options:

* awareness of the need to draw on research
* all nurses doing some research during an education programme
* nurses being able to decide whether and how to implement research findings of which they are aware.

A mere awareness of research is not considered sufficient to result in the ability to critique and use research (Mander 1988). While learning by critiquing can be useful, it also depends, as we saw in Chapter 9, on the nurse acquiring skills to do this well. The second option is currently the most widely used approach to teaching research in degree programmes. As the numbers of people undertaking these programmes increase, so the effects of inexperienced researchers producing mediocre research and exposure of vulnerable groups (patients, students, staff) to this research also increase.

Clark & Sleep (1991) discuss two main approaches to teaching research:

- facilitating an awareness of research with the aim of increasing the use of research findings in practice
- learning about research by doing.

These authors identify different competencies required by each approach.

■ **BOX 10.7** (Clark & Sleep 1991, p. 174)

Research awareness

Aim: to improve standards of care and enhance the professional status of nurses, midwives and health visitors

Practitioners need to be able to:
- identify the main sources of knowledge underpinning professional practice
- seek and identify relevant information sources including those drawn from other disciplines
- provide a sound rationale for clinical decisions and actions through a process of critical and reflective thinking
- understand the research process in order to evaluate research
- use research in practice
- protect the rights of patients/clients and colleagues in the conduct of health care research.

Learning by doing

Aim: to conduct research and contribute to the body of nursing knowledge

Practitioners need to be able to:
- identify researchable questions
- identify appropriate supervision and mentorship
- conduct a literature search and review
- select a design appropriate to the research question
- develop a research proposal
- collect, analyse and interpret data
- write a research report and disseminate findings.

Clark & Sleep (1991) provide ways of implementing Mander's (1988) second and third options for making nursing practice research based. If we also consider the Taskforce Report recommendations (DoH 1993) we have the components for an ethical debate regarding how research is taught in nurse education, related to the following questions and ethical principles:

- Who benefits from the completion of a small-scale research project? (beneficence)
- Is any harm done by the completion of a small-scale research project? (non-maleficence).

If there is a 'double effect' (i.e. a good outcome accompanied by a harmful process), who or what takes precedence: the individual (deontology); the institution (utilitarianism); the profession (utilitarianism); or the consumer—patient, student, teacher or practitioner—(deontology)?

■ **BOX 10.8**

To complete a degree programme, a practitioner is required to submit a small-scale research project. Phenomenology (see Ch. 5) is the methodology considered by the student as the most appropriate way of exploring the chosen topic. There is one lecturer with experience of this methodology and of supervising research students. The lecturer is already supervising several students and feels unable to offer sufficient time to provide adequate support. Another lecturer has some knowledge of the methodology but no experience of supervising research students at this level. Another lecturer has limited knowledge of this methodology while having experience of research supervision.

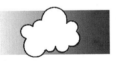

Consider what decisions you would make as the student, and then as each of the lecturers if approached for supervision. You can use the following guidelines:

1. *Can you identify moral theory (e.g. utilitarianism or deontology) influencing your decision making?*
2. *Consider the effect of emotion (your feelings; knowing the student/lecturer; interest in the topic) on the topic.*
3. *Does the emotional impact alter if you consider this situation from an individual perspective and then an institutional perspective?*
4. *Can you suggest a compromise (e.g. co-supervision) and provide justification in terms of greatest good for greatest number; duty to self; student; institution; emotional stability?*

Undertaking research has traditionally been considered the only way to develop an appreciation of the process that allows the newcomer to understand its complexities and the possible hurdles that need to be overcome. The individual who undertakes research benefits in a way that is difficult to articulate to anyone who has not undergone a similar experience. Teaching research through doing is fraught with the potential for making mistakes. The result might be a project which does not provide **reliable** or **valid** data that can be generalized for subsequent use by practitioners. The data obtained may have great interest to and benefit for the individual researcher but the learning process involved in their collection may not be transferable to other prospective researchers. Considerable knowledge may be gained from the chosen methodology but no appreciation of other methodologies, so that the researcher has a limited ability to critique and utilize research generally.

As already stated, research subjects may be requested by several novice researchers to take part in individual small-scale research projects which take a lot of time but offer little benefit. Such projects will not be viewed sympathetically by managers committed to a cost-efficient health service, where 'time is money'.

Researcher autonomy can be influenced by the place of work and its potential for attracting funding. The amalgamation of colleges of nursing with higher education establishments has put greater emphasis on research activities in order to achieve higher ratings in the university research assessment exercise (RAE). Rating is determined by the number and perceived value of declared research projects, with funding being more readily available for 'topical' areas (an issue explored in greater detail in Ch. 11). University nursing departments are likely to focus on developing specialist research areas (as recommended by the DoH 1993) in an attempt to achieve a higher rating and attract funding. This may limit the individual researcher's autonomy in choosing a topic, but it may be possible to incorporate aspects of individual interest into a departmental research programme that covers topics which are likely to attract funding.

For research to be ethical, competent supervision is essential. Nursing research is a developing discipline and nurse researchers and teachers with the knowledge and expertise to supervise research projects may receive numerous requests for assistance. This can place unrealistic demands on them and may result in students receiving either insufficient time and support or being allocated supervisors with limited skills. How can nurse researchers and teachers gain the knowledge and experience of providing supervision? One way to do this is to co-supervise with researchers from allied disciplines such as sociology, anthropology, psychology and physiology who have a long tradition of academic research.

When research is being carried out in the clinical areas, questions arise regarding the practitioner's role as patients' advocate. The nurse's function may be to empower and emancipate subjects. In order to act as an advocate, the nurse needs to be aware of what the research process entails, or have easy access to someone who does, in order to develop the confidence and ability to express these views.

The concept of informed consent is of prime concern to the practitioner. As discussed in some detail above, the person requesting consent is obliged to provide sufficient accurate information for the other person to make an autonomous decision about participating in the research. Munhall (1988) considers consent in qualitative research to require renegotiation throughout the research process, because projects change as they progress and the rights of participants require protection by seeking ongoing consent to such changes. She refers to participants as 'collaborators' because, by consenting, they have joined the research project. This notion of renegotiation of consent may need also to be considered by researchers using quantitative methodologies, to allow subjects to opt out of the study at any time.

Oakley (1989), for example, describes the different **study designs** used in **randomized controlled trials** in which subjects are divided into experimental and **control** groups. In some instances, the control group may be unaware that they are part of a research study because only the experimental group are asked to sign a consent form following randomization to that group. In the more ethically sound trials, informed consent is obtained at the outset of the study so that nobody enters the trial without knowing that they could potentially end up in an experimental or control group. The subjects can then withdraw from the study whatever their allocation. Informed consent is a big issue for many researchers who undertake clinical trials because some of them contend that as a procedure it may lead to high non-participation rates which bias the final results of the study and limit their **generalizability**.

Beside the ethical implications involved in the completion of a research project, there are also ethical aspects integral to the dissemination and use of the completed research project.

Ethical aspects in disseminating and using research

Ethical aspects related to the dissemination and use of completed research projects may be explored from the following perspectives: the journal article where the majority of nurses read about research; the author/researcher presenting the research; and the reader/consumer of the research.

Journal articles

Nurses are being encouraged to publish. However, the journals in which articles are published carry differing amounts of kudos and reach a variety of audiences. Some journals are widely read by nurses with a variety of backgrounds and experiences; other journals are read by a specialist audience. Articles range from a report of results, with little or no discussion of research methodology or how the results were obtained, to detailed discussion regarding all aspects of the research process. Such articles may raise questions regarding the limitations of the results. Journals may have differing aims. The intention of some may be to inform the reader of potentially useful information regarding practice which would otherwise remain known only to a limited number of people. Others may intend to invite debate and discussion within the profession regarding appropriate research methodologies.

Credit is given to individuals and institutions not only according to the number of articles published but also the prestige attached to the journal in which the article appears. Some journals appear to attach great importance to academic writing style (such as use of the third person) or particular research styles. This may be at the expense of encouraging debate about a range of research methodologies and their contribution to the development of a nursing knowledge base.

Competition to achieve publication may have contributed to the proliferation of nursing journals. Does this increase in quantity equate to an increase in quality? Journals publishing small-scale research projects that are not generalizable may meet the individual's and institution's needs for an increased number of publications, but may not add significantly to the nursing knowledge base. Alternatively, there may be a rapidly growing amount of research which should be made available for critique and potential benefit to patients and staff. Editors and referees of journals, therefore, have a responsibility to exercise judgement over what is and is not published in an ethical manner. Both hold considerable power to influence what is known or remains unknown, which has vast implications for the development of nursing.

Author/researcher

The researcher has a responsibility to publish findings. Subjects have given time and effort to provide the researcher with data to complete the project. The researcher has to decide whether completion of the project for his/her own individual development is ethically justifiable. Publication can also be ethically justified if aspects learnt during the process will benefit other researchers. Furthermore, results that are made available can be critically evaluated by researchers, educationalists and practitioners for the benefit of patients and to contribute to nursing's developing knowledge base.

Readers/consumers

Readers or consumers of published articles also have responsibilities. These responsibilities include reading widely and critically in order to stay up to date with changes. Akinsanya (1994) suggests that while research may be disseminated through publication, it remains unknown to most nurses. Clause 3 of the UKCC Code of Conduct (1992) requires registered practitioners to maintain and improve professional knowledge and competence. Nurses have a duty of care to patients and to be unaware of information is not considered sufficient defence by the profession or in a court of law for bad practice.

In order to make an informed decision about the usefulness of the research, the reader requires sufficient, accurate information from the author, as well as knowledge of the various aspects of the research process. It should then be possible to estimate the value of the article to the reader's practice setting. Implementation of research can have wide-ranging effects. These can be short term in that they can be used to inform the allocation of resources. Long-term effects are more difficult to predict and may only be realized at a later date. One example of this may be the developing and expanding role of paramedics/nurses in the emergency treatment of sudden illness, such as myocardial infarction, and accidents. Advanced training is undertaken with the intention of transferring people to hospitals in a better condition. However, it has become apparent that such interventions can result in the survival of people with extensive injuries who formally would have died at the scene of the accident. Sadly they may never recover and end up in a 'persistent vegetative state', as in the case of Tony Bland referred to earlier in this chapter. The importance of researching the long-term effects of such interventions needs to be considered in order to reduce future ethical dilemmas.

CONCLUSION

We hope that having read this chapter you will have increased your ability to recognize the ethical theories and principles involved in everyday clinical practice as well as in research. Exploration of the values that guide practice can facilitate more equal interdisciplinary discussion and debate of issues surrounding patient care and research. If this comes from a sound knowledge base, practitioners will be more articulate and confident.

We have endeavoured to demonstrate how ethical theory, research and clinical practice are inextricably linked. Therefore, while within the chapter we have concentrated on the ethical issues associated with research, readers need to view them holistically in the context of the research process, individual practice and this book as a whole.

REFERENCES

Akinsanya J 1994 Making research useful to the practising nurse. Journal of Advanced Nursing 19: 174–179

Bage B 1992 Ethics committees and their general responsibilities and liabilities in law. Health Law Bulletin 17 (June): 1–2

Beauchamp T, Childress J 1989 Principles of biomedical ethics, 3rd edn. Oxford University Press, New York

Caplan A L, Edgar H, King P A, Jones J H 1992 Twenty years after—the legacy of the Tuskegee syphilis study. Hastings Centre Report 22(6) (November–December)

Clark E H, Sleep J 1991 The what and how of teaching research. Nurse Education Today 11: 172–178

Department of Health 1992 The Children Act 1989: an introductory guide for the NHS. HMSO, London

Department of Health 1993 Report of the Taskforce on the Strategy for Research in Nursing, Midwifery and Health Visiting. DoH, London

Department of Health and Social Security 1972 Report of the Committee on Nursing (Chair: Professor Asa Briggs). HMSO, London

Eraut M 1985 Knowledge creation and knowledge use in professional contexts. Studies in Higher Education 10(2): 117–133

Gilligan C 1982 In a different voice: psychological theory and women's development. Harvard University Press, Cambridge, Mass

Gillon R 1986 Philosophical medical ethics. Wiley, Chichester

Harbison C 1992 Gilligan: a voice for nursing? Journal of Medical Ethics 18: 202–205

Hunt G 1992 Local research ethics committees: a critical look. British Journal of Nursing 1(7): 349–351

Hutton W 1995 The state we're in. Jonathan Cape, London

Jasper M 1994 Issues in phenomenology for researchers of nursing. Journal of Advanced Nursing 19: 309–314

Kiikkala I, Munnukka T 1994 Nursing research: on what basis? Journal of Advanced Nursing 19: 987–995

Lelean S 1975 Ready for report nurse. RCN, London

Mander R 1988 Encouraging students to be research minded. Nurse Education Today 8: 30–35

Munhall P L 1988 Ethical considerations in qualitative research. Western Journal of Nursing Research 10(2): 150–162

Neuberger J 1992 Ethics and health care: the role of research ethics committees in the United Kingdom. King's Fund Institute, London

Oakley A 1989 'Who's afraid of the randomised controlled trial?' Some dilemmas of the scientific method and 'good' research practice. Women and Health 54(4): 25–39

Pollack L, Tilley S 1988 Submitting for approval. Senior Nurse 8(5): 25

Popkin R H, Stroll A 1993 Philosophy: made simple books, 3rd edn. Butterworth-Heinemann, Oxford

Royal College of Nursing Research Advisory Group 1993 Ethics related to research in nursing. Scutari, London

Royal College of Physicians 1990 Research involving patients. RCP, London

Seedhouse D 1988 Ethics: the heart of health care. Wiley, Chichester

Shevrell M I, Evans B K 1994 The 'Shaltenband experiment' Wurzberg 1940: scientific, historical and ethical perspectives. Neurology 44 (Feb): 350–356

Smith L 1994 An analysis and reflections on the quality of nursing research in 1992. Journal of Advanced Nursing 19: 385–393

Thompson I, Melia R, Boyd K 1988 Nursing ethics, 2nd edn. Churchill Livingstone, London

Traynor M, Wade B 1994 The morale of nurses working in the community: a study of three NHS trusts: year 3. The Daphne Heald Research Unit, RCN, London

United Kingdom Central Council for Nursing, Midwifery and Health Visiting 1986 Project 2000—a new preparation for practice. UKCC, London

United Kingdom Central Council for Nursing, Midwifery and Health Visiting 1992 Code of Professional Conduct, 3rd edn. UKCC, London

Webb C 1993 Feminist research: definitions, methodology, methods and evaluation. Journal of Advanced Nursing 18: 413–416

Research proposals and funding

Stevan Monkley-Poole

11

KEY ISSUES

- **Strategies for developing proposals**
- **The essential elements and costs of a research proposal**
- **The relative merits of preparing proposals which take different research approaches**
- **Strategies for obtaining funding**
- **Implications of the move into higher education and the research assessment exercise**

INTRODUCTION

This chapter is concerned with the awareness, skills and knowledge required to write successful proposals and obtain funds for a range of activities. The proposals I discuss are primarily concerned with gaining approval to undertake research and/or obtaining funding to do so. Proposal writing is an important element in the range of skills necessary to be able to call oneself research minded and develop practice that is based on an understanding of research and its political context. I draw on previous chapters in this book to explore strategies for developing proposals.

There can be many reasons for writing a proposal apart from 'pure' research. For example, similar principles can be applied to writing proposals to obtain resources to introduce change into clinical practice or undertake an audit of services. Proposals can also be submitted to request funding to support study leave or attendance at a conference. You may be able to think, either now or as the chapter progresses, of other examples of how the skills used in writing research proposals can be utilized elsewhere in your professional practice.

This chapter will assist you to identify the essential elements and costs of a research proposal. It will also discuss the relative merits of preparing proposals which take different research approaches. Various strategies are explored for ways of obtaining funding. Finally, the move of nursing and other health care professions into higher education and the implications of the research assessment exercise on the need to obtain postgraduate degrees and funding of research is addressed.

RESEARCH MINDEDNESS AND PROPOSAL WRITING

As you have found from previous chapters in this book, the number of authors who have written on the subject of research mindedness is now very numerous. Tierney (1993) uses the Department of Health's Taskforce Report on the strategy for research in nursing, midwifery and health visiting to make a very strong case for the instilling of research literacy and research mindedness in students and registered practitioners.

The recent move of nurse education into the university setting is another reason why nurses, midwives and health visitors need to become research minded, since one of the traditional tasks of universities is to undertake research. The research assessment exercise (RAE) carried out by the Higher Education Funding Council for England (HEFCE) has raised the profile of university research even further. Because the RAE requires university departments to put their research under the scrutiny of their peers, the need to attract research funding and improve the number of studies being successfully completed has increased since its inception in 1986. To move into a research-oriented environment clearly offers many advantages for the development of research mindedness and nursing research. Nurse educators in particular are being encouraged to undertake research degrees such as MPhils and PhDs, in which case they will be required to submit their research proposals to the university's higher degrees committee.

In the health service, the move to the market with its emphasis on evidence-based health care, supported by the recommendations made by the Culyer Report (DoH 1994a, Culyer 1995) referred to in Chapter 1, suggests the need for practitioners to be able to attract monies to fund research and to clearly identify and document research activities being undertaken in the clinical areas.

Both the RAE and Culyer recommendations suggest that research will be rewarded by allocations of monies to undertake further research, but baseline research activities, including education and training, are clearly required in the first place. Furthermore, the Taskforce and Culyer Reports emphasize the need for more multidisciplinary research between different types of health professionals and academics. The ability to have good ideas and write successful proposals, therefore, is clearly an important skill for practitioners and teachers to acquire as part of research mindedness and political awareness, if they are to take their place as equal partners in multidisciplinary research programmes.

RESEARCH PROPOSALS

So, what is a research proposal? A proposal puts forward the argument for why a piece of research will add to the body of knowledge in a particular area, in other words why it is worth doing. Included in this is how the research will be undertaken. The proposal can be seen as answering many questions such as:

- Will the project add to the body of knowledge and is the individual competent to undertake the data collection?
- Has the applicant identified sound procedures with which to analyse the findings?
- Has the project been carefully planned and can it be successfully executed?
- If funding is being sought, has the individual demonstrated that it is a good financial risk in which funding bodies can confidently place their money?

Also, by developing the skills necessary to write an effective proposal by which you have to clarify on paper each stage of your intended study, you may find that your ability to critique other people's research is enhanced.

RESEARCH APPROACHES
AND PROPOSAL WRITING

Many key texts, such as Bond (1991), offer advice regarding a framework for writing research proposals. Anyone who has already explored this area will be aware that such frameworks are often oriented towards the quantitative research approach (Field & Morse 1985, Marshall & Rossman 1989). Furthermore, as we saw in Chapter 10, medical ethics committee members who traditionally scrutinize nursing research proposals tend to have a greater understanding and respect for the rigours involved in research associated with the physical rather than the social sciences.

The research **approaches** and **methods** of the physical and social sciences and their association with a **quantitative** or **qualitative** orientation has been the focus for discussion throughout this book. By now you will be beginning to form some preferences of your own. It is important to be aware, therefore, that the move of nurse education into higher education may influence the nature and development of nursing and health services research. This is because the philosophical orientation of the higher education establishment may differ depending on whether nursing and its associated discipline of health studies come under the aegis of the physical sciences, such as physiology and biology, or the social sciences, such as sociology or anthropology. As we saw in Chapter 2, the physical sciences tend to have a quantitative orientation whereas the social sciences are more likely to demonstrate a qualitative orientation. Psychology as a discipline is less clear cut and draws on both quantitative and qualitative approaches.

It may be the case that different nursing specialities go separate ways in their alliance with the physical and social sciences. For example, it is possible that adult and child nursing may come under the management and philosophy of the physical sciences while mental health and learning disabilities nursing are located within social sciences. If this is the case, is it a problem? The short and optimistic answer is no if (and it is a big and as yet unforeseeable 'if') nursing has access and encouragement to immerse itself in the richness offered by both quantitative and qualitative orientations to research.

If an institution such as a university department or health care facility has a particular research orientation (be it qualitative or quantitative), then mechanisms are likely to be in place to support that particular orientation. These mechanisms will provide the necessary framework for writing proposals to obtain funding and guide the research from conception to execution. Examples of support mechanisms to ensure successful research outcomes include experienced colleagues who have a depth of knowledge and understanding of the fundamental principles involved in particular research approaches and who are able to act in a supervisory capacity to novice researchers. The accessibility of suitable supervisors for health care professionals wishing to undertake research is thus crucial to the development of research mindedness.

There may, however, be frustrations when individuals new to research are unable to identify researchers experienced in their preferred approach. Because of the traditional dominance of quantitative research in medicine and health care, many nurses report working in institutions unfamiliar with qualitative approaches. At worst, this situation may result in conflict for those individuals who want to take a qualitative orientation in preference to a quantitative one.

Since nursing encompasses a wide body of knowledge and associated research questions, it is important to recognize that many different research philosophies, approaches and methods are necessary. Nursing's wide knowledge base emphasizes the need to be familiar with writing research proposals from both the quantitative and qualitative stance.

At this point, you may like to refer back to Chapter 2 to reconsider the philosophies, approaches and methods associated with quantitative and qualitative research to prepare you for writing proposals.

Quantitative proposals

The proposal with a quantitative orientation is highly structured and serves as a predictable guide to the research process. Generally speaking, as described in Chapter 3, quantitative methods, such as experiments and **clinical trials**, are employed to test **hypotheses** and **theories** following set procedures.

Qualitative proposals

The main purpose of qualitative research is to discover important questions, processes and relationships as the research progresses, in order to generate knowledge and theory about little-known topic areas. Consequently, by its very nature, qualitative research is adapted as the study proceeds. Examples of qualitative research approaches such as phenomenology and ethnomethodology can be found in Chapters 5 and 6.

Quantitative or qualitative?

When writing any proposal it is important to consider the membership of the panel or committee who will be taking decisions based on its content, since each member will have a different background and bias. As noted above, ethics committee members are usually drawn from a largely medical background so that they tend to be more familiar with quantitative research. Similarly, the membership of research degrees committees in universities can also be dominated by physical and some social scientists who have only undertaken quantitative research. However, this should not deter individuals from submitting a proposal that adopts a qualitative approach. It is important, however, to be clear and explicit when putting together the proposal, especially if the people making decisions about it are unfamiliar with its approach.

One of the reasons qualitative research is often criticized is because it is seen by traditional scientists to lack rigour. Many texts have now been written for ensuring appropriateness and rigour in qualitative research and you are referred to these for further reading (Sandelowski 1986, Koch 1994). In particular, Cobb & Hagemaster (1987) suggest 10 criteria for ensuring the soundness of qualitative research proposals. These criteria include:

- evidence that the researcher has appropriate expertise in the approach, or supervision by someone who has
- a clearly stated research problem usually in the form of broad questions rather than hypotheses
- a literature review that highlights appropriate areas but is flexible enough to incorporate new literature as the research proceeds
- explicit techniques for **sampling**, data collection and analysis
- guidelines for how access and **ethics** will be handled
- the significance of the study to nursing and health care.

It could be argued that the rigid separation between quantitative and qualitative research is not helpful. Indeed Haase & Myers (1988) state that both approaches share the common purpose of gaining understanding about nursing and the world about us. Furthermore, Cobb & Hagemaster's criteria for qualitative research proposals demonstrate the areas of overlap between the two approaches in relation to rigour of data collection and analysis, ethics and significance of the research to nursing and health care. Quantitative and qualitative research approaches might be better seen, therefore, as different ends of the same continuum (Rolfe 1994). Nevertheless, in reality, the orientations of the two approaches have implications for how proposals are written and applications made for funding. Whatever the approach, the researcher may benefit from having a supervisor or colleague who has a key role in defending, explaining and supporting the work in its passage through the committee stage.

I now provide you with a case study based on classroom discussion with colleagues to assist you to identify the implications of writing proposals from a quantitative or qualitative stance.

CASE STUDY

In an attempt to tease out some of the issues involved in writing a proposal using either a quantitative or qualitative approach to a research problem, an exercise was carried out with a group of postgraduate students. The group was divided into two subgroups, each of which was given the task in Box 11.1. While both subgroups had the same population group, issue and focus to consider, one was to take a quantitative orientation, the other a qualitative one.

■ BOX 11.1

You are a group of nurse researchers working in a university department of nursing. You are setting out a research proposal to seek funding for a project exploring the following:

Population group: 65 years and over
Issue: Promoting continence
Focus: Service provision

You are asked to identify and detail the content of a proposal in the light of the research orientation you are following.

On evaluating the exercise, some interesting issues were raised. The writing of the research proposal appeared to be relatively easy for the subgroup taking a quantitative approach who managed to complete the activity in the 45 minutes available. Interestingly, the subgroup taking a qualitative approach did not complete the task within the time allocated. They spent considerable time debating the merits of the various philosophical stances that could be adopted within the realms of the qualitative approach. As you saw in Chapters 5 and 6, different philosophical stances underpin phenomenology and ethnomethodology. The 'qualitative' subgroup felt that debate was essential before they were able to proceed and develop a research proposal. This debate emphasizes the importance of spending time on clarifying approaches and methods before writing a qualitative research proposal.

In contrast, it appeared that the 'quantitative' subgroup found writing their proposal rather like building a structure in which all the pieces were available and ready to be assembled in the right order with the right nuts and bolts. The 'qualitative' subgroup members were still in the process of formulating what was implied by the building materials because they were exploring and challenging the philosophies and methods of their approach. Their 'quantitative' colleagues took the philosophies and methods of their approach as given, assuming that they would set up a **randomized controlled trial** based on an intervention (e.g. testing a new drug to improve bladder tone) to promote continence.

What was also interesting was that the values and assumptions held about the target population and the topic differed between the two subgroups. The quantitative subgroup accepted that a population of 65 years and over was a reasonable choice for their proposed study, given that continence problems were more likely to arise in this age group. Whilst acknowledging that they would need to define their population in order to decide sample size and whether to include men and women, they accepted that they would randomly allocate their sample into experimental and control groups.

The 'qualitative' subgroup had more problems in taking at face value the assumption that the population of choice should be 65 and over. The midwives, for example, pointed out that the promotion of continence was a serious concern for their client population of childbearing women. They had difficulties, therefore, in assuming that the 'over-65s' should be the population of choice for the exercise.

When it came to discussion of the topic, both subgroups assumed that they were looking at the promotion of urinary rather than faecal continence. However, the 'quantitative' subgroup asked different questions, looked for different outcomes and had different emphases from their 'qualitative' colleagues. They wanted to find out about the number of times the experimental and the control group went to the toilet, the types of aids they used to assist their continence (such as sheaths for men and pads for women) and, if they were in the experimental group, whether they experienced any side effects from the drugs.

The 'qualitative' subgroup were more interested in issues of self-esteem and body image and whether men and women differed in this respect. They considered in-depth interviewing of people in an old people's home compared with people who attended a luncheon club to be the method and sample of choice. The exercise ended before they were able to commit their ideas to paper.

This exercise may offer some pointers to the planning and timing of proposal construction and submission in relation to different research orientations. This is even more pertinent if more than one individual is involved in the project. The philosophical nature of the proposal needs to be explored by the team so that a consensus view about the approach and methods to be used and understanding of the population and topic being investigated can be reached.

Similarly, if one is undertaking the study on one's own, the importance of being able to talk to experienced research and clinical colleagues cannot be overestimated.

WRITING PROPOSALS

We now look at some of the nuts and bolts of writing a proposal.

Bond (1991) suggests that a proposal may have the following elements:

- Title
- Summary or abstract
- Aims and objectives
- Justification or rationale
- Literature review
- Plan of investigation
- Ethical considerations
- Resources including the budget
- Curriculum vitae.

To arrive at the point of writing a proposal, a great deal of work will already have been undertaken by the applicant. For example, decisions will already have been taken on the philosophical approach and methods to be adopted.

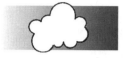

Before reading further you may like to identify an area of interest for research or practice and draw up your own proposal as we work through each section.

Valiga & Mermel (1985) give a number of examples from clinical practice such as: the patient admission process to a paediatric unit; the evaluation of a structured cardiac teaching programme; care of leukaemia patients in reverse isolation; the complex technical care of patients being nursed at home. They state that although there are no shortages of research questions in clinical practice, nurses need to develop a routine for identifying them through a combination of 'intellectual curiosity, familiarity with the literature and a habit of observing events carefully and systematically' (p. 4).

If you cannot think of your own example of a research question, in order to get yourself started refer to Smith's account of applying for a Fulbright Scholarship Grant (1994). She describes how she went about writing a successful proposal to obtain funding for study leave to do research.

The Fulbright programme was founded by the US senator of that name to promote overseas educational exchange. There are different categories of award and Smith chose the one most appropriate to her needs, which allowed her to be at a US School of Public Health to research health care and the market. She tells us when and which journals to scan to obtain information about the scholarship. As we discuss later, this advice applies to any fund since you need to know which ones are available, for what purposes, and when and where they are advertised.

Smith also describes the specific information required by the Fulbright programme organizers, which came as a four-page application form, and the institutional commitments she needed to obtain before even submitting the proposal. These commitments had to be obtained in writing from her employers and the host institutions she wished to visit. Smith then goes into some detail about the information required on the application form and the benefits associated with obtaining a Fulbright Scholarship.

Having read this account, you can now apply it or your own example to the following format.

The title

The title should be explicit but relatively brief and flexible enough to accommodate any changes in the evolution or direction of the project. Where possible, the title should also give an indication of the underlying philosophy and approach used. It may be that at the planning stage you have a working title which helps you to focus your ideas but may change as what you want to do becomes clearer. The title is very important for a number of reasons. First, it may be read by many people, whilst relatively few will read the entire proposal (Day 1989). Second, the title has to attract attention, not least because it is the first item read by the committee assessing the proposal for its ethical, research and funding soundness. Smith (1994), for example, entitles her proposal 'Contracting for Care or Contracting for Health? Primary Health Care and Nursing in the United States: Lessons to be Learnt'. This title is long but it does sum up the main components of the proposal, which aimed to investigate and learn from the impact of the market on the delivery of US health care and nursing's specific contribution. The title suggests that Smith's study will be descriptive.

Summary or abstract

In practice, this section may be easier to write last. The summary or abstract allows the researcher to draw together the most significant information on the objectives of the project and its implementation. It is an important indicator of the quality of the proposal that is to follow. It may therefore be prudent to give the summary or abstract careful consideration and probably several redrafts to ensure the 100–200 words give a relevant and concise synopsis (Field & Morse 1985, RCM 1989).

Justification or rationale

At this point in the proposal the justification or usefulness of the project needs to be stressed. This section must convince the reviewer that the proposed work is important in adding to the body of knowledge. It will suggest how the proposal will add to previous work in the area and how it relates to relevant theory. Further justification can be made by putting the research question into a context that identifies the importance of the problem. It may be a useful tip to consider highlighting a succinct statement to catch the reader's attention. Smith's rationale for studying health care in the US related to the shift in the UK system towards an American-style market approach. She noted that a number of commentators were uneasy with this shift and advised caution. Her rationale for studying nurses in this process was that they were the largest occupational group within the delivery of health care.

In summary, this section must demonstrate that the project will contribute to knowledge, will be useful and meaningful to policy development and can be used by practitioners (Marshall & Rossman 1989). Smith suggested that her work would meet these requirements by showing how cost containment, which accompanied market reforms in the US, left nurses 'no time for a caring attitude' (Collins 1988). She wanted to show that cost containment could be seen as a false economy since patients chose particular types of health care on the basis of quality of nursing. If that quality was deteriorating in some facilities, then patients would look for alternatives.

Literature review

The literature review is always an important feature of the proposal. What purposes do you think it serves? Marshall & Rossman (1989) suggest it has four broad functions:

- to demonstrate the underlying assumptions of the general research question
- to demonstrate that the individual is knowledgeable about the related research and the intellectual traditions that surround and support the project
- to identify gaps in previous research and show that the proposed project adds to the body of knowledge
- to define and refine the question to be explored and the related tentative hypotheses by embedding them in larger research traditions.

The literature review includes the key studies forming the basis of the project. The applicant, using non-specialist language, outlines how these key studies are relevant and how this project moves beyond them. The review should relate to substantive concerns and methods regarding the subject under study and be in sufficient detail to inform the reviewer of its relevance. Similarly, the applicant should indicate his or her knowledge of studies in the topic area currently being undertaken. This demonstrates an appreciation of the theoretical aspects of the project and firmness of the theoretical base and also shows the applicant's ability to manipulate the complex issues involved. However, there are differences of opinion as to what extent the literature should be examined in certain qualitative approaches (Field & Morse 1985). These issues are dealt with in more depth in Chapter 8. Smith's literature review was used to substantiate her rationale for her proposal. She drew on her own research on emotional labour (Smith 1992) and the impact of the NHS reforms (Smith et al 1993). Finally she referred to British Government policy documents and critiques of the US health care system.

Aims and objectives

Articulating the purpose of the project clearly is crucial (Cobb & Hagemaster 1987). The aims and objectives should arise from the literature review and the author's experience and are listed and numbered in order of importance, using a sentence or two for each. The criteria should be defined as specifically as possible. It may be possible to state objectives in the form of a hypothesis that can be tested, such as the example from our case study in which the 'quantitative' subgroup wanted to test whether a specific intervention promoted the continence of the experimental group compared with the control group.

The aims and objectives of the proposal can also be expressed as a research problem or question(s). This process can be challenging. Problems and questions come most often from 'real world' observation, dilemmas and situations, which may be difficult to frame in the 'if–then' form of hypothesis used in traditional quantitative approaches. It is permissible to use a hunch as a starting point. Smith, for example, stated that: 'The US had devised a number of new roles and functions for nurses (such as primary nursing, nurse practitioners and clinical nurse specialists)' which led her to speculate as to whether 'the "market" had favoured such developments'. This hunch can be used as a guiding hypothesis to generate questions and search for patterns. These guiding hypotheses may develop into the more substantive and formalized questions presented in the proposal but also as the project gets underway. Smith, for example, asked: 'Is nursing care costed into the contract?'; 'What specific roles and skills do nurses perform in community (rather than acute hospital) facilities? Are these specific roles and skills reflected in district nursing and health visiting roles in Britain and if so how?'.

Plan of investigation

The plan of investigation outlines the process by which the research will be undertaken. What benefits can you see from the plan of investigation being detailed at the proposal stage? It may identify the researcher's over-all understanding and capacity to undertake and complete the project. It will also give some indication of the resources that need to be available, for example study leave requirements. This is important for researchers, employers and those who may be awarding time and funding for the research. The plan of investigation may follow the format outlined below.

If you would like to refresh your memory regarding the terms used to describe the plan you can refer to a number of chapters in this book, in particular Chapter 3 on experimental methods; Chapter 5 on phenomenology and Chapter 6 on ethnomethodology as examples of qualitative approaches; and, for a general review and revision, Chapter 9 on research critique.

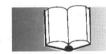

Population and sample

The criteria used to identify populations and select samples will vary according to the approach taken. Sampling in most qualitative projects uses selection criteria which seek individuals with special knowledge or unique experiences to increase the researcher's understanding of the topic studied. Generally, there will be fewer subjects involved compared to a quantitative approach. The proposal writer needs to be aware of the rationale for such sampling techniques and defend them as purposeful rather than haphazard (Cobb & Hagemaster 1987).

In quantitative research, because **representativeness** is a desired goal, issues concerning subjects' accessibility/availability, criteria for inclusion and exclusion, sample recruitment and management and how the issue of non-participation will be dealt with are explored and resolved in this section.

Design

The research design will vary according to the approach taken. Therefore, it is important that the introduction to this section outlines the intended research approach. It will serve as a starting point for the research and convey information about its nature to the committee(s) making decisions about the proposal. Examples of experimental research design are given in Chapter 3 and case study design in Chapter 9.

Qualitative research design is less clear cut than in quantitative research studies. The progress of the research tends to be dependent on the close integration of data collection and analysis which guides ongoing research.

Data collection

This section identifies the method(s) of data collection to be used, within the particular philosophical orientation and research approach adopted. As we saw in Chapters 5 and 6, phenomenology and ethnomethodology, in common with other qualitative research approaches, have specific techniques for collecting data such as in-depth interviews and observation.

Issues of **reliability** and **validity**, or their qualitative equivalents of 'credibility' and 'dependability' as discussed in Chapter 9, must always be addressed in the proposal (Cobb & Hagemaster 1987). The committee reviewing it need to be reassured that the researcher has thought about ways of ensuring rigour in the study.

Research proposals should be accompanied by appendices which contain examples of the proposed data collection tools such as a questionnaire, an interview or observation schedule.

Pilot study

As we saw in Chapter 3, the notion of a pilot study is of particular relevance to quantitative research, where tools are being tested for their validity and reliability. The pilot study should be described in some detail and identify the steps taken to ensure that the project is workable, acceptable to the subjects and manageable by the individual(s) undertaking the project. In qualitative research, the pilot study may be less specific and described as the exploratory phase where the researcher visits a number of potential research settings and subjects to decide on future directions of the study.

Recording data and analysis

Regardless of the philosophical approach taken, it is useful at an early stage of the project to consider how data will be recorded and analysed. An indication of how these activities will be undertaken should be outlined in the proposal. It is also worth noting that data analysis often takes twice as long as you might expect.

In quantitative research, how data will be recorded and analysed should be considered in conjunction with designing tools such as questionnaires. Questionnaires are standardized forms for the collection and recording of data. If statistical methods are to be used to analyse the data, they must be consistent with the specific objectives and design of the study. Any statistical computer packages (such as SPSS—Statistical Package for the Social Sciences) that the researcher intends to use should be outlined. Further information on quantitative data analysis is given in Chapter 4.

The process of qualitative analysis must also be described in the proposal. The author must convey how qualitative data are usually recorded in the form of field notes or interview transcripts and that interpretation and analysis begin in parallel with data collection. This process is necessary to guide the ongoing direction of the research. Examples of how qualitative data are coded and categorized into themes and concepts for the purposes of analysis in phenomenological research are given in Chapter 5. Computer packages such as 'Ethnograph' and 'Nud*ist' now exist to assist the researcher to code, categorize and analyse qualitative data.

Work plan

The proposal should include a work plan. The work plan identifies a timescale and plan of the project to show the anticipated duration of each stage of the study. Generally, time is underestimated, especially for the data collection and analysis, gaining entry to subjects and ethical approval. The individual's competence in proposal writing will be reflected in the identification of a clear and realistic time schedule. A realistic timetable will help the researcher to meet deadlines during the study and allow for unexpected events such as sickness or postal strikes.

A proposal entitled 'Early post-natal transfer home provides the best start together for the mother and her new babe' submitted by senior midwife Jo Whelton (1989), whilst a student on a research awareness course, shows her intended timetable for taking her study forward (Fig. 11.1). Her submission to the Royal College of Midwives/Maws Research Scholarship for Midwives was successful.

Outcomes

Specific outcomes expected from the research should be stated in the proposal. Expected outcomes may include a final report; new research tools and techniques; innovative teaching interventions and clinical aids. Smith (1994), for example, stated the expected outcomes and benefits of her study as 'publications, scholarly collaborations, and exchanges with US colleagues and informing my teaching'.

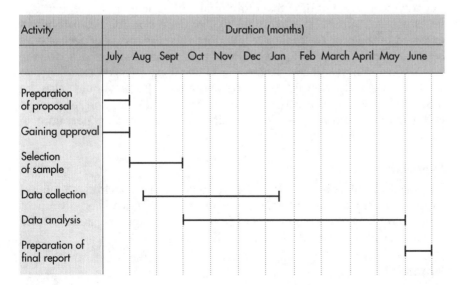

Figure 11.1 Time line submitted by Jo Whelton to summarize her work plan (reproduced by permission).

Dissemination of results

It is useful to make specific suggestions in the proposal regarding dissemination of information and recent research findings (DoH 1993) as there is
little merit in undertaking research if it only reaches a small audience.
Feedback to the participants should also be considered since the research
could not have taken place without their cooperation.

Ethical considerations

In writing a proposal it is important to indicate the major ethical issues
and state clearly how these will be handled. A research proposal must
always be submitted to an ethics committee. Some funding bodies will
only release funds subject to ethical approval having been obtained.
Higher degrees committees will not allow students to proceed with their
studies unless their proposal has also been passed by the local ethics
committee.

It is essential to show that consent will be obtained from all the relevant
parties who are involved in the project. A proposal must contain a standard information letter and consent form guaranteeing that participants in
the research can withdraw at any time. These issues are dealt with in more
detail in Chapter 10.

Resources

This section gives an outline of necessary resources, whether they be
human, material or financial, demonstrating that they have been realisti-
cally appraised.

Human

It is important that the applicant clearly identifies who will direct the project and the amount of time this individual will be able to devote to it. It is
necessary to outline the relationships and responsibilities of others
involved in the project. If it is a team effort, then the mix of expertise may
be an important element: for example, it may be necessary to describe the
active consultation and assistance offered by an experienced researcher to
someone less experienced. Any collaborative efforts should also be
described in detail. The consideration of the amount of time the project
will demand is important, especially if it is being undertaken 'part time' in
addition to full-time work commitments.

Material

You need to identify support and additional services such as secretarial
support, access to computers, library facilities, and work environment
considerations. Letters of agreement from relevant agencies, such as those
described by Smith (1994), should be included.

Financial

In some circumstances the preparation of the financial plan (budget) of the
project needs as much, if not more, skill than any other part of the project.

In preparation, consider research staff salaries, secretarial staff salaries, data collection costs, data processing costs, book purchases, conference attendance, travel and dissemination costs. A useful ally is someone in the finance department who can give an indication of the costs to be added in relation to 'overheads'. Overheads are the costs of running a research study from a particular institutional base. Overheads can add as much as an extra 25% to a budget. For example, a salary is often costed at more than that paid to the individual because of pension and other entitlements. It is a false economy to underfund the project as the reviewers can take this as a sign of inexperience. It is useful to bear in mind that, within limits, budgets for projects can be, and are, negotiable if unexpected costs are incurred.

Curriculum vitae

Curriculum vitae (CV) comes from the Latin and can be translated as 'the way your life has run'. A CV is not always essential but, if required, it should normally include: name; age; qualification; education; work experience; research experience; and recent relevant publications. In it you are trying to demonstrate why you are an appropriate person to undertake this research.

FUNDING

Although funds are not normally sought until the proposal is complete, funding should be considered at an early stage of the project and certainly before any purchase is made, as retrospective funding is rarely available. Interestingly, although it is normally stated in the literature that funding is calculated to fit the proposal (Hodgson 1989), discussions with experienced nurse researchers suggest that it is often the other way around. In other words, researchers with an interest in the area will apply for funding when tenders are advertised. Such advertisements are found in a variety of places, for example nursing journals such as the *Nursing Times* or *Nursing Standard*. Newspapers like *The Guardian* or *The Times Higher Education Supplement* (where the Fulbright Scholarships are advertised) are also good sources of information about funding.

In addition, the Charities Aid Foundation annual publication entitled the *Directory of Grant Making Trusts*, will help you to find out about funding sources and their purposes.

Guidelines supplied by the funding organization will contain the relevant information to inform the applicant. These guidelines may also suggest the philosophical approach to be employed with regard to the research approach. For example, the Department of Health Research and Development Division is particularly keen on funding the setting up of randomized controlled trials. This purchaser-led approach to funding may lead to the market dictating research topics and approaches, rather than researchers' and practitioners' preferences.

Individual funding bodies invite submissions at different times of the year and may offer varying degrees of financial support. It is important, therefore, for the project proposer to be realistic when estimating the budget and to request resources which will satisfy anticipated need as 'top-up' funds after the event may not be forthcoming. In addition to the Department of Health, funding bodies currently include the English National Board for Nursing, Midwifery and Health Visiting, and the United Kingdom Central Council for Nursing, Midwifery and Health Visiting. Funding is also available through higher education establishments. Most universities have a research committee which will allocate monies to local staff. It is also worth investigating health service opportunities for funding since most trusts will have a research budget. As stated earlier, the RAE and Culyer recommendations aim to increase research budgets by rewarding staff who are already 'research active'.

Submission of the funding proposal should be delayed until presentation of the documentation is of a high standard. The focus of the project should match that of the sponsoring organization: for example, it would be inappropriate and probably unsuccessful to seek funding for a clinically based study from organizations offering support for studies of an educational nature. It will add increased weight to the argument for financial support if the project can be shown to fit in with local, regional and national research priorities such as those outlined in *Working in Partnership* (DoH 1994b). When seeking funding, it may be a more effective strategy to seek smaller amounts from a larger number of organizations rather than put all the 'eggs in one basket'. However, conditions attached to the awarding of funding should always be checked carefully as there may be restrictions on obtaining funding from more than one source. If funding is sought from several sources, this should be clearly stated on the submission forms, and a copy should be kept of each application for reference. It may be several weeks before it is known whether an application has been successful. If the submission has been unsuccessful, then it is time to refine, develop the proposal in the light of any comments received, and try again.

■ **BOX 11.2**

Funding check list

- Does your topic match the interests of the funding body?
- Do the conditions for funding confirm whether or not you are eligible to apply?
- How much money is available and for what?
- Check submission dates and set yourself deadlines for preparing the proposal.
- Use the telephone to seek preliminary information.
- Where possible, get a named person who is involved in administering the fund to guide you through the application process.

The funding of nursing research has come under scrutiny and the Taskforce Report (DoH 1993) offers some useful recommendations. It identifies a 'need for more high quality research in nursing, midwifery and health visiting, particularly stable, long-term programmes of work on the efficacy and efficiency of clinical, organizational and managerial practices' (p. 14).

At best, the Report's call for nursing research programmes that are coherent and focused, forming part of regional and national NHS research strategies, should ensure the future funding of projects. At worst, the identification of particular issues and topics may limit their theoretical and methodological scope.

THE MOVE INTO HIGHER EDUCATION:
SOME IMPLICATIONS

Nursing aspires to be a research-based yet practical profession. With the integration of the majority of colleges of nursing into higher education structures, there may be pressure exerted by the new host institutions for nursing education to conform to the existing framework. There are many benefits to be gained from entering an institution with an established research strategy but it could be an awkward and painful process which results in both short- and long-term change. Moving nurse education into higher education offers nurses both opportunities and constraints. An example of this is the research assessment exercise (RAE) carried out by the Higher Education Funding Council for England (HEFCE). The implications of the RAE are significant and might benefit from some exploration.

The RAE formalizes the link between research ratings and future funding of research grants within higher education (UFC 1992a, b, c). This exercise began in 1986 and has since taken place periodically. The most recent assessment is taking place as we write (1996). The report in 1992, which included the 'new' universities (i.e. the former polytechnics) for the first time, identified only three out of the 29 university departments who submitted as performing nursing research in several areas that was of national excellence (Robinson 1993).

The focus of nursing research can be divided into two broad categories:

1. the study of social, economic, political and practical **phenomena**
2. the development and evaluation of specific interventions.

The criteria for research assessment are complex and are changed only with substantial consultation. They include, for example, research active staff, publications, external research income and research plans. It may be significant that the specific criteria by which excellence is assessed are not made public (Robinson 1993). Some of the categories of assessment carry higher prestige than others. One area surrounded by uncertainty is that of journal publication. It is not made explicit which nursing journals are considered academic and which are viewed as professional. There is a suggestion, however, that academic journals have higher currency than professional ones and therefore increase the research rating (Robinson 1993).

For nurses in education it seems that it is not simply a matter of 'publish or perish' but also necessary to ensure that you publish in the 'right' place. Such an approach may mean that, for practitioners, valuable information is less accessible both physically and linguistically. This reinforces the need for practitioners to be research minded.

As a result of the RAE, departments are graded on a scale of excellence with 5 being the highest and 1 the lowest. A rating of 5 identifies a department with work of international and national excellence.

The RAE is used to assist the allocation of funding from the HEFCE, using funding as a reward for excellence (Kiger 1994). This linkage of research rating to funding may encourage institutions to attempt to play the system by adopting the following strategies:

- elect to be known as a 'teaching-only' institution and rely on student income for resources
- declare certain departments within the institution to be 'teaching-only' and allocate internal resources disproportionately
- withdraw support entirely from departments which fail to improve their RAE rating over a given period of time.

This form of rationalization has been observed as the result of earlier RAEs where, for example, not a single chemistry department that achieved the lowest rating of 1 in 1989 had maintained an unadulterated existence until the subsequent exercise in 1992. In other words, low-scoring departments did not survive (Robinson 1993).

For the foreseeable future, the majority of funds for pre-registration nursing education will continue to come from central government, but will inevitably be affected by the higher education institutions with which it is associated. Opting out of the RAE by nursing and midwifery educators may not be a viable solution in the long term as students become increasingly sophisticated in their choice of training establishment.

Additionally, universities which aspire to high research ratings will not tolerate non-research-producing departments in their midst. It is not surprising that, as a general rule, the most recent newcomers to the university structure achieved the lowest ratings. Within nursing, the longer a department had been established within a university structure the higher its rating. For example, King's College London, the University of Surrey and Manchester University departments of nursing all gained high ratings. Members of these departments also tended to be on the RAE panel. Overall, in a rating of academic cost structures, nursing came bottom.

CONCLUSION

This chapter has discussed writing research proposals and funding sources. Many of the principles involved can be transferred to applications for study leave and the marketing of new ideas for clinical practice. The discussion has led to several issues being raised. These include the differences arising from quantitative and qualitative approaches, as well as the effects of the NHS research and development strategy, the association between nursing and higher education and the research assessment exercise. By addressing the insights, skills and knowledge required to compile a research proposal, the relationship of research mindedness and political awareness has been demonstrated.

REFERENCES

Bond S 1991 Preparing a research proposal. In: Cormack D F S (ed) The research process in nursing, 2nd edn. Blackwell Scientific Publications, Oxford

Cobb A K, Hagemaster J N 1987 Ten criteria for evaluating qualitative research proposals. Journal of Nursing Education 26(4): 138–143

Collins H L 1988 When the profit motive threatens patient care. RN 51(10): 74–80

Culyer T 1995 Cure at a cost. Synthesis, Times Higher Education Supplement, January 20, p i

Day R A 1989 How to write and publish a scientific paper, 3rd edn. Cambridge University Press, Cambridge

Department of Health 1993 Report of the Taskforce on the Strategy for Research in Nursing, Midwifery and Health Visiting. DoH, London

Department of Health 1994a Support for research and development in the NHS (Chair: Professor T Culyer). HMSO, London

Department of Health 1994b Working in partnership. HMSO, London

Field P A, Morse J M 1985 Nursing research: the application of qualitative approaches. Chapman & Hall, London

Haase J E, Myers S T 1988 Reconciling paradigm assumptions of qualitative and quantitative research. Western Journal of Nursing Research 10(2): 128–137

Hodgson C 1989 Tips on writing successful grant proposals. Nurse Practitioner 14(2): 44, 46, 49, 53–54

Kiger A 1994 Nursing education and the research assessment exercise. Nurse Researcher 1(3): 85–95

Koch T 1994 Establishing rigour in qualitative research. The decision trail. Journal of Advanced Nursing 19: 976–986

Marshall C, Rossman G B 1989 Designing qualitative research. Sage, London

Robinson J 1993 Nursing and the research assessment exercise: what counts? Nurse Researcher 1(1): 84–92

Rolfe G 1994 Towards a new model of nursing research. Journal of Advanced Nursing 19: 969–975

Royal College of Midwives 1989 Writing a research proposal and applying for funding. RCM, London

Sandelowski M 1986 The problem of rigor in qualitative research. Advances in Nursing Science 8(3): 27–37

Smith P 1992 The emotional labour of nursing—how nurses care. Macmillan, Basingstoke

Smith P 1994 Fulbright Scholarship: an opportunity for UK nurses. Nurse Researcher 1(4): 87–92

Smith P, Mackintosh M, Towers B 1993 Implications of the new contracting system for the district nursing service in one health authority: a pilot study. Journal of Interprofessional Care 7(2): 115–124

Tierney A 1993 Research literacy: an essential pre-requisite for knowledge led practice. Nurse Researcher 1(1): 79–83

University Funding Council 1992a Research assessment exercise: circular letter. UFC, Bristol

University Funding Council 1992b Research assessment exercise 1992: membership of assessment panels. Circular 24/92. UFC, Bristol

University Funding Council 1992c Research assessment exercise 1992: the council outcome. Circular 26/92. UFC, Bristol

Valiga T M, Mermel V M 1985 Formulating the researchable question. Topics in Clinical Nursing 7(2): 1–14

Epilogue

Pam Smith

PREAMBLE

The use of literature and art to inform the research process has been an important element within this book. It is not surprising therefore that in coming to write this epilogue, a line from a poem by the American poet Thom Gunn entitled 'On the Move' came to mind. Writing in the 1960s about the motorbike riders of California, Gunn concludes his poem with the line: 'One is always nearer by not keeping still ...' (Gunn 1962). You might ask why did I recall this particular line? Partly I think because the production of this book has been about 'not keeping still'. First, it originated as a series of teaching sessions which took the participants on a voyage of discovery about research, teaching and practice. Second, the process of turning the spoken word into a written text required another shift, which was achieved during a series of interactive discussions between individuals and groups. Third, although the book is coming to an end, the world of health care, education and research has moved on. This would seem to suggest therefore that the research-minded practitioner, like the motorbike riders in Gunn's poem, will get nearer to the meaning of life (in this case the heart of practice) by not keeping still.

INTRODUCTION

If you refer back to the introduction to this book you will note that its purpose is to:

- start you on a journey of becoming research minded
- assist you to decode research jargon
- explore and explode myths associated with research
- increase your confidence to ask questions and think critically and analytically
- recognize what you already know and do as part of being research minded
- apply research mindedness to practice.

In other words, we hope that the book has assisted you to identify the links between research and practice and recognize your own store of knowledge and experience including your own unique database and expertise in techniques such as story telling, observation and recording of patients' and clients' physical and psychosocial states.

Getting nearer

In each chapter, the authors chose topics which interested them and which they saw as offering an opportunity to explore the meaning of research mindedness and its relationship to seeing, thinking and knowing as practitioners and teachers. They were in a unique position to bridge those two worlds, many of them just having left practice to undertake teacher training.

Things have moved on since the idea for the book was first conceived and there are many aspects of the current NHS research and development culture which have since gained prominence. Of particular importance has been the growth of the evidence-based health care movement and associated information technology to support it. The purpose of evidence-based health care is to encourage practitioners to use evidence-based findings in their daily practice by making them more accessible. One way of making research accessible is for systematic reviews to be undertaken of a variety of topics. Reviewers critically assess the methods and findings of the studies (usually clinical trials) in order to synthesize them, publish them and store them on computerized databases such as those housed at the Cochrane Centre in Oxford and the Centre for Reviews and Dissemination at York University. The long-term aim for the NHS information systems strategy is to build up a national and international database which, as well as systematic reviews, stores local and regional information about research initiatives and projects. There are even plans to use these databases with patients so that they can study the evidence of various treatment options with their doctor or nurse and make informed decisions about their care (Moore 1996).

Information systems are very important to the success of the Culyer initiative mentioned in Chapter 1, so as to ensure that research activities carried out by practitioners are recorded and accessible. Like the research assessment exercise (RAE) in the universities, the NHS will also be expected to provide evidence that they are 'research active' if they are going to attract research funding. While we are on the topic of the RAE, you may be interested to know that another assessment has come and gone. Information has been collected by university departments, including nursing, about their research funding, projects and publications since 1992 and will be reported at the end of this year 1996. It will be interesting to see the extent to which nursing departments have managed to improve their rating from the rather low scores the majority achieved in the last exercise.

In terms of the media, topics have also come and gone and surfaced a second and third time since Wladyslawa Czuber-Dochan, Linda McBride and Julie Wilson wrote Chapter 7. For example, the killer bug story has raised its head as a repeated theme in the ugly guise of meningitis. The interesting point about these stories is that the press 'discover' diseases that have always been present (i.e. endemic) in the community. It is likely, therefore, that the press coverage of diseases such as the killer bug or meningitis has increased rather than the number of cases. It is also worth noting that sensational stories about exotic and deadly diseases such as Ebola fever also sell newspapers.

But we also see that the press has an important role in exposing evidence that may be in the interest of a range of institutions such as pharmaceutical companies and even governments to distort, conceal or even ignore. We saw the example of the thalidomide crisis in Chapter 7. More recently, journalists have reported the possible food chain link between bovine spongiform encephalopathy (BSE or 'mad cow disease') and a form of the fatal Creutzfeldt–Jakob disease in humans which is due to an infectious agent that affects the brain. It has been the press rather than the British Government who have taken on the responsibility of systematically and accurately reporting the scientific evidence to the public. The BSE story illustrates the fine balance between social responsibility, sensitive news reporting and the relationship between scientists, the media and the Government in keeping the public adequately informed.

In relation to the central theme of Chapter 7, 'Miracle cures for AIDS', yet another story has come to light recently. The source of the story is Kenya where a top government medical scientist is claiming a product called 'Pearl Omega' will treat people with HIV or AIDS (McGreal 1996). There are reports that sick and dying people are spending their scant life savings in the hope of buying a reprieve from the killer disease.

So the world moves on, but being research minded is to be both aware of change but also sensitive to its implications for teaching, practice and patient care. A fundamental question which presents itself is about the nature of evidence, whose interests and agendas is it serving and how is it being incorporated into the body of knowledge and applied to policy and clinical decision making?

The process of production

What perhaps is not transmitted in these pages is that the approach adopted both for the module and book emphasized collective rather than individual learning as a means of using research mindedness to encourage collaboration and advocacy to empower health professionals and their clients, not only through the acquisition of new knowledge but also by recognizing the knowledge that they already have.

The process of writing this book has been an exciting one. In our meetings, the same magic that kept alive our Friday afternoon seminars was transferred to our contributors' get-togethers. It is much easier to discuss and debate amongst a group who you know well than commit these ideas to the written word. But we have tried to keep the spirit of our enquiry alive in the pages of this book.

RESEARCH MINDEDNESS FOR PRACTICE

Since the key purpose of this book was to start you off on a journey to promote research mindedness for practice you might like to review each of the chapters and consider their contribution to your understanding of this endeavour. For example, has your definition of research mindedness changed from how you defined it while reading Chapter 1? Is there any one definition presented in the book which you prefer more than others?

You may recall that we looked at a definition that was used by the authors of a textbook for social workers to describe the characteristics of the research-minded practitioner (Everitt et al 1992).

To refresh your memory research-minded social work practitioners were described in the following way:

- [they] will be constantly defining and making explicit their objectives and hypotheses;
- [they] will treat their explanations of the social world as hypotheses—that is, as tentative and open to be tested against evidence;
- [they] will be aware of their expertise and knowledge and that of others;
- [they] will bring to the fore theories that help make sense of social need, resources and assist in decision making with regard to strategies;
- [they] will be thoughtful, reflecting on data and theory and contributing to their development and refinement;
- [they] will scrutinize and be analytical of available data and information;
- [they] will be mindful of the pervasiveness of ideology and values in the way we see and understand the world

We liked the definition of research mindedness adopted by these authors because of the integrated approach they took to research-based practice.

In revisiting those characteristics you will be reminded that the emphasis for Everitt and colleagues was clearly not on doing research but on using its theoretical perspectives and methods to think analytically about and inform practice. We have encouraged the development of these characteristics throughout the chapters of our book. For instance, the characteristic to 'be mindful of the pervasiveness of ideology and values in the way we see and understand the world' is addressed by a number of authors. Margaret Harper and Nina Hartman use critical theory and feminism, and Benny Goodman and Frank Strange ethnomethodology, to encourage us to challenge our values and beliefs. Nina's story, for example, is a powerful indictment of racism, stereotyping and hierarchical relationships within midwifery and nursing.

Chapters 4, 7 and 9 encourage you to 'scrutinize and be analytical of available data' be it in the form of statistics, print and TV journalism or written reports. Although all the chapters encourage you to be reflective of specific research approaches and techniques, Chapters 2 and 5 in particular encourage 'theory development and reflection from practice'. Chapter 3, in the spirit of experimental method, and Chapter 7, in terms of getting behind the media, assist you to 'constantly define and make explicit your objectives and hypotheses and treat explanations of the social world as tentative and open to be tested against evidence'. Chapters 8 and 11 will assist you to acquire the characteristic to 'bring to the fore theories that help make sense of social need, resources and assist in decision making with regard to strategies' through reviewing the literature and considering how to write research proposals. The ethical implications of research as discussed in Chapter 10 is a core theme which informs each characteristic of the research-minded practitioner. Finally, all the chapters emphasize the need to be 'aware of your expertise and knowledge and that of others'.

An underpinning theme throughout the book has been the ongoing debate within nursing and health services research about the appropriateness of adopting qualitative and quantitative approaches and methods. Nurses, like social workers, feel uneasy with the so-called and assumed objectivity of quantitative scientific research which categorizes and numbers clients as opposed to capturing the warmth and spontaneity of their relationships (Everitt et al 1992). Everitt and colleagues go so far as to suggest that social work as a practice discipline has disengaged from research because of its association with positivist science. Such an approach is seen as inappropriate to a world that is 'uncertain, complex, spontaneous and concerned with individual difference' (p. 8). Qualitative approaches therefore are seen as more appropriate for capturing the nuances of this world.

However, as we have endeavoured to show in Chapters 3 and 4, the quantitative approach to research offers important tools for addressing clinical issues. Furthermore, because of the current orientation of the NHS research and development strategy towards the accumulation of evidence using randomized controlled trials, all health care practitioners need to have a critical understanding of the use of these tools. The claims for miracle AIDS cures as discussed in Chapter 7, and the need for systematic scientific evidence, is a case in point. Furthermore, as we suggested in Chapter 1, it may be that a number of factors influence a researcher's decision to select a particular research approach. You will recall that these factors include items such as the topic of study, resources available, including time and money, and the experience and preferences of the person conducting the research. Indeed, the topics selected for each chapter of this book are based on each author's experiences and preferences.

Our message to you is that the research-minded practitioner will be able to critically assess the repertoire of research approaches and methods currently available rather than reject either qualitative or quantitative research out of hand.

'ON THE MOVE' OR 'NOT KEEPING STILL': DISSEMINATION, IMPLEMENTATION AND ACTION

We are all familiar with the human reaction to ignore so-called scientific evidence. On the smoking and lung cancer debate, for instance, many stalwart smokers will point out that they know lots of people in their eighties who, despite a lifetime of smoking, are happy and healthy and cancer-free. Similarly, many nurses greet new initiatives in wound or pressure area care with scepticism and opposition to existing treatments, pointing out that 'we've always done it this way!' Doctors too, despite the Government's crusade to promote evidence-based medicine, continue to ignore research findings (Moore 1996). Using research therefore requires attitudinal and behavioural changes (in other words the adoption of Sapsford & Abbott's research stance referred to in Ch. 1) as part of the social process of dissemination and implementation (Bond et al 1996).

The reasons why people do not incorporate evidence into their practice are many and various, not least because of a lack of access not just to findings but also to the time and space to critically consider their relevance. Furthermore, there may be a power issue, since if a ward sister or consultant does not agree with the evidence, junior staff are placed in a difficult position in trying to implement new practices. A much quoted example is the use of EUSOL (Edinburgh University solution of lime) for cleansing wounds. Research showed that the substance was actually harmful but nurses reported that consultants were still ordering it to be used for their patients (Walsh & Ford 1989, Farrow & Toth 1991).

In principle, the introduction of systematic reviews should make it more difficult for practitioners, even powerful consultants, to resist the pressure of evidence, especially if they are used to develop practice guidelines. The GRIPP initiative (Getting Research into Practice and Purchasing) is addressing the issue of how to incorporate research evidence into both practice and buying health care proven to work (Dunning et al 1994). GRIPP, an initiative of the former Oxford Regional Health Authority, involved the setting up of seminars to examine the evidence related to the following topics: the use of corticosteroids in pre-term delivery; management of services for stroke patients; dilatation and curettage (D & C) for women under 40 years; the use of grommet surgery for children with suspected glue ear. The first two areas were concerned with effectiveness; the second two with appropriateness. Evidence showed that corticosteroid use reduced the incidence of pre-term delivery whilst better multidisciplinary coordination of care reduced morbidity and mortality. Evidence revealed for the second two areas that the use of such interventions had very little benefit in the long run in relieving symptoms and, in the case of D & C, detecting disease.

You will note that with the exception of the management of stroke patients, the majority of these studies are concerned with medical practice. This bias, however, is beginning to change. In Chapter 3, Jane Say and Julie Cumpper drew your attention to one of the first systematic nursing reviews undertaken by Nicky Cullum on the management of leg ulcers. The York Centre is currently extending the scope of their activities to undertake a survey of practice and service developments amongst the nursing and therapy professions (NHS CRD 1995).

But, as was recently reported by the Derbyshire Royal Infirmary's chief executive about an initiative involving doctors, nurses and physiotherapists in jointly developing 'care pathways' of best practice for back pain, the secret lies in organizational commitment by managers and practitioners and multidisciplinary collaboration (Moore 1996).

Indeed, you may now well be wondering how to sustain a research-minded perspective for practice, given the demands on your time and the constant changes within the NHS. As Luker & Kenrick (1995) point out, the organizational and policy context is a major factor for creating the climate for good practice. Participants at a research-awareness workshop, for example, felt that for their stimulation and interest to be sustained in practice they needed increased access to and availability of local experts to advise them on the practical application of research in their own settings. They also identified the importance of supportive managers to promote and sustain a research culture as part of practice development and innovation

(Cook et al 1992). Put another way, the individual practitioner alone may face an uphill struggle to implement good practice, as the EUSOL example above illustrates.

Thus, research and practice are integrally linked, but for one to inform the other a number of organizational attributes are necessary. You might like to see if these attributes (outlined in Box 12.1) are present in your organization, be it ward, hospital, health centre, clinic, college or classroom. Even better, you might be in a position to create them as a teacher, ward sister, or practice development nurse.

■ BOX 12.1

Organizational attributes for successful service-based nursing research programmes (adapted from Snyder-Halpern 1991):

- an organizational mission compatible with research
- the availability of local nurse experts who are 'dynamic facilitators' with research training and experience
- organizational commitment to and support of grassroots research
- the Chief Nurse values research and sees it as integral to sound nursing practice
- the Chief Nurse ensures financial commitment to research activities
- access to a range of consultation services including computers, statistics, statisticians, qualitative and quantitative research experts
- flexible work structures to allow research activities to take place.

In Chapter 2 and again in Chapter 9, the authors gave you practical ideas for how to implement research in practice. Margaret Harper and Nina Hartman began Chapter 2 with stories, to represent their ideas about research mindedness and the use of narrative to generate ideas, make sense of events and learn from practice. They suggest that in order to substantiate proposed nursing action there must be a willingness to think critically and clearly and a willingness to enter into dialogue with other nurses and members of the multidisciplinary team. Telling stories helps us to rehearse our arguments and our logic. In Chapter 9, Donna Lewis and Charmagne Barnes suggested the use of posters, journal clubs, resource folders, peer group discussion and writing practice standards based on research and experience.

Bond and colleagues (1996) suggest the need to expose users and researchers to each others' needs and complementary ways of thinking. One way of doing this, according to Bond and colleagues, is to forge links between academic departments and clinical nurses so that they can work together in carrying out and participating in projects of mutual interest. One such example involved psychiatric nursing service users, their carers and other mental health disciplines investigating the fundamental question: 'What do people in care need nurses for?'. This type of research not only aims to improve the effectiveness of a service but also cuts across the interdisciplinary and professional/client divide.

As discussed in Chapter 11, some of the best ideas for research come from everyday practice. Nursing development units (NDUs), which have increased in number since the first ones were set up by the King's Fund in the late 1980s, are an ideal base from which to develop research and research-based practice. When I was a district director of nursing research and development, for example, I was called in by clinical nurses and their managers involved in an NDU, to investigate the impact of primary nursing on the quality of patient care and the effects of ward-based handovers on nurse–patient communication (Bamford et al 1990, Bamford & Jones 1997). The NDU worked well because the managers supported the clinical nurses in their endeavours by giving them time and flexibility to develop their ideas. The nurses themselves sought advice and developed skills from working with local researchers such as myself and Shelagh Sparrow, the ENB 870 Research Course Tutor. Members of staff enrolled on the course and worked with myself and Shelagh to develop research proposals to attract local regional research monies, which were then available specifically to encourage novice nurse researchers.

Bond and colleagues (1996) also give a number of examples of how nurse academics have worked with NDU staff on projects such as patient self-medication, continence promotion and discharge planning. One outcome of these initiatives has been an increase in the number of funded studies involving practitioners and nurse researchers. Bond and colleagues refer to a specific research approach known as **action research** as a means of bringing about change and improvements in practice. There are many different ways of developing an action research project, but its hallmarks are collaboration and participation between researchers and researched in defining issues, questions and solutions (Hart & Bond 1995). Often, the researcher takes on the role of change agent on behalf of the participants. Bell (1993) concludes: 'The essentially practical, problem-solving nature of action research makes this approach attractive to practitioner-researchers who have identified a problem during the course of their work, see the merits of investigating it, and if possible, of improving practice'. The use of action research in nursing is growing and a recent user of the approach, Julienne Meyer (1993), describes some of the issues for participants as they attempted to move away from professionally dominated care to an increased role for patients and their lay carers.

The importance of education in promoting research mindedness cannot be overestimated and it is significant that this book began life in the classroom. It was there we began to explore our future roles as teachers in this process. The objectives of pre- and post-registration nursing curricula clearly state the need to prepare students to evaluate the literature critically and to incorporate research into practice. But, as noted in Chapter 1, teachers need to be competent in research skills themselves to develop them in students. The experience of preparing the seminars and writing the chapters demonstrated the need for teachers to view research in two ways. First, as the knowledge that informs teaching and, second, as a series of approaches and techniques to generate new knowledge and encourage critical thinking.

We endeavoured in each chapter, therefore, to reflect on our experiences of using particular approaches and techniques for promoting research mindedness. Through our reflections we hope we have achieved our purpose in exploding myths, decoding jargon and confirming that you are your own unique database with knowledge, expertise and stories worth telling. And those stories are an integral part of being research minded and being you. In Gunn's words, they also prevent you from keeping still.

REFERENCES

Bamford O, Dinean L, Pritchard B, Smith P 1990 Change for the better. Nursing Times 86(23): 28–33

Bamford O, Jones A 1997 Researching nursing development units. In: Smith P (ed) Nursing research: setting new agendas. Edward Arnold, London (in press)

Bell J 1993 Doing your research project: a guide for first-time researchers in education and social science, 2nd edn. Open University Press, Buckingham, p 7

Bond S, Barker P, Pearson P, Procter S 1996 Forging links between academe and practice through research. Nursing Standard 10(27): 45–47

Cook S, Ghazy F, Smith P 1992 Nursing and midwifery research: making it happen. Nursing Practice 5(4): 27–28

Dunning M, McQuay H, Milne R 1994 Getting a grip. Health Service Journal (28 April): 24–25

Everitt A, Hardiker P, Littlewood J, Mullender A 1992 Applied research for better practice. Macmillan, Basingstoke, pp 4–5

Farrow S, Toth B 1991 The place of EUSOL in wound management. Nursing Standard 5(22): 25–27

Gunn T 1962 On the move. In: Gunn T, Hughes T (eds) Collected poems. Faber & Faber, London

Hart E, Bond M 1995 Action research for health and social care. Open University Press, Buckingham

Luker K A, Kenrick M 1995 Towards knowledge-based practice; an evaluation of a method of dissemination. International Journal of Nursing Studies 32(1): 59–67

McGreal C 1996 Professor turns Aids into lucre. The Guardian, May 25, p 11

Meyer J 1993 New paradigm research in practice: the trials and tribulations of action research. Journal of Advanced Nursing 18: 1066–1072

Moore W 1996 Lives in the balance. The Guardian Society, May 1996, pp 2–3

NHS Centre for Reviews and Dissemination 1995 Practice and service development. University of York, CRD, York

Snyder-Halpern R 1991 Service-based nursing research programs organisational attributes for success. Conference paper, ANA Research Conference, Los Angeles

Walsh M, Ford P 1989 Nursing rituals: research and natural action. Butterworth Heinemann, Oxford

FURTHER READING

The Foundation of Nursing Studies 1996 Reflection for action: an exploration of national and local nursing research implementation cultures; barriers, expectations and achievements; identifying opportunities for the future. The Foundation of Nursing Studies, London

Kitson A, Ahmed L B, Harvey G, Seers K and Thompson D R 1996 From research to practice: one organisational model for promoting research-based practice. Journal of Advanced Nursing 23: 430–440

Glossary

Absolute variation. See under variation.

Accounting procedure. An accounting procedure is the process we use to make sense of the world, drawing on everyday theories and common-sense, taken-for-granted knowledge to 'socially construct' a phenomenon such as suicide. See also ethnomethodology.

Action research. Research involving a planned cycle of social interventions and an evaluation of their effects. Action research aims to solve practical problems and increase knowledge.

Applicability. The qualitative equivalent of generalizability in quantitative research. It is also associated with 'fittingness' since a study is judged to be transferable if the findings are able to 'fit' into other contexts. See also transferability.

Approach/approaches. Refers to the research approach used within a specific paradigm. Methodology and approach can be used interchangeably. Both terms are used to denote the overall research enterprise which incorporates theories, philosophies and methods. See also methodologies and methods.

Auditability. Auditability is achieved when the researchers give a clear account of the research process to allow the reader to assess whether they and the project are dependable. Sandelowski (1986) devised the notion of the 'decision trail' as a means of assisting researchers to indicate clearly how their findings emerged. A decision trail allows the reader to follow the progression of events in a study and understand their underlying logic. See also dependability.

Autonomy. Autonomy, derived from the Greek for self and rule, refers to a person's ability to choose freely for him/herself and be able to direct his/her own life.

Bar chart. Gives a visual representation of nominal data in which the height of the bars is used to represent the frequency of occurrence of different values.

Beneficence. Beneficence builds on the principle of nonmaleficence in that it goes beyond preventing or removing harm to actually doing or promoting good.

Bias. A general research term used to describe how the perceptions and interpretations of researchers are influenced by their preconceptions and experiences. Bias also refers to the effects researchers may have on research settings and subjects. Phenomenologists use bracketing to reduce bias. See also bracketing.

Biomedicine/biomedical paradigm. Refers to the application of positivist science to medicine by which the mind and body are regarded as separate parts which can be 'fixed' like a machine when affected by illness. Biomedicine emphasizes the importance of objective evidence such as the outward signs of disease, rather than the subjective (i.e. the social, cultural and historical) aspects of patients' lives. See also positive paradigm/positivism.

Bracketing/bracket. Processes used by phenomenologists to reduce bias by temporarily suspending preconceptions, assumptions, values, beliefs and feelings in order to focus on the experience under study and hold prior knowledge, theory and facts at bay. Some interpretive studies attempt to retain a sense of objectivity about the subjective meanings of others by 'bracketing' their own assumptions about the phenomenon. See also bias.

Clinical trial. A scientific test or trial carried out in a laboratory is an experiment. Since it is simply a means of testing a theory, it can also be carried out in many different areas including clinical practice. In this case it is referred to as a clinical trial. See also randomized controlled trial.

Concept. A general summary of the abstract aspects of life such as care, goodness, stress which have acquired meaning through common recognition, lay usage or formal definition.

Confident. See levels of confidence.

Construct. A construct is a concept that has been given a more systematic definition to enable scientific hypothesizing and measurement in the 'real' world. Therefore a construct has qualities that allow it to be measured. The use of the word construct is to point out that concepts do not have independent existence and meanings outside of human beings. We collectively and individually 'build' or construct meanings and concepts whether as lay persons or scientists. Social scientists often use the terms construct and concept interchangeably.

Schutz (1972) divides constructs into first and second degree constructs. For example, stress is a lay concept that has many meanings in everyday speech. As such it is defined as a first degree construct. The everyday actor operates in the commonsense world of first degree constructs.

Schutz refers to the constructs used by scientists as second degree constructs by which they proceed to measure and analyse theoretical terms. Attachment and quality of life are examples of second degree constructs which researchers devise to try to explain the concept of stress. See also operationalization.

Control. The researcher attempts to eliminate or minimize the effects of extraneous variables on the dependent variable. This is achieved by exerting control over the experimental conditions. A control group is a group of people with similar characteristics to the experimental group except they do not receive the intervention. They can be used therefore as a baseline against which the effects of the intervention can be measured.

Content validity. See under validity.

Convenience sample. Subjects who meet the criteria for inclusion in a study are recruited because they are conveniently available to the researcher. The sample may be limited by time constraints and distance, and the likelihood of bias is great. This is an example of non-probability sampling.

Correlation. The term is used when variables appear to vary together, i.e. a relationship (called correlation) exists between the two variables. We can use the value of one variable to predict or infer the value of the other variable. However, correlation does not necessarily mean causation. See also negative and positive correlations.

Correlation coefficient. A numerical index to look at the degree of fit between two variables. Correlation coefficients range from + 1.0 (which indicates a perfect positive relationship) to − 1.0 (which indicates a perfect negative relationship). See also Pearson product-moment correlation and Spearman's correlation coefficient.

Credibility. See also trustworthiness/validity. Credibility with its connotations of 'truth' can be compared with internal validity in quantitative research. A study's credibility is said to be confirmed when readers recognize the situation being described in a research report as closely related to their own experience. Another interpretation of credibility is when a reader subsequently recognizes an experience after only having read about it in a research report.

Critical theory (also referred to as critical social theory). See also feminism. Generally acknowledged to have evolved out of a critique of the technological knowledge developed by positivist science which contributed to the oppression of the working class. The focus of this work took place in Frankfurt, Germany in the late 1920s and was inspired by Marxist ideas. The group, who became known as the Frankfurt School, consisted of a range of interdisciplinary scholars, including Erich Fromm, psychologist; Herbert Marcuse, philosopher; Max Horheimer, philosopher and social psychologist; and Friedrich Pollack, economist. Critical social theory acknowledges and integrates subjective forms of knowledge, so that both human perceptions and experiences, as well as 'objective' observations, are considered of scientific worth. Feminists criticize critical social theory because it accepts the male world-view as the social norm, taking it as the frame of reference for all research.

Critical social theory and feminism go beyond positivism and interpretivism to make us conscious of the bias and political agendas that may inform research. Critical social theory and feminism therefore have the actual or potential power to improve and transform the situations under study and empower the clients and consumers of health care as well as the health professionals themselves.

Deductive. A form of reasoning which proceeds from the general to specific hypotheses for testing by observation. Often follows induction.

Deontology. There are two generally accepted ethical theories in western society: utilitarianism and deontology. Deontology (from the Greek *deon*—duty) suggests that some actions are right or wrong in themselves, not merely as a result of their consequences but because of their actual characteristics; for example, telling lies is always wrong irrespective of the consequences.

Dependability. Dependability is the qualitative equivalent of reliability. It is achieved as the researchers become increasingly familiar with the research setting. As the study proceeds, they are able to check the accuracy and recurrence of the data over time in a number of different settings and from a variety of participants' perspectives. The dependability of a study is evaluated according to whether it fulfils the associated criterion of auditability. See also auditability.

Dependent variable. The variable to be explained or predicted which is 'dependent' on the independent, causal or explanatory variable. Examples are smoking cessation following health education; healing time of leg ulcers dependent on type of dressing.

Descriptive statistics. Statistical methods used to organize, describe, summarize or display data in order to give a sense of their main features. See also univariate statistics.

Ecology. The science or study of plants, animals and people in relation to their environment.

Empiricism. Scientific method is based on empiricism (a word closely related to experiment and experience) in order to establish the factual basis of knowledge through careful, detached, objective measurement, followed by replication and the confirmation of recurring patterns and relationships within the data. Empirical refers to data generated by trial, experiment or field experience.

Epistemology. Refers to the study of the theories of knowledge; assumptions about knowledge and truth; ways of knowing—i.e. 'how do we know what we know?'—and the 'knowledge-producing system' that each individual learns to develop from early childhood.

Ethics. The term ethics refers to the study of morals. The two terms are often used interchangeably to refer to a code or set of principles which provide a framework of norms, values, beliefs, right, wrong, good and bad.

Ethical issues. Issues of daily life, which require both specific and general levels of ethical decision making. General levels of ethical decision making are not necessarily recognized.

Ethnography. A subdiscipline of anthropology, ethnography is the detailed study of small groups of people such as gangs, nurses, patients and their subcultures in a range of settings such as hospitals and housing estates. It has traditionally taken a broader approach than ethnomethodology.

Ethnomethodology. A branch of sociology created by Howard Garfinkel (1967), and a relatively new approach to the study of the production of knowledge in the social sciences. The term literally means 'the study of people's methods' and its aim is to understand the everyday world in which we live by the use of accounting procedures.

Extraneous variable. An accidental connection or incidental factor which appears to explain a relationship between variables. Extraneous variables are more likely to occur if standard experimental conditions have not been applied to control them. See also control.

First degree construct. See under construct.

Face validity. See under validity.

Feminism. Has similarities with critical theory. Feminism requires feminists to do the work for women that the Frankfurt School researchers began and continue to do for men. The aim of feminist theory is to research or investigate women's lives and experiences in their own terms, by creating theories grounded in the actual experiences and language of women. Feminist approaches to theory and research reflect 'woman-centredness' by making women's experiences the major focus of study.

Fittingness. See under transferability.

Generalizability. An experiment should be designed to allow the results to be generalized beyond the sample to the wider target population. Generalizability of research results is important if the findings are going to be applied to the population from which the sample has been drawn. See under validity; see also representativeness, transferability.

Grounded theory. An inductive qualitative research approach popular amongst sociologists and nurse researchers. Grounded theory provides a framework for collecting, coding and analysing data in order to develop concepts and hypotheses from the data by means of theoretical sampling of participants and settings to guide ongoing data collection. The ultimate goal of grounded theory is theory development.

Hermeneutic. See under interpretive paradigm/interpretive hermeneutic approach.

Histogram. Used to visually present interval or ratio data as apparently continuous. The definition of a histogram is that the area of the bar (rather than its height) represents the value of the frequency.

Hypothesis. A proposition, a question or a predicted relationship between variables which we try to confirm by means of a statistical test.

Ideology. Belief and value systems that are presented as 'facts' by society's most powerful groups, in order to control or exert power over other groups.

Independent variable. A variable which is thought to produce or cause changes in another variable. In experiments, the independent variable (e.g. an educational intervention, type of drug or dressing) is systematically varied or manipulated by the researcher.

Indexicality. A central concept within ethnomethodology. It refers to the need to take into account the context around words and phrases to give us meaning. See also reflexivity and social constructionist perspective.

Inductive. Specific events are observed and analysed for patterns in the data, then used as a basis to formulate general theoretical statements (specific to general). May precede deduction.

Inferential statistics. A form of statistical activity to make inferences or predictions about the population as a whole from which a sample has been drawn. Statistical activities include the calculation of correlations between variables and significance tests.

Inter-rater reliability. The extent to which two raters observing the same phenomenon (e.g. nurses recording a patient's blood pressure) and using the same measures (e.g. sphygmomanometer) obtain the same results. See also reliability.

Interpretive paradigm/interpretive hermeneutic approach. Interpretivism has been embraced by many nurses and midwives as being preferable to positivism because it aims to discover meaning and promote understanding. Furthermore, the researcher's subjective involvement is positively valued. The interpretive paradigm provides health care research with increased reflectivity and improved communication, and thus a point from which to implement enhancements in care itself.

The interpretive hermeneutic approach is both a theory of and a method for interpreting the meaning of human actions. It is concerned with obtaining an authentic version of actions created through behaviour, books or pictures. The approach originates from interpreting biblical text.

Interval. See under levels of measurement. The interval level of measurement allows the researcher to measure data on a scale in which the intervals between adjacent levels of measurement are assumed to be the same, as illustrated by the gradations on a thermometer which measure temperature.

Justice. The principle of justice (being fair) is based on Aristotle's concept that how individuals are treated relates to their position and worth within a given society. Individuals will be treated, therefore, in proportion to their standing (Beauchamp & Childress 1989). This is a complex principle, since it suggests that not all individuals are equally valued within society.

Levels of confidence. A test can be applied that states statistically that you can be 99% confident or 95% confident that a treatment worked. In other words, there is only a 1% or a 5% possibility that the results of the treatment are due to chance. P is the symbol for the level of confidence or the probability that the results have not occurred by chance, i.e. the treatment did make a difference. $P < 0.01$ means that the P or probability that the difference occurred by chance rather than as a result of the treatment is < (less than) 1 in 100.

Levels of measurement. It is usual to identify four levels or scales of measurement—nominal, ordinal, interval, ratio. See measurement.

Logical positivism. See under positivist paradigm.

Mean. The mean is the most familiar and useful measure used to describe the central tendency or average of a distribution of scores for any set of data. The mean (μ) is computed by dividing the sum of the scores (ΣX) by the total number of scores (N). See also mean absolute deviation.

Mean absolute deviation. The means of all the absolute deviations, i.e. the sum of the values obtained by subtracting the mean from each score (treating negative values as positive; $\Sigma |X - \mu|$) divided by the total number of scores (N).

Measure of central tendency. Data can be summarized by one single result, i.e. its central or average mark. In statistical terms this is accomplished by finding a measure of central tendency. There are three different ways to calculate a measure of central tendency which are the mean, median and mode. See also mean, median and mode.

Measure of variance. Summarizes the variability of the data, which is the way that the data spread out from the measure of central tendency. See also variability.

Measurement. A procedure for classifying individuals, groups or other units and putting them into predetermined categories to which a number can be attributed. There are four levels or scales of measurement; see under nominal, ordinal, interval and ratio.

Median. Another useful measure of central tendency is the median or middle score. To find the median you need to (1) put the data in order and (2) find the middle score, or rather the score that has exactly the same number of scores above it as below. If there is an even number of scores, i.e. there is no middle point, then the median is calculated by taking the two middle scores and finding the score half way between them.

Methodology/methodologies. The study of the theories, philosophies and values which inform research designs and methods. See also approaches.

Methods. The techniques of doing research: asking questions, observing people and groups, analysing case records, historical documents and newspapers. A variety of research methods can be used independently of methodology or approach. This is a useful distinction since it differentiates between the paradigms, i.e. philosophies and values, that drive the research and its implementation in the field.

Mode. The mode is the score that occurs most frequently in a set of data.

Nascent. See also theory. Nascent theory is referred to by feminists as an 'emancipatory' version of 'the truth'. Theory is described as 'nascent' not only in the sense of being a (relatively) recent theoretical perspective, but also because it conveys the sense of being unusually reactive or volatile, as in 'nascent hydrogen' (Oxford English Dictionary 1981). This sense reflects the frequently hostile reaction that much feminist theory has engendered, not only from men, but often amongst women themselves, often 'just' for desiring the knowledge.

Negative correlation. Means that high scores on one variable tend to be associated with low scores on the other and vice versa, i.e. as one variable increases, the other decreases.

Nominal/categorical. See under levels of measurement. Using the nominal level of measurement allows you to allocate your measure into a named category only, such as male or female, professional or working class. The data are in no particular order and implications/judgements cannot be made about their size or value.

Non-parametric. Describes statistical techniques that are not dependent on the normal distribution curve. They are used to test differences in data derived from samples that are not assumed to be from normally distributed populations. The data have usually been measured on nominal or ordinal scales.

Non-random sampling. Also known as non-probability sampling, this occurs when a non-probability procedure is used for selecting a sample. The likelihood of bias is quite high. Such samples are known as non-random or non-probability samples. See also convenience, opportunistic, purposive and snowballing.

Nonmaleficence. The notion of nonmaleficence, is defined as the duty of not inflicting harm.

Normal distribution. A distribution with the following properties: (1) symmetrical; (2) bell-shaped; (3) its mean, median and mode fall in the same place on the curve; (4) the two tails never actually touch the horizontal axis.

Null hypothesis. Mathematicians believe that it is far better to state the hypothesis in terms of there is *no chance*, there is *no relationship*, there is *no improvement* and then to prove that this hypothesis, now called a null hypothesis, falls down. A null hypothesis is also know as a statistical hypothesis of no difference.

Objective. Quantitative research approaches require researchers to be objective and maintain objectivity during their study. They must be impartial and unbiased when carrying out the research and avoid including their personal views and interpretation of what is occurring. See also bias, quantitative research.

Observation. In order to collect data in experimental research, a means of obtaining, recording and quantifying the data is needed. This is achieved through observation and measurement. Careful observation using one's senses is required to allow accurate measurements to be performed.

Ontology. The assumptions that describe reality are known as ontology.

Operationalization/operational definition/operationalizing. Operationalization means that researchers devise indicators of abstract concepts (such as social class, quality of care) so that they can be observed and measured in the field using a variety of methods. See also concept, construct and reductionist.

Opportunistic sample. A sample in which participants are selected according to the quality of their relationship and their willingness and ability to act as informants. An example of non-probability sampling.

Ordinal. See under levels of measurement. In the case of ordinal measurement, data can be put into discrete categories, ordered and ranked as illustrated by six-point postoperative pain scales which range from 'excruciating' to 'no pain'. The intervals between points, however, do not have the same value.

Paradigm. A paradigm is a world-view based on a set of assumptions and values and shared by a particular research community. Methodologies and approaches are informed by these paradigms. A variety of research methods can be used irrespective of paradigm.

Parametric. Describes statistical techniques that are dependent on the normal distribution curve. They are used to test for significant differences in data derived from samples assumed to be drawn from normally distributed populations whose parameters (e.g. mean, median, standard deviation) of different characteristics can be estimated. The data have usually been measured on an interval or ratio scale.

Pearson product-moment correlation coefficient. A measure of the strength of the relationship between variables, each of which must be measured on an interval or ratio scale. See also coefficient.

Phenomenology. A complex research approach which uses rigorous and effective research methods to collect and analyse rich data to illustrate another person's world. Phenomenology was developed by Husserl (1859–1938) and Heidegger (1889–1976).

Phenomenon/phenomena. Anything that is apparent to the senses or directly observed. It is used to describe the human lived experience of a particular aspect of life.

Philosophy. Leddy & Pepper (1993), two American nurse academics, define philosophy as 'a science that comprises logic, ethics, aesthetics, metaphysics and the theory of knowledge'. It is popularly regarded as the pursuit of wisdom and knowledge.

Pie chart. In a pie chart the 'pie' is divided into slices, the size of which represents the frequency distribution of the data. The size of the slice is proportional to the middle angle of the slice; the total angle for the complete pie is 360°.

Positive correlation. Means that variables vary with each other in such a way that high scores on one variable tend to be associated with high scores on the other and low score with low scores, i.e. as one variable increases so also does the other.

Placebo. A drug or treatment which looks identical to the genuine intervention in a clinical trial. It is given to a control group in order to rule out the possibility that a different outcome in the experimental group is due to expectation or belief rather than therapeutic effect.

Positivist paradigm/positivism. The positivist paradigm, also referred to as the positivist philosophy of science, is attributed to the French philosopher Comte (1789–1857). It was refined and developed by the Vienna Circle of scientists in the 1920s and known as logical positivism. Scientists who subscribed to logical positivism believed that the only true knowledge was that gained by the application of logic to data derived from sensory experience. Logical positivism, later referred to as logical empiricism, engendered a new certainty in the power of science to solve human problems. It became synonymous with the scientific method and what 'counted' as knowledge. Positivism is based on the assumption that an independent, objective reality exists based on natural laws and amenable to observation and measurement. Phenomena are reduced to their component parts as a means of understanding the whole. It has influenced the development of medical science, known as biomedicine and nursing. See also biomedicine.

Purposive sample. A sample which includes individuals specifically chosen for their possession of special knowledge or characteristics which are required to increase the researcher's understanding of the phenomena under study. An example of a non-probability or non-random sample.

Qualitative. A general term used to describe particular types of research and their processes. Qualitative research approaches are believed to embody an idealist philosophy, which holds that the world is known through human perceptions and subjectivity; this is seen to be more closely associated with the interpretive and critical paradigms. Qualitative research methods allow for reflection. Key methods include: participant observation, small purposive samples, in-depth interviewing and the use of literary descriptions and analyses. This approach is also referred to as naturalistic.

Quantitative. A general term applied to describe particular types of research and their processes. Quantitative approaches have been closely associated with the positivist paradigm and are taken to represent a realist philosophy, which assumes an independent reality existing independently of perception. Quantitative approaches require researchers to be objective in their approach to the research. Traditionally the methods used in quantitative research have been viewed as a scientifically superior means of data collection, useful for theory testing and the development of law-like generalizations. Quantitative methods include hypothesis testing, measurement and observation, experiments, statistics, numbers, visual presentations in tables and graphs. Quantitative research is also viewed as being reductionist. See also objective, reductionist.

Random sample. A sample in which probability sampling ensures that all members of the population have an equal chance of selection. It should contain individuals with characteristics similar to the population as a whole, i.e. they should be representative. See also sampling.

Randomization. In experiments, clinical trials or any type of controlled intervention, subjects are assigned to a control or experimental group by using a randomization procedure. This requires the researcher to use a table of random numbers or to toss a coin to assign them to their groups. Randomization ensures that the two groups have similar characteristics and are therefore not significantly different in factors such as age, sex, mobility, work or smoking status.

Randomized controlled trial. Randomized controlled trials (RCTs) are a type of experimental research that have become increasingly popular within clinical practice and as such offer a means of replication and generalizability. As with any 'true' experiment this method must demonstrate a means of exerting control over the research situation, manipulation of independent variable(s) and random allocation of clients between the control and experimental groups.

Range. The simplest measure of spread. The range is the difference between the highest and lowest scores in a set of data.

Ratio. See under levels of measurement. The ratio level of measurement differs from the interval level of measurement in that zero has an absolute value on the scale. For the purpose of statistical work, the interval and ratio levels of measurement can be put together in one category and treated the same.

Reductionist. A term used to describe quantitative research because systems are 'reduced' to their component parts for the purposes of the study. For example, the venous ulcer study reproduced in the appendix 'reduced' patients' assessment of their experience of wound dressings in terms of pain, quality of life, comfort and convenience to measures on a scale for each of these abstract concepts.

Reflexivity. Together with indexicality is central to the ethnomethodological approach. Reflexivity of accounts refers to the process whereby our knowledge of our social world explains and is explained at one and the same time. See also social constructionist perspective.

Relativism. Relativism argues that all knowledge is bound by culture and theoretical and/or historical contexts. Thus ethnomethodology's account is just another way of describing the world and is therefore no more or less valid than anybody else's view. This is referred to as the infinite regress of 'relativism' by which we cannot accept anything as 'real'.

Reliability/reliable. Reliability is concerned with consistency and replicability, i.e. that the research methods being used will always give the same answers over time, across groups and by whoever is administering them. Within this broad definition two types of reliability can be identified: 'internal' reliability which refers to the internal consistency of a measure; and 'external' reliability which refers to applying the measure to a variety of settings and groups.

Replication/replicated. The overall design of research is important to enable other researchers to replicate an experiment. Replication of a study allows the results of the original to be verified and it also allows results to be obtained from different settings.

Representativeness. This is required to fulfil one of the main aims of quantitative research approaches, which is to generalize from the findings. One of the ways to do this is to ensure that the samples selected for the research are representative of the population as a whole by using probability sampling. See also sampling.

Sample. A group selected for study from a larger population using a variety of sampling procedures which depend on the type of research approach.

Sampling. A procedure for selecting a sample from the designated study population. The two main types are: probability and non-probability sampling. Probability sampling is the procedure of choice to ensure representativeness. This requires the researcher to have access to a list of the entire population from whom the sample will be drawn. Probability sampling reduces the risk of selecting a biased sample.

Scatter graph. A quick visual way to analyse the possibility of a relationship between variables is to plot the two sets of data on a scatter graph with one variable along the horizontal axis and the other along the vertical axis.

Second degree construct. See under construct.

Snowballing. Identification of a small number of individuals with required characteristics who are then used as informants to identify others for inclusion in the study. In turn, these informants are used to identify further participants until sufficient numbers are reached. An example of non-probability sampling. See also sampling.

Social constructionist perspective. Views the individual as the builder of perceptions that are strongly culturally influenced and fits comfortably with the view that situations are both indexical and reflexive. See also indexicality and reflexivity.

Spearman's correlation coefficient. A non-parametric statistical test used to assess the degree of association between variables. It is used to test observed differences between groups of data in which a normal distribution is not assumed, or which have not been assessed using an interval scale. See also correlation coefficient.

Spread. See under range and variability.

Standard deviation. The square root of the variance. The formula is given on page 95. However, in most cases a button on your calculator or a command on a computer can be used to calculate it.

Structured interview. An interview conducted with set questions which have a predetermined range of possible replies.

Study design. Refers to all aspects of the study, including sampling procedures, study size, methods of allocating subjects to experimental and control groups, statistical techniques and outcome measures.

Theory. A theory highlights and explains something by providing a set of explanatory concepts to answer a 'Why?' question. It is often provisional and subject to reformulation and revision at any time. A theory can also provide predictions.

Transferability. Transferability is the equivalent of external validity in quantitative research. It may also be referred to as 'applicability'. A study is judged to be transferable if the findings are able to 'fit' into contexts outside the study situation, i.e. it is judged on the 'fittingness' of the findings. To transfer the findings elsewhere, the reader needs to have enough information to be able to assess whether the research context in which the study took place is applicable to other settings.

Triangulation. A strategy which draws on a variety of data sources, methods, theories and researchers to study a phenomenon. It provides different perspectives on the same phenomenon. The term is geographical or nautical in origin, meaning to ascertain one's position by comparing it to more than one other known location.

Trustworthiness. This term is used to assess the 'truth value' of qualitative research. It suggests that the research has been conducted in such a way as to give the reader confidence in the findings. Trustworthiness can be judged on three criteria; see under credibility, transferability and dependability.

Typifications. Ethnomethodologists define 'typifications' as 'recipes for action that exist in the culture as a whole'. Take the example of 'the ward round'. How do you describe a 'typical' ward round? Your descriptions or 'typifications' may include behaviours that are taken for granted, such as the nurse or junior doctor pushing the notes trolley behind the consultant.

Univariate statistics. Describes the world in terms of one variable at a time. The three main statistics describe the frequency and distribution of a variable as rates (proportions—percentages); levels (central tendency—the mean, mode and median) and variability (dispersions, standard deviation and variance). See also descriptive statistics.

Unstructured interview. An interview that allows for spontaneity and freedom of response.

Utilitarianism. There are two generally accepted ethical theories in western society: utilitarianism and deontology. The utilitarian viewpoint considers that the end justifies the means, suggesting that an action is justified if it produces the greatest good (and also happiness) for the greatest number.

Validity/valid/face and content validity. Validity refers to the extent to which a test, questionnaire or other operationalization is really measuring what the researcher intends to measure. In other words, validity is defined as the extent to which a research method or technique actually measures what it purports to. Textbooks list a number of different ways of assessing validity. These include face validity and content validity. Their labels give some sense of what criteria are being used to judge the validity of methods and techniques. For example, 'face validity' suggests that the researcher judges at 'face value' that a measure is actually measuring what it says it is. Content validity is similar to face validity but more extensive. The researcher may ask colleagues who are experts in the topic area to give their opinions on the validity of the measure. There are other types of validity known as criterion and construct validity.

Validity criteria apply to the internal consistency of a study in relation to the measures taken by the researcher to ensure that data collection instruments are valid as a prerequisite for yielding valid findings. Such studies are said to have internal validity. External validity relates to whether the research findings are generalizable beyond the immediate study sample and settings.

Qualitative researchers seek alternative ways of defining validity and reliability; see under trustworthiness, credibility, transferability and dependability.

Variable. Any characteristic, factor or trait under study. The factors that are being investigated are known as the variables.

Variability. See under measure of variance.

Variance. The mean square deviation. To calculate the variance you calculate the deviation of each value (X) from the mean (μ) and find the mean of the sum of the squares of the deviations ($\Sigma(X - \mu)^2 / N$).

Variation. The stage following the calculation of the range. To calculate the variation you take the mean of a set of data (μ) as the central score and calculate how much each score (X) varies or deviates from the central score ($X - \mu$). Since values of $X - \mu$ above and below the mean will cancel each other out if they are added together, a measure called absolute variation is used.

In the calculation of absolute variation we avoid the problem of negative and positive deviations cancelling each other out by the process of ignoring the minus sign and treat all deviations as positive. In mathematical terms we calculate $|X - \mu|$.

REFERENCES

Beauchamp T, Childress J 1989 Principles of biomedical ethics, 3rd edn. Oxford University Press, New York

Garfinkel H 1967 Studies in ethnomethodology. Prentice-Hall, New Jersey

Leddy S, Pepper J M 1993 Conceptual bases of professional nursing, 3rd edn. J B Lippincott, Philadelphia

Sandelowski M 1986 The problem of rigor in qualitative research. Advances in Nursing Science 8(3): 27–37

Schutz A 1972 The phenomenology of the social world. Heinemann, London

The following texts have been drawn upon in compiling this glossary:

Jupp V, Miller P for The Course Team 1979 Glossary, research methods in education and the social sciences (DE304 G). Open University, Milton Keynes

Smith P for the Course Team 1996 Research methodology (MIM61U) study guide. Royal College of Nursing, London, especially Addendum to Unit 1, Unit 2 and Unit 6

Appendices

The dressing makes the difference: trial of two modern dressings on venous ulcers

Appendix

1

Barbara A. Smith RGN

Clinical Nurse Specialist in Dermatology, Bradford Royal Infirmary

Reproduced with permission from Professional Nurse (1994) 9(5): 348–352.

Despite the plethora of modern dressings available for leg ulcers, and the huge financial and social cost of inappropriately treated ulcers, many are still left virtually untreated. This comparison of two modern dressings illustrates the benefits of using appropriate dressings.

KEY POINTS

1. **The choice of modern wound dressings should suit both the needs of the patient and the practitioner.**
2. **Occlusion can aid pain relief.**
3. **Participation in a clinical trial serves to motivate nursing staff and cultivate an interest in wound care.**
4. **Modern dressings can have a positive effect on even long-term ulceration.**

Chronic venous leg ulceration remains a distressing and depressing problem for sufferers and a substantial drain on nursing time and resources—particularly within the community. Remarkable improvement can be achieved in individual cases, however, by a relatively short period of good and carefully monitored wound care, using high quality dressing material. There is not a great deal of scientific evidence available to allow those involved in wound care to decide which of the many modern dressings best suits their needs and those of their patients; this article describes a trial which was intended to increase that body of knowledge. It was an open, randomised, parallel group trial to compare the performance, convenience and cost-effectiveness of two such dressings—an alginate and a hydrocolloid (Improved Granulation Granuflex) in the treatment of patients with chronic venous leg ulcers. For the purposes of this article, Improved Granulation Granuflex is referred to as 'Granuflex'.

MODERN DRESSINGS

Turner (1979) proposed that an ideal dressing should fulfil eight functions (Table 1), and manufacturers of modern dressings have generally followed these proposals, although there is currently no product which meets all eight criteria. The manufacturers' claims for the two products compared in this trial were, at the time of the trial, as follows:

Table 1 Properties of the ideal wound dressing (Turner 1979)
1. Allow excess exudate removal from the wound surface.
2. Maintain a moist micro-environment at the wound/dressing interface.
3. Allow its removal from the wound surface without causing trauma to newly formed granulation tissue and capillary buds.
4. Be impermeable to micro-organisms.
5. Be free from contamination.
6. Not shed fibres into the wound.
7. Allow gaseous exchange and act as a semipermeable membrane.
8. Provide thermal insulation.

Alginate dressings have the capacity to absorb a considerable amount of wound fluid. A soft gel is formed as a result of ionic exchange between dressing and exudate, keeping the wound moist. Alginate dressings are supplied in a sterile pack and do not constitute a barrier to fluid, gases or bacteria. It is necessary, therefore, to apply a secondary dressing [such as the gauze used in this study] over them in addition to compression bandaging as required. The patient cannot take a bath under these circumstances with the dressing in place. However, occlusive dressings may be used later in the healing process when exudate levels have reduced, permitting the patient to bathe.

Granuflex is a modified form of the standard Granuflex dressing, with improved capacity to contain wound fluid. Each dressing consists of a hydrocolloid matrix backed with semi-open cell polyurethane foam and impermeable polyurethane film. A gel is formed by interaction between the hydrocolloid layer and wound exudate which keeps the wound moist. Each dressing is supplied in a sterile pack and the polyurethane film is impermeable to fluid, gases and bacteria. It is thought that this impermeability to gas exchange leads to an increase in acidity of the wound surface which is bacteriostatic (Varghese et al 1986). No additional dressing is necessary and compression bandaging as advised. Patients are able to take a bath with the dressing in place. The trial examined these properties as well as such practical points as convenience and cost.

METHOD

Consenting adult patients with a venous leg ulcer of greater than 2.5 cm diameter were recruited to the trial, which was conducted in the Department of Dermatology at Bradford Royal Infirmary. Patients were excluded from the trial if they had any condition which might affect wound healing (including infection, immune deficiency, treatment with steroids, malignant disease), if the ulcer was not clearly venous in origin, if they were receiving systemic treatment which might affect ulcer healing (fibrinolytic or anticoagulant therapy) or if it was thought they would be better treated in another way.

Eligible patients were allocated randomly to treatment with either the alginate or Granuflex. Wounds were cleaned with physiological saline and dressings were applied according to the manufacturers' instructions with compression bandaging in each case. Patients reattended the dermatology clinic for dressing whenever necessary and a costing sheet was completed at each dressing change, listing all materials used, to allow a total approximate materials cost to be calculated. Trial dressings were to continue for six weeks unless the ulcer healed before this time. The degree of pain suffered by the patient over the previous two weeks was assessed at the beginning of the trial, then at two, four and six weeks, using a visual analogue scale from 0 = no pain to 10 = the worst possible pain. The following factors were assessed after two, four and six weeks: disturbance of sleep due to ulcer pain (often, sometimes, rarely or never), pain during dressing change (visual analogue scale as before), change in quality of life over the previous two weeks (deteriorated markedly, deteriorated somewhat, no change, improved somewhat or improved markedly), frequency of dressing changes per week (mean over two weeks) and convenience at dressing changes (visual analogue scale from 0 = least convenient to 10 = most convenient). A final assessment of dressing performance was made for each patient in terms of ability to contain exudate, wear time, patient comfort, positive effect on healing, ease of application and ease of removal using a six-point scale (excellent, very good, good, fair, poor, awful). Subjective comments from nurses and patients were also solicited.

An acetate tracing of the ulcer was made on the first and last day of the trial and the ulcer area was calculated in each case using an image analyser. Statistical analysis was carried out on results from patients who completed the trial, using the Wilcoxon Rank Sum test, Kruskal–Wallis test or Fischer's exact test as appropriate. All adverse events were recorded, including severe pain and suspected infection of the ulcer. Patients could be withdrawn from the trial at any time.

RESULTS

A total of 40 patients entered the trial; 18 were randomised to the alginate and 22 to Granuflex. Twelve patients were withdrawn before completion, six on the alginate and six on Granuflex; reasons for withdrawal are shown in Table 2. In addition, two adverse events were recorded on Granuflex which were not thought to warrant withdrawal—one case of wound infection and one of pain and erythema at the final trial visit. There were no statistically significant differences between treatment groups in terms of sex, age, mobility, work or smoking status for those patients completing the trial. The mean ulcer area at enrolment was considerably larger in the Granuflex group (22.17 cm²) than the alginate group (12.74 cm²).

Table 2 Reasons for withdrawal from the trial

Reason	Granuflex	Alginate
Adverse events		
Pain	1	4
Ulcer infection	1	2
Possible allergy	1	0
Other causes		
Dressing leakage	1	0
Misdiagnosis	1	0
Subject default	1	0

The mean score for pain experienced due to the ulcer over the previous two weeks fell from 4.86 on enrolment to 2.15 after six weeks in those patients treated with the alginate, and from 4.74 to 1.46 in those on Granuflex. There was no statistically significant difference between dressings in this result, but four patients withdrew from the alginate treatment due to pain, compared to only one on Granuflex.

Disturbance of sleep due to ulcer pain was not assessed on enrolment, but the proportion of patients reporting no sleep disturbance increased from 8.3% at two weeks to 40% at six weeks on the alginate and from 31.25 to 78.6% on Granuflex. The difference between treatment groups in this assessment approached statistical significance ($P = 0.0721$). There was little change from week two to week six in the degree of pain experienced at dressing changes in either treatment group, and the mean pain score at week six was low in both cases (2.16 alginate; 1.73 Granuflex). Quality of life was reported to have improved remarkably after six weeks treatment with both dressings (in 40.0% of patients on alginate and 42.9% on Granuflex).

It was found necessary to use either one or two alginate dressings and between one and three Granuflex dressings per week. The mean of the dresser's scores of the convenience of the dressing at changes was 7.03 for the alginate and 9.31 for Granuflex, but there was again no statistically significant difference between groups.

On final evaluation, the alginate and Granuflex were found to be equivalent in terms of wear time and patient comfort; the alginate was slightly superior in terms of ability to contain exudate, and Granuflex was slightly superior in terms of positive effect on healing and ease of application. Granuflex was statistically significantly superior in terms of ease of removal of the dressing ($P < 0.001$)—the alginate dressings often needed to be soaked off the ulcer.

Ulcers healed completely in six of the 40 patients during the six weeks of trial treatment, two using the alginate and four using Granuflex. Since the mean ulcer size at enrolment was considerably higher in the Granuflex group, the effect of treatment was expressed as percentage change in size from enrolment of final visit. There was a 34.9% decrease in mean ulcer area after the alginate and a 57.1% decrease after Granuflex, but no statistically significant difference between groups. The mean total approximate cost of materials to achieve this improvement was £364.08 for the alginate and £431.73 for Granuflex.

DISCUSSION

This trial compared two types of modern wound dressing—one an alginate and one a hydrocolloid—directly in terms of performance and convenience and indirectly in terms of Turner's criteria for an 'ideal' wound dressing listed above. Table 3 highlights the respects in which the alginate and Granuflex were found to differ. From the patients' point of view, both dressings brought about a decrease in the degree of ulcer pain suffered; there was slightly less pain reported after six weeks by those in the Granuflex group, and considerably less sleep disturbance due to their ulcer. It has been suggested that exclusion of oxygen from a wound, as

Table 3 Summary of differences between dressings after six weeks

Assessment	Alginate	Granuflex
Pain suffered from ulcer*	2.15	1.46
No sleep disturbance	40.0%	78.6%
Pain during dressing change*	2.16	1.73
Convenience on dressing change*	2.97	0.69
Decrease in ulcer area	34.9%	57.0%
Excellent ease of removal	8.3%	56.3%
Approximate materials cost	£364.08	£431.73

(* scale 0–10 where the higher score is worse)

brought about by Granuflex, may be a factor in rapid alleviation of pain (Silver 1985). In this study the difference in the degree of pain experienced may also have been associated with the degree of wound hydration. The larger wounds in the Granuflex group may have been more heavily exuding and hence remained more moist than the smaller wounds in the alginate group.

From the dressers' point of view, Granuflex was judged to be somewhat more convenient to use, since an additional dressing is not required. It was also significantly easier to remove from the wound—the alginate often needed to be soaked off. The cost of materials involved in treatment with Granuflex was greater than that for the alginate, but no account was made in the cost calculation of the amount of nursing time spent, nor of the potentially shorter healing time.

Twice as many ulcers healed completely after Granuflex as after the alginate, and the percentage reduction in ulcer area was considerably higher after Granuflex, despite the fact that mean ulcer area on enrolment was almost double that in the alginate group. The better healing rate with Granuflex may have been partly due to ease of removal; since newly formed granulation tissue and capillary buds are not damaged. The difference between treatment groups in ease of removal could be explained, as above, by a difference in the amount of wound exudate in the two groups. The wounds in the alginate group may have become dehydrated, resulting in dressing adherence and a reduced healing rate. The degree of hydration of the alginate dressing has been shown to affect the consequent healing rate (Barnett and Varley 1987). Porter (1991) suggests that alginates are particularly suited to dressing heavily exuding wounds, and Thomas (1990) states that alginates need to be occluded over lightly exuding wounds to enable complete hydration of the dressing.

Clinical observations of the team conducting the trial suggest that larger wounds tend to produce more exudate than do smaller ones; those observed in this trial tended to be lightly to moderately exuding, which was to be expected from their size. It is possible that the alginate dressing group might have performed better if their wounds had been larger and more exuding, but at the same time this might have increased the frequency of dressing change, so increasing the material cost.

Both nurses and patients were delighted by the marked improvement in some cases where venous ulceration had been a long-term and intractable problem. The level of interest and motivation of nurses caring for these patients was increased by the evidence that carefully controlled and rigorous trial treatment brought about noticeable improvement in ulcer healing and patients' quality of life.

Despite the fact that Granuflex was found to be substantially better than the alginate in terms of reduced sleep disturbance and decrease in ulcer area, the only statistically significant superiority was in ease of removal. This is likely to be because the sample size was too small: the subjective opinion of the team conducting the trial was that Granuflex was the better dressing because of more rapid healing rates and ease of use, even over awkward sites such as the ankle.

Referring back to the 'ideal' qualities of a wound dressing described previously, both dressings removed excess exudate from the wound surface, maintained a moist micro-environment, were free from contamination and provided thermal insulation. Neither shed fibres, as such, but the alginate was often difficult to remove from the wound surface. The fact that Granuflex is impermeable to gases and micro-organisms, while the alginate is not, did not seem to greatly affect infection rates in this study: two patients in each group developed wound infection.

CONCLUSION

This study demonstrated that remarkable improvement in rate of healing and patients' quality of life can be achieved by means of intensive and carefully controlled use of modern wound dressings.

In the wounds studied, a significant difference was found between alginate and Granuflex, in that the latter was easier to remove from wounds at dressing changes. Granuflex was also found to be superior in terms of pain relief, convenience of use and healing rates. The subjective conclusion was that Improved Formulation Granuflex was the preferable dressing and it is likely that increased healing rates and decreased nursing time taken at dressing changes counteract the somewhat higher material costs for this product.

This trial was supported by ConvaTec Ltd.

REFERENCES

Barnett, S.E. and Varley, S.J. (1987) The effects of calcium alginate on wound healing. *Ann Royal Coll Surgeons Eng*, **69**, 153–55.

Porter, J.M. (1991) A comparative investigation of re-epithelialisation of split skin graft donor areas after application of hydrocolloid and alginate dressings. *B.J. Plastic Surgery*, **44**, 333–37.

Silver, I.A. (1985) Oxygen and tissue repair. *Royal Society of Medicine International Congress and Symposium Series*, **88**, 15–19.

Thomas, S. (1990) Alginates in wound management. In: Wound Management and Dressings. Pharmaceutical Press, London.

Turner, T.D. (1979) Hospital usage of absorbent dressings. *Pharm. J.*, **222**, 421–22.

Varghese, M.C. *et al* (1986) Local environment of chronic wounds under synthetic dressings. *Arch Dermatol*, **122**, 52–57.

Helping people to stop smoking: a study of the nurse's role

Appendix

2

Jill Macleod Clark BSc PhD RGN

Senior Lecturer

Sheila Haverty BA RGN

Project Officer, Department of Nursing Studies, King's College, London

Sally Kendall BSc RGN RHV

Lecturer in Nursing, Buckinghamshire College of Higher Education, Chalfont St Giles

Reproduced with permission from Journal of Advanced Nursing (1990) 16: 357–363.

Accepted for publication 1 March 1989

Helping people to stop smoking: a study of the nurse's role

Sixteen trained nurses from various clinical backgrounds participated in a project designed to describe the process and assess the outcome of their attempts to help a range of patients and clients to stop smoking. A case-study approach was employed and the nurses initiated 68 health education interventions related to smoking cessation. All interventions were tape-recorded and data on patients' and clients' characteristics, smoking history, health beliefs and motivation to give up smoking were also collected. Forty-two patients were followed up 1 year post-intervention. Data collected at this time revealed that 17% had successfully given up smoking, while a further 12% had substantially reduced their cigarette consumption. These findings compare very favourably with those of previous studies in which general practitioners have attempted to help patients stop smoking. The results of the research reported here therefore suggest that nurses have enormous potential for fulfilling a highly effective health education function.

INTRODUCTION

Smoking continues to be the largest cause of preventable disease in the United Kingdom (UK). One in four of all smokers will die from a smoking-related disease such as lung cancer, heart disease or chronic obstructive lung disease (Doll & Peto 1981). Currently, an average of 33% (about 18 million) of the population of the UK smoke. Although smoking rates among men have been declining over the past 20 years, the decline in smoking among women has been neither fast nor continuous. Young people, especially women, continue to take up smoking, and 25% of adolescents will smoke by the time they leave school (Murray et al 1983). Smoking prevalence continues to be higher among manual workers than non-manual groups (Office of Population Censuses and Surveys 1988).

Attention is often drawn to the high numbers of nurses who smoke, and there is concern that as health professionals, nurses should be aiming to substantially reduce their smoking rates. A review of recent research studies (Haverty et al 1986) found that, taken as a whole, nurses are no more likely to smoke than the rest of the female population. Moreover, the studies showed that there are variations in smoking rates when looking at specific categories of nurse. Smoking patterns appear to be broadly similar to those in the general population, with nurses with higher professional status and responsibility, such as ward sisters and health visitors, smoking less than other groups, such as pupil nurses and auxiliaries.

It is estimated that two-thirds of the 18 million current smokers in the UK want to stop smoking and will have made one or more unsuccessful attempts to do so. There are several smoking cessation strategies and approaches available, as well as a range of mass media approaches, but there is an overall need to develop appropriate smoking cessation strategies which will reach the social groups most resistant to current measures. The range of smoking cessation methods has been comprehensively reviewed by Schwartz (1987), and the discussion here will be limited to the strategy which has most bearing on this study.

The Minimal Intervention Approach

The Minimal Intervention Approach (MIA) was developed by Russell et al (1979) in order to enable general practitioners to give smoking prevention education to patients within normal consultation time. It is based on a simple routine of the general practitioner giving advice to smokers, giving them a leaflet, and warning the smoker that there would be a follow-up to monitor change in smoking behaviour. Jamrozik et al (1984) added the use of a measurement of expired-air carbon monoxide to the MIA protocol. Fowler (1983) summarized the role of the primary care practitioner with a seven-point approach, and suggested that such an approach can be used by all members of the primary health care team, within the normal course of their work. The prescription of nicotine chewing gum was available as a supplement to the intervention. A later study by Russell et al (1987) has also suggested that a brief intervention can be effective although as Goldstein & Niaura (1988) have noted there was no description of the actual process and content of each intervention.

Success rates in terms of smoking cessation using this approach vary from 5% (Russell et al 1979) to 15% (Jamrozik et al 1984). To date very little research has been undertaken to explore the effects of nurses fulfilling a health education role in relation to smoking cessation, although a few studies have pointed to the potential value of nurses taking such a role. For example, a study conducted by Burt et al (1974) yielded a 62% cessation rate among patients following myocardial infarction who were visited at home by health visitors. A large community project in North Karelia, Finland, involving nurses is reported to have reduced smoking prevalence from 52% in 1972 to 38% in 1982 (Vartianen et al 1986). However, although nurses were involved in this project, little is known of their specific impact.

Other evidence suggests that, although nurses feel very positively about their health education role (Syred 1981), they are also aware of their limitations and lack of appropriate training in terms of both knowledge and skills (Macleod Clark et al 1985). In the context of these findings the study reported here was therefore designed to explore in detail the process and outcome of nurses' interventions in relation to smoking cessation, and thus broaden the approach taken in the studies described above.

THE STUDY

A training programme consisting of two 1-day workshops was developed. This built on trained nurses' existing abilities and aimed to equip them with the additional knowledge and skills they would need to undertake an effective health education role in relation to smoking cessation. Twenty nurses were recruited to the programme, all of whom had expressed an interest in helping smokers to give up the habit. They included hospital nurses, health visitors and midwives. The teaching input was spread over 2 study days, the main aims of which were to provide a sound knowledge background on which nurses could base their health education input related to smoking cessation, to suggest a framework around which nurses could base their interventions and to help nurses develop the communication skills required to be effective health educators.

The first study day essentially consisted of lectures on the physiological and pathological effects of smoking, statistics and cessation strategies. Each session was followed by discussion. There was also some debate about the usefulness of theories and models of health education, and feelings about non-smoking policies in health service premises were explored.

There was a 2-week gap between the 2 study days and during this period the nurses were asked to audio-record themselves talking to someone who wanted to give up smoking. The aim was to provide baseline data on a health education intervention before any skills training had been given. The second study day was concerned with the framework for health education and developing the participants' communication skills.

THE FRAMEWORK

The research team felt strongly that nurses need a framework on which to base their health education interventions and this was supported by findings from researchers such as Syred (1981). The framework (Table 1) was devised by the researchers and was based partly on the health belief model (Becker 1974) and partly on the nursing process. It was felt to be important that the nursing process was used as a basis as nurses are already familiar with its principles and an *individualized* approach is essential to effective health education. Putting the framework shown in Table 1 into action demands certain communication skills from nurses. These skills were first explored in theory and then in practice using role-play and analysis of the baseline tapes. Although the importance of non-verbal skills was acknowledged, verbal skills were the focus of the training. The particular skills needed to carry out each stage of the framework were identified and practised.

The nurses analysed their own tape-recorded 'baseline' interventions, identifying the positive use of skills and also where communication was not effective. Not surprisingly, at this stage there were many examples of

Table 1 Framework for health education

Assessment
Assess the smoker in terms of motivation to give up, health beliefs and fears or worries about continuing to smoke or giving up. Information should relate to the individual's health beliefs.

Planning
Plan a course of action to stop smoking *with* the smoker not *for* him/her. Utilize knowledge of cessation techniques and outside agencies, such as smokers' clinics, constructively. Suggest coping strategies.

Implementation
Client attempts to implement plan: nurse's role is one of support and encouragement. The nurse can act as referral agent if continued support is impractical.

Evaluation
Evaluate intervention in terms of client attitude and behaviour and your own approach. If plan has failed, look at where it went wrong and start again. Reinforce positive changes in smoking behaviour.

ineffective communication in the baseline interventions. These included an inability to listen, the use of more closed or leading questions than open questions and a lack of structure within the interventions.

DATA COLLECTION

Ethical approval to undertake the study was obtained from the three health authorities in which patients and clients would be approached. Following the 2 study days the nurses were asked to talk to up to five of their patients or clients about giving up smoking. A tape-recording was made of each intervention and data were collected from all the patients and clients involved. The informed consent of these patients and clients was obtained at the outset.

A total of 16 of the 20 nurses who had attended the study days completed one or more intervention (Table 2). The interventions took place either in the nurse's place of work or, in the case of the health visitors, in the client's home. The nurses were asked to identify patients/clients on the basis of the following criteria: they smoked regularly, they were motivated to give up smoking, and they were aged between 16 and 60.

Data were collected from a total of 68 patients and clients and the researchers used radio microphones linked to a portable cassette recorder to record each intervention. This was found to be less intimidating for the nurses, patients and clients, and less intrusive as the researcher did not need to be present during the intervention.

Table 2 Nurses in study who carried out one or more interventions

	n
Ward nurses	3
Health visitors	7
Midwives	6

Table 3 Data collected

A. Demographic data from patients and clients
B. Patients' and clients' smoking history
C. Patients' and clients' motivation to stop smoking
D. Patients' and clients' beliefs and worries related to smoking and giving up smoking
E. Expired carbon monoxide measurements
F. Outcomes of interventions in terms of change in smoking behaviour, motivation, beliefs and worries at 6 months and 1 year follow-ups
G. Analysis of audio-tape recorded interventions
H. Relationship between process of health education interventions and outcomes
I. Patients' and clients' perceptions of nurses' interventions
J. Nurses' perceptions of their involvement in study days and project

Each patient/client was asked to read and sign a consent form explaining the study, and complete a checklist which was aimed at assessing their level of motivation and determination to stop smoking, worries about the health consequences of continuing to smoke, and their feelings about the implications of stopping smoking for their health. Their level of carbon monoxide (in expired air) was also measured using a 'Bedfont' carbon monoxide monitor. This was intended as a health education tool (Jamrozik et al 1984), and also for use as a validation measure of smoking cessation at follow-up.

At 1-year follow-up a measurement of urinary cotinine was taken from all patients and clients who claimed to have stopped smoking to validate such claims. Patients and clients were followed-up at 6 months and 1 year, to collect data on any change in smoking behaviour, or motivation change. Data were also collected on their recollections and perceptions of the nurse's intervention (Table 3).

Data from the study were analysed using SPSS (Nie et al 1975). The tape-recordings of the nurses' health education interventions were meticulously transcribed for detailed analysis of the process of the interviews.

FINDINGS

A comprehensive account of the analysis and findings can be found in the Project Report (Macleod Clark et al 1987). A brief summary of some of the results is presented here. Of the 68 patients and clients in the study, 54 (80%) were followed-up at 6 months and 42 (62%) of these respondents were followed-up 1 year after the interventions. Those not followed-up could not be contacted due to moving away, and moving abroad, and two were unwilling to continue in the study for personal reasons.

Analysis of data obtained from the patient/client data form completed by all participants showed that the sample of patients and clients were from a wide range of backgrounds with an age range of 16–76 years, the majority (72%) being between 21 and 40 years old. A total of 61 (90%) of the sample were female. The majority (41%) of the sample were in social class 3 with 25% being in social class 4 and 19% in social class 2 (as defined by the Registrar General's Classification of Occupations, OPCS 1970).

All patients and clients were 'smokers' and had agreed to discuss smoking with the nurse. With regard to smoking history, 34% of the sample had smoked for 10 years or less, 34% for 11–20 years, and 12% had smoked for between 21 and 30 years. Expired-air carbon monoxide measurements taken from each patient/client at intervention showed that all were smokers, with readings ranging from 12 to 56 parts per million. Variations in the readings reflected the number of cigarettes smoked, and the amount of time between the last cigarette and the carbon monoxide measurement.

Beliefs and worries about smoking

Patients and clients were questioned in some detail about their beliefs and worries about smoking, if they continued to smoke. The most common worries expressed were in the areas shown in Table 4.

These findings were interesting in that people were less worried about heart disease than about breathlessness or lung cancer. The high percentage who were worried about the effects of smoking on their babies reflected the fact that some of the sample were pregnant at the time of intervention and/or had young children. Patients and clients were also asked about what might happen if they managed to give up smoking. As might be predicted, there were both positive and negative reactions. The majority (81.4%) felt that they would feel a sense of achievement, and would feel physically fitter (76.9%). At the same time over two-thirds were concerned that they might put on weight (70.3%) and feel irritable (66.6%). Some of the negative reactions may well have been due to previous experience of stopping smoking.

Changes in smoking behaviour

At 1-year follow-up all patients and clients were asked if they had changed their smoking behaviour since the initial interview. As can be seen in Table 5, seven were still non-smokers, five claimed to have cut

Table 4 Beliefs and worries about effects of smoking

		%	n
1	Effects on health of baby	68.5	47
2	Breathlessness	66.7	45
3	Lung cancer	66.6	45
4	Heart disease	59.2	40
5	Effects on health of family	57.4	39

Table 5 Outcomes of nurses' interventions in terms of change in smoking behaviour at 1-year follow-up ($n = 42$)

Smoking behaviour	n	%
Stopped smoking	7	17
Cut down substantially	5	12
Made at least 1 attempt to give up	13	31
No change in behaviour	17	40

down substantially, 13 had made at least one attempt to stop, and 17 had not changed their behaviour in any way.

Expired-air carbon monoxide measurements were repeated and, in order to validate all claims either to have stopped or to have substantially cut down smoking, urine samples were collected for urinary cotinine measurement.

Relationship between motivation fears and worries and changes in smoking behaviour

It was of interest to learn whether there was any relationship between level of motivation to stop smoking and level of concern about the health consequences of continuing to smoke or stop smoking. The Spearman's Correlation Coefficient was applied to the 42 cases who remained in the study for both follow-ups. As may be predicted, there was a highly significant ($P \leq 0.01$) relationship between level of motivation and concern about health consequences, such as breathlessness or bronchitis, and level of motivation and likelihood of feeling a sense of achievement. There were also negative relationships between the desire to stop smoking and concern about resulting feelings of stress.

Cross-tabulations of smoking behaviour at 1 year by the variables of breathlessness, bronchitis, and sense of achievement, indicated that the only factor related to actually stopping smoking was concern about breathlessness but this was not a significant relationship. A high level of confidence in ability to give up smoking was related to successfully stopping ($P \leq 0.03$).

Analysis of tape-recorded interventions

Analysis of the interventions was carried out using a skill-based analysis, closely linked to the health education intervention 'Framework'. The aim of this analysis was firstly to accurately measure the use of the communication skills and the 'Framework' taught in the study days, and assess their use in practice.

The tape-recordings ranged in length from 4 to 45 minutes, but most were between 10 and 20 minutes in length. In 58% of the recordings, nurses talked substantially more than the patients/clients (sometimes twice as much), and exercised considerable 'control' of the conversation. In 21% of the recording the patients/clients talked more, and in the other 21% nurses and patients/clients talked about equally.

Analysis demonstrated that the nurses were generally able to make a detailed assessment of the clients, through their use of open and closed questions about smoking history, daily smoking pattern, and clients' everyday lives. The hospital nurses were less able to do this as they often had only just met the patient/client, whereas the health visitors and midwives often had a more established relationship with their clients. The nurses were able to assess their clients' desire to be healthier, but sometimes did not find out a great deal about their true level of motivation to stop smoking. However, some tape transcripts show clearly that talking with the nurse was influential in raising the client's level of motivation, and this was borne out by the smoking cessation and smoking reduction rates from this study.

The nurses were asked to plan with the patient or client, how to go about stopping smoking. Information about cessation strategies and ways of coping with stopping smoking had been discussed in detail at the first study day. In practice, however, they found this part of the approach quite difficult. One or two clients with strong motivation to stop smoking participated to some extent in working out a cessation strategy. In general, though, the nurses tended to fall back on prescriptive advice, telling the clients what was 'best', not focusing on the client's needs, or allowing the client to think about what would work best for them.

The health visitors and midwives found it easier to offer support and follow-up as they would have the opportunity to see the client again. The hospital nurses found this more difficult, although one of them telephoned the patients a week or so after they had left hospital to see how they were getting on. Clients were not often in practice referred to other agencies— for example a smokers' clinic, or to see a health visitor after leaving hospital.

Relationship between process of health education interventions and outcomes

Very few previous studies to date have attempted to demonstrate any relationship between outcome following an intervention and the process of the intervention. Since in this study audio-tape recordings were collected of every health education intervention as it occurred, it was possible to explore the relationship between interventions and outcomes.

Given the limitations in terms of sample size it is difficult to draw anything but tentative conclusions. However, there did appear to be some relationship between the use of specific skills such as the use of open questions, listening and positive response to cues and successful outcomes in terms of smoking cessation. Moreover, successful interventions were also characterized by clear evidence of patient/client involvement in the planning process and, most markedly, by a high ratio of patient/client talk to nurse talk. In other words, in successful interventions the patient and client fully participated in the interaction. This is clearly an area which requires further investigation.

DISCUSSION

The very positive findings from this study of nurses' attempts to help their patients and clients to give up smoking have important implications for nursing education and practice.

The case study approach taken in this research project enabled us to build a rich and detailed picture of the group of patients and clients involved. The patients and clients in the sample were predominantly female and ranged in age from 16 to 76 and the majority were classified as social economic groups 3 and 4. Most had been smokers for between 10 and 20 years and the majority smoked between 20 and 30 cigarettes a day. In general, they were relatively well informed about the effects of smoking.

Half admitted that they were worried about the effects of smoking on the health of their babies and family and effects of smoking on their own health in terms of breathlessness, lung cancer and heart disease.

When asked to predict their reactions if they were able to give up smoking the majority felt they would enjoy better physical health as a consequence. Just over half anticipated that giving up would result in extra stress. Interestingly, over two-thirds believed that they would put on weight.

These findings have important implications for the way in which nurses may need to tackle the issue of smoking cessation with their clients. Attempts to help people give up smoking are unlikely to be successful unless the individual's very real concerns about the negative effects of cessation are addressed.

Seventeen per cent of the sample who were followed-up after 1 year had successfully given up smoking. These figures compare very well with previous studies carried out in the UK which have primarily concentrated on the general practitioner's influence on smoking cessation. For example, a study by Russell et al (1979) used a minimum intervention approach and achieved a cessation rate of 5%. Later work which included the carbon monoxide monitor as part of the intervention increased the cessation rate to 15% (Jamrozik et al 1984) and to 13% where a supported brief intervention was offered (Russell et al 1987).

In this study of nurses' interventions there was, perhaps predictably, a significant relationship between the patient's or client's confidence and motivation to give up and subsequent success. Again this emphasizes the wisdom of concentrating attempts to help people give up smoking upon those who are truly motivated to succeed. Where individuals are not yet motivated to stop smoking, energies could more profitably be directed towards increasing motivation to stop rather than the stopping process *per se*.

Analysis of the tape-recorded conversations in this study revealed the importance of assessment in health education interactions. With hindsight it is clear that many patients and clients were not really strongly motivated to give up even though, at the outset of the intervention, they had claimed to be so. Using a nursing process framework, accurate assessment could lead to a plan of intervention which would focus either on increased motivation or the facilitation of smoking cessation.

It is important to recognize that success in smoking education interventions need not be judged solely in terms of smoking cessation figures. As was discussed previously many of the patients and clients in the study attempted to change their smoking behaviour subsequent to the nurses' interaction with them. Forty-three per cent of them made at least one serious attempt to give up smoking and a further 12% reduced the amount they smoked substantially. This means that 60% of the sample may have been influenced in some way by the nurses' attempts to help them stop smoking.

These influences were particularly apparent in the health visitors' and midwives' interventions with their clients. Two-thirds of the clients seen by health visitors subsequently changed their behaviour. Four clients gave up smoking and a further 12 reduced their cigarette consumption or made an effort to stop. Similarly, nearly half of the pregnant women seen by midwives subsequently made an attempt to stop smoking. These findings suggest that if contacts and support were increased by these groups of nurses even higher smoking cessation rates may result.

CONCLUSION

Through this analysis of case studies of nurses' attempts to help their clients and patients to stop smoking we have gained considerable insight into the nurse's potential as a health educator. At a simple outcome level it is clear that nurses can be highly effective in helping and supporting their patients to stop smoking. The proportion of patients and clients who changed their smoking behaviour following the nurses' intervention compares very favourably with the results of studies using other groups of health professionals such as general practitioners. There is a need to undertake further research studies in this area, investigating nursing interventions using controlled trials and larger samples.

This research project has also illuminated the fact that the nurse–patient/client relationship provides an ideal basis from which to develop a health promotion approach to nursing care. However, it is also quite clear that such an approach differs radically from the ones that nurses, and indeed other health professionals such as doctors, are trained to adopt. A certain amount of 'unlearning' must therefore take place and it would be naive to expect nurses or other health professionals to become effective in their new roles without appropriate training.

Acknowledgement

This research was funded by the Health Education Council.

REFERENCES

Becker M.H. (1974) The health belief model and sick role behaviour. *Health Education Monographs* 2, 409–419.
Burt A., Illingworth T., Shaw P., Thornley P., White P. & Turner R. (1974) Stopping smoking after myocardial infarction. *Lancet* 1, 304–306.
Doll R. & Peto R. (1981) *The Causes of Cancer.* Oxford University Press, Oxford.
Fowler G. (1983) Advice against smoking: the attitudes of general practitioners. UICC Workshop on Smoking Cessation, Belfast, Union Internationale Centre de Cancer, Geneva.
Goldstein M. & Niaura R. (1988) Intervention by general practitioners to reduce smoking. *British Medical Journal* 296, 358–359.
Haverty S., Macleod Clark J. & Kendall S. (1986) Nurses and smoking education: a literature review. *Nurse Education Today* 6, 237–243.
Jamrozik K., Fowler G., Vessey M., Wald N., Parker G. & Van Vunakis H. (1984) Controlled trial of three different antismoking interventions in general practice. *British Medical Journal* 288, 1499–15.
Macleod Clark J., Haverty S., Elliott K. & Kendall S. (1985) *Helping People to Stop Smoking — The Nurses' Role.* Phase 1. Reports A, B and C.; Department of Nursing Studies, King's College, University of London, London.

Macleod Clark J., Haverty S. & Kendall S. (1987) *Helping Patients and Clients Stop Smoking*. Phase 2, Assessing the Effectiveness of the Nurses' Role. Research Report No. 19, Health Education Authority, London.

Murray M., Swan A.V., Johnson M.R.D. & Bewley B.R. (1983) The development of smoking during adolescence — the MRC/Derbyshire smoking study. *International Journal of Epidemiology* 12, 3–9.

Nie N.H., Hadlai Hull C., Jenkins J.G., Steinbrenner K. & Bent D. (1975) *Statistical Package for the Social Sciences*. MacGraw Hill, New York.

Office of Population Censuses and Surveys (1970) *Registrar General's Classification of Occupation*. HMSO, London.

Office of Population Censuses and Surveys (1977) *Smoking and Professional People*. HMSO, London.

Office of Population Censuses and Surveys (1988) *General Household Survey* 1972–1986. HMSO, London.

Russell M.A.H., Wilson C. Taylor & Baker C.D. (1979) The effect of general practitioners' advice against smoking. *British Medical Journal* 2, 231–235.

Russell M.A.H., Stapleton J.A., Jackson P.H., Hajek P. & Becker M. (1987) District programme to reduce smoking: effect of clinic supported brief intervention by general practitioners. *British Medical Journal* 29J, 1240–1244.

Schwartz J.L. (1987) *Review and Evaluation of Smoking Cessation Methods*. US Department of Health & Human Services, Washington, DC.

Syred M.E.J. (1981) The abdication of the role of health education by hospital nurses. *Journal of Advanced Nursing* 6, 27–33.

Vartianen E., Puska P., Koskela K., Nissenen A. & Toumilehto J. (1986) Ten year results of a community based anti-smoking programme (as part of the N. Karelia Project in Finland). *Health Education Research* 1(3), 175–184.

Index

Page numbers in bold type refer to illustrations and tables.